Ruminant Surgery

Editors

ANDREW J. NIEHAUS
DAVID E. ANDERSON

VETERINARY CLINICS OF NORTH AMERICA: FOOD ANIMAL PRACTICE

www.vetfood.theclinics.com

Consulting Editor
ROBERT A. SMITH

November 2016 • Volume 32 • Number 3

ELSEVIER

1600 John F. Kennedy Boulevard • Suite 1800 • Philadelphia, Pennsylvania, 19103-2899

http://www.vetfood.theclinics.com

VETERINARY CLINICS OF NORTH AMERICA: FOOD ANIMAL PRACTICE Volume 32, Number 3
November 2016 ISSN 0749-0720, ISBN-13: 978-0-323-47697-3

Editor: Katie Pfaff
Developmental Editor: Meredith Clinton

Veterinary Clinics of North America: Food Animal Practice (ISSN 0749-0720) is published in March, July, and November by Elsevier Inc., 360 Park Avenue South, New York, NY 10010-1710. Subscription prices are $240.00 per year (domestic individuals), $361.00 per year (domestic institutions), $100.00 per year (domestic students/residents), $265.00 per year (Canadian individuals), $476.00 per year (Canadian institutions), $335.00 per year (international individuals), $476.00 per year (international institutions), and $165.00 per year (international and Canadian students/ residents). To receive student/resident rate, orders must be accompanied by name of affiliated institution, date of term, and the signature of program/residency coordinator on institution letterhead. Clinics subscription prices. All prices are subject to change without notice. POSTMASTER: Send address changes to Veterinary Clinics of North America: Food Animal Practice, Elsevier Health Sciences Division, Subscription Customer Service, 3251 Riverport Lane, Maryland Heights, MO 63043. Customer Service (orders, claims, online, change of address): Elsevier Health Sciences Division, Subscription Customer Service, 3251 Riverport Lane, Maryland Heights, MO 63043. Tel: 1-800-654-2452 (U.S. and Canada); 314-447-8871 (ouside U.S. and Canada). Fax: 314-447-8029. E-mail: journalscustomerservice-usa@elsevier.com (for print support); journalsonlinesupport-usa@elsevier.com (for online support).

Reprints. For copies of 100 or more, of articles in this publication, please contact the Commercial Reprints Department, Elsevier Inc., 360 Park Avenue South, New York, NY 10010-1710. Tel.: 212-633-3874; Fax: 212-633-3820; E-mail: reprints@elsevier.com.

Veterinary Clinics of North America: Food Animal Practice is covered in Current Contents/Agriculture, Biology and Environmental Sciences, MEDLINE/PubMed (Index Medicus), and Excerpta Medica.

Contributors

CONSULTING EDITOR

ROBERT A. SMITH, DVM, MS
Diplomate, American Board of Veterinary Practitioners; Veterinary Research and Consulting Services, LLC, Greeley, Colorado

EDITORS

ANDREW J. NIEHAUS, DVM, MS
Diplomate, American College of Veterinary Surgeons, Large Animal; Associate Professor, Farm Animal Surgery; Associate Professor, Food Animal Surgery, Department of Veterinary Clinical Sciences, College of Veterinary Medicine, The Ohio State University, Columbus, Ohio

DAVID E. ANDERSON, DVM, MS
Diplomate, American College of Veterinary Surgeons; Professor and Head, Department of Large Animal Clinical Sciences, College of Veterinary Medicine, University of Tennessee, Knoxville, Tennessee

AUTHORS

DAVID E. ANDERSON, DVM, MS
Diplomate, American College of Veterinary Surgeons; Professor and Head, Department of Large Animal Clinical Sciences, College of Veterinary Medicine, University of Tennessee, Knoxville, Tennessee

AUBREY N. BAIRD, DVM, MS
Associate Professor, Large Animal; Chief-of-Staff, Department of Veterinary Clinical Sciences, Purdue University College of Veterinary Medicine, West Lafayette, Indiana

LIONEL J. DAWSON, BVSc, MS
Diplomate, American College of Theriogenologists; Professor, Veterinary Clinical Sciences, Center for Veterinary Health Sciences, Oklahoma State University, Stillwater, Oklahoma

ANDRÉ DESROCHERS, DMV, MS
Diplomate, American College of Veterinary Surgeons; Diplomate, European College of Bovine Health Management; Professor, Department of Clinical Sciences, Faculty of Veterinary Medicine, Université de Montréal, St-Hyacinthe, Quebec, Canada

THOMAS J. DOHERTY, MVB, MSc
Diplomate, American College of Veterinary Anesthesia and Analgesia; Professor, Department of Large Animal Clinical Sciences, College of Veterinary Medicine, University of Tennessee, Knoxville, Tennessee

MISTY A. EDMONDSON, DVM, MS
Diplomate, American College of Theriogenologists; Associate Professor, Department of Clinical Sciences, Auburn University College of Veterinary Medicine, Auburn, Alabama

DAVID FRANCOZ, Dr Vet, MSc
Diplomate, American College of Veterinary Internal Medicine; Faculté de Médecine Vétérinaire, Université de Montréal, St-Hyacinthe, Quebec, Canada

JOSEPH W. LOZIER, DVM
Farm Animal Surgery; Resident, Large Animal Surgery, Department of Veterinary Clinical Sciences, College of Veterinary Medicine, The Ohio State University, Columbus, Ohio

PIERRE-YVES MULON, Dr Vet
Diplomate, American College of Veterinary Surgeons; Assistant Professor in Farm Animal Medicine and Surgery; Department of Large Animal Clinical Sciences, College of Veterinary Medicine, University of Tennessee, Knoxville, Tennessee

SYLVAIN NICHOLS, DMV, MS
Diplomate, American College of Veterinary Surgery; Associate Professor, Department of Clinical Sciences, Faculté de Médecine Vétérinaire, Université de Montréal, St-Hyacinthe, Quebec, Canada

ANDREW J. NIEHAUS, DVM, MS
Diplomate, American College of Veterinary Surgeons, Large Animal; Associate Professor, Farm Animal Surgery; Associate Professor, Food Animal Surgery, Department of Veterinary Clinical Sciences, College of Veterinary Medicine, The Ohio State University, Columbus, Ohio

KARL NUSS, Prof Dr med vet
Diplomate, European College of Veterinary Surgeons; Farm Animal Department, Vetsuisse Faculty University of Zurich, Zurich, Switzerland

REBECCA PENTECOST, DVM, MS
Veterinarian and Partner, Coldwater Animal Clinic, Coldwater, Ohio

TULIO M. PRADO, DVM, MS
Diplomate, American College of Theriogenologists; Associate Professor, Theriogenology; Department of Large Animal Clinical Sciences, College of Veterinary Medicine, University of Tennessee, Knoxville, Tennessee

JENNIFER A. SCHLEINING, DVM, MS
Diplomate, American College of Veterinary Surgeons, Large Animal; Associate Professor, Lloyd Veterinary Medical Center, Iowa State University, Ames, Iowa

JIM SCHUMACHER, DVM, MS
Diplomate, American College of Veterinary Surgeons; Professor, Equine Surgery; Department of Large Animal Clinical Sciences, College of Veterinary Medicine, University of Tennessee, Knoxville, Tennessee

REZA SEDDIGHI, DVM, MS, PhD
Diplomate, American College of Veterinary Anesthesia and Analgesia; Associate Professor, Department of Large Animal Clinical Sciences, College of Veterinary Medicine, University of Tennessee, Knoxville, Tennessee

SAREL VAN AMSTEL, BVSc, MMedVet
Diplomate, American College of Veterinary Internal Medicine; Professor, Large Animal Clinical Sciences, College of Veterinary Medicine, University of Tennessee, Knoxville, Tennessee

RICARDO VIDELA, DVM, MS
Diplomate, American College of Veterinary Internal Medicine; Clinical Assistant Professor, Large Animal Clinical Sciences, College of Veterinary Medicine, University of Tennessee, Knoxville, Tennessee

Contents

Local, regional, and spinal anesthesias are safe, effective, often more desirable procedures for ruminants than general anesthesia. Many procedures can be performed safely and humanely in ruminants using a combination of physical restraint, mild sedation, and local, regional, or spinal anesthesia. This article focuses on the use of local anesthetics for providing anesthesia for dehorning, procedures of the nose and eye, laparotomy, reproductive procedures, teat repair, and procedures on the distal limb. Local, regional, and spinal anesthesia techniques are safe effective methods for providing anesthesia for common surgical procedures and analgesia for painful conditions in cattle and small ruminants.

Many surgical procedures on ruminants can be performed humanely and safely using local or regional anesthesia and physical restraint, but sedation and general anesthesia are necessary in order to perform some procedures. Although anesthesia-associated risks are greater in ruminants than monogastrics, ruminants can be anesthetized relatively safely in a field setting if the risks are understood, and adequate planning and precautions are in place. This article discusses the important features impacting sedation and anesthesia of cattle and small ruminants, and describes some commonly used drug protocols.

Conditions of the head requiring surgery in cattle are not uncommon when considering the incidence of conditions such as ocular squamous cell carcinoma and requests for surgical dehorning. Surgery involving the eyes in cattle is relatively common, whereas surgery of the paranasal sinuses is less common. Generally speaking, however, surgery for conditions of the head tend to have a more favorable prognosis when there is early intervention.

Diseases of the bovine digit remain the major cause of painful lameness in cattle and commonly constitute a diagnostic and therapeutic challenge for clinicians. Prompt surgical wound revision is critical in acute injuries. Deep infections may be treated with debridement, resection of tendons, synovioscopy, joint lavage, arthrotomy and facilitated joint ankylosis. Postoperative care is more involved, lameness persists longer, and cost of treatment is higher after salvage techniques than after amputation of the digit. Luxations and fractures of the digits often are amenable to conservative treatment but may be treated surgically if indicated.

 Video content accompanies this article at http://www.vetfood. theclinics.com.

Lameness related to synovial infection needs to be addressed promptly because rapid degradation of the synovial homeostasis results in permanent cartilage alterations detrimental to complete recovery. Diagnosis is based on clinical signs, synovial fluid analysis, and imaging. Commonly affected joints are the fetlock, carpus, tarsus, and stifle; shoulder, elbow, and hip may also be infected. Knowing the source of infection is essential in cases of remote septic arthritis. Antimicrobials should be administered; local delivery systems may be used. Therapy relies on the removal of inflammatory mediators. Pain management is critical throughout the surgical procedures and the recovery period.

Long bone fractures and disorders of tendons and ligaments represent a significant proportion of surgical orthopedic cases presented to ruminant veterinarians. The presentation of these patients, their diagnostic workup, surgical treatment, and expected outcome will be discussed. The outcome of these cases depends largely on the presenting problem; however, accurate diagnosis and prompt surgical intervention can greatly improve the outcome of many of these cases.

Lacerations of the teat should be treated as emergency. First-intention repair should be attempted under sedation in lateral or dorsal recumbency. Surgeons should pay attention to the atraumatic manipulation of the tissue and the anatomic reconstruction using small-diameter absorbable suture material. Hand milking should be prohibited for 10 days postoperatively after laceration repair; prognosis is overall good. Ultrasound evaluation of the teat allows excellent understanding of the internal lesions and should be performed before planning any elective surgery. Milk outflow impairment originating from the rosette of Fürstenberg or the streak canal is best treated using minimally invasive surgery (theloscopy).

VETERINARY CLINICS OF NORTH AMERICA: FOOD ANIMAL PRACTICE

ISSUE OF RELATED INTEREST

Veterinary Clinics of North America: Equine Practice
December 2015 (Vol. 31, Issue 3)
Equine Neonataology
Pamela A. Wilkins, *Editor*

THE CLINICS ARE NOW AVAILABLE ONLINE!
Access your subscription at:
www.theclinics.com

Preface

Ruminant Surgery

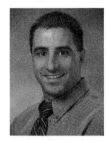 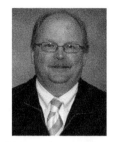

Andrew J. Niehaus, DVM, MS   David E. Anderson, DVM, MS
Editors

Surgical management of disorders of ruminants continues to evolve with time. Improvements in chemical restraint, surgical technique, and pain management require the ruminant surgeon to remain vigilant in their professional development so that the client and patient can be afforded the best care possible. Constraints experienced by the ruminant surgeon often involve economics, regulatory prohibitions, and dogma. Limitations of ruminant surgery often occur because of patient size, weight, and mentation; because of surgeon knowledge, training, or skills; and because the client may lack the ability to fully comply with needs during the convalescent period. Dogma, knowledge, skills, and training all can be changed through continuing education, research, and innovation. We hope that the contents of this Ruminant Surgery issue of the *Veterinary Clinics of North America: Food Animal Practice* series will enable ruminant surgeons to advance their knowledge of the science and that this will result in personal development in the art of surgical practice.

We have tried to provide some depth of surgical details in as broad a cross-section of clinical practice as possible. As such, expert authors were invited to cover topics including surgery of the head and neck, respiratory, abdominal, musculoskeletal, and urogenital tissues. Surgical correction of problems nearly always requires anesthesia. In fact, advancements in the clinical practice of surgery often follow improvements in anesthesia: spinal, perineural, regional, local, or general anesthesia. A critical component of perioperative management of surgical patients includes pain management. Although specific recommendations for pain management are provided for each of the surgical techniques described herein, we recommend that you explore the *Veterinary Clinics of North America: Food Animal Practice* issue on Pain Management published in March of 2013 for a detailed review of analgesic drugs, techniques, and regulatory issues.

Our hope is that this issue on Ruminant Surgery is sufficiently focused on clinical practice so that it can be of value as a daily resource. We have asked the authors to emphasize techniques that can be implemented on the farm or in typical private

Vet Clin Food Anim 32 (2016) xiii–xiv
http://dx.doi.org/10.1016/j.cvfa.2016.08.001
0749-0720/16/© 2016 Published by Elsevier Inc.   **vetfood.theclinics.com**

practice settings. However, you will find a variety of advanced techniques in surgery and anesthesia for those who enjoy a challenge or are motivated to try new techniques.

Andrew J. Niehaus, DVM, MS
Department of Veterinary Clinical Sciences
College of Veterinary Medicine
The Ohio State University
Columbus, OH 43210, USA

David E. Anderson, DVM, MS
Department of Large Animal Clinical Sciences
College of Veterinary Medicine
University of Tennessee
Knoxville, TN 37931, USA

E-mail addresses:
niehaus.25@osu.edu (A.J. Niehaus)
dander48@utk.edu (D.E. Anderson)

Local, Regional, and Spinal Anesthesia in Ruminants

Misty A. Edmondson, DVM, MS

KEYWORDS

- Anesthesia • Local • Regional • Spinal cattle • Sheep • Goats

KEY POINTS

- Local, regional, and spinal anesthesia techniques are safe and effective methods for providing anesthesia for common surgical procedures and painful conditions in cattle and small ruminants.
- These techniques are inexpensive and easy to perform and offer a safe alternative to general anesthesia, in some cases.
- Many surgical procedures can be performed safely and humanely in ruminants using a combination of physical restraint, mild sedation, and local, regional, or spinal anesthesia.

INTRODUCTION

Although general anesthesia is commonly used in cattle and small ruminants, there are some risks associated with using general anesthesia. An alternative in some cases may include the use of local, regional, or spinal anesthesia. Local, regional, or spinal anesthesia is safe, effective, and often a more desirable procedure in many situations. Many surgical procedures can be performed safely and humanely in ruminants using a combination of physical restraint, mild sedation, and local, regional, or spinal anesthesia. Local anesthetic techniques are popular and used commonly because they are usually simple and inexpensive and provide a reversible loss of sensation to a relatively well-defined area of the body. Local and regional anesthesias also offer some advantages over general anesthesia, which include a lower risk of toxic effects, decreased risk associated with placing an animal in recumbency (bloat, regurgitation), and the need for less equipment. Before local or regional anesthesia is performed, the animal should be adequately restrained. The type of restraint used depends on the temperament of the animal and the anesthetic technique to be used. However, sedation may be necessary in some cases. The site of injection should be prepared by clipping or shaving the hair and scrubbing and disinfecting the skin.

The author has nothing to disclose.
Department of Clinical Sciences, Auburn University College of Veterinary Medicine, 1500 Wire Road, Auburn, AL 36849, USA
E-mail address: abramms@auburn.edu

Vet Clin Food Anim 32 (2016) 535–552
http://dx.doi.org/10.1016/j.cvfa.2016.05.015
0749-0720/16/$ – see front matter © 2016 Elsevier Inc. All rights reserved.

LOCAL ANESTHETICS

There are many local anesthetic agents that may be used for these procedures. These anesthetic agents vary in their potency, toxicity, and cost.[1] Two percent lidocaine hydrochloride and 2% mepivacaine hydrochloride have become the most commonly used local anesthetic agents in cattle because of low cost and limited toxicity. Lidocaine is 3 times more potent than procaine and diffuses more widely in the tissues. Lidocaine also has an intermediate duration of action from 90 to 180 minutes, is 3 times more potent than procaine, and diffuses into tissues more widely.[2,3] A vasoconstrictor, such as epinephrine (5 mg/mL), added to the local anesthetic solution (0.1 mL of epinephrine [1:1000] to 20 mL of local anesthetic) increases the potency and duration of activity of both regional and epidural anesthesia. However, anesthetic agents containing epinephrine (1:200,000) should not be used in wound edges or in the subarachnoid space because of the risks of producing tissue necrosis and spinal cord ischemia.[3] In cattle, procaine (1%–2%) is expected to have a longer time to onset of anesthesia when compared with lidocaine and a shorter duration of action at no more than 60 minutes. Alternatively, mepivacaine (1%–2%) is expected to have a similar time of onset of anesthesia but longer duration of activity at 120 to 180 minutes when compared with lidocaine. Bupivacaine (0.25%–0.5%) is a long-acting local anesthetic lasting up to 360 minutes. However, bupivacaine can be toxic to cattle if it is given intravenously. Hence, bupivacaine is not recommended for routine clinical use because of the risk of inadvertent intravenous injection (5 = 1[4]).

It is imperative for the clinician to be conscious of toxicity and preventative measures to ensure that overdosage does not occur. Avoiding an overdose is critically important when local anesthesia is being performed in a large area, such as for cesarean section. The maximum safe dose of lidocaine hydrochloride in cattle is 10 mg/kg of body weight. Small ruminants are exquisitely more sensitive to anesthetics with a maximum safe dose of lidocaine hydrochloride of 4 mg/kg (5 = 1[4]). In some cases where a larger area is to be covered and thus a larger volume is needed, the standard 2% lidocaine hydrochloride may be diluted to 1% with sterile saline.

ANESTHESIA FOR DEHORNING

The cornual nerve block is used for anesthesia for dehorning cattle and small ruminants. The horn and the skin around the base of the horn are innervated by the cornual branch of the lacrimal or zygomaticotemporal nerve, which is part of the ophthalmic division of the trigeminal nerve. The cornual nerve passes through the periorbital tissues dorsally and runs along the frontal crest to the base of the horns. Approximately 5 to 10 mL of a local anesthetic agent (in cattle) is deposited subcutaneously and relatively superficially midway between the lateral canthus of the eye and the base of the horn along the zygomatic process (**Fig. 1**). Complete anesthesia may take 10 minutes. Larger cattle with well-developed horns require additional anesthetic infiltration along the caudal aspect of the horn, in the form of a partial ring block, to desensitize subcutaneous branches of the second cervical nerve.[2,5,6]

Because of anatomical differences, the cornual nerve block in goats requires at least 2 injection sites per horn versus the aforementioned one site in cattle. In goats, the cornual nerve is a branch of the zygomaticotemporal nerve and lies halfway between the lateral canthus of the eye and the lateral base of the horn. The horn base in goats is also heavily innervated by the cornual branches of the infratrochlear nerve, which exits the orbit at or in close proximity to the medial canthus. Because of the widespread branching, the nerve is best blocked using a line block midway

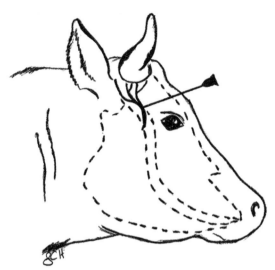

Fig. 1. Needle placement for desensitizing the cornual branch of the zygomaticotemporal nerve in cattle. (*From* Edmondson M. Local and regional anesthesia in cattle. Vet Clin North Am Food Anim Pract 2008;24:211–26; with permission.)

between the medial canthus of the eye and the medial horn base.[7] Alternatively, a ring block around the base of the horn may also be used for anesthesia for dehorning.

NASAL ANESTHESIA

The infraorbital nerve block may be used for the repair of nasal lacerations and the placement of a nose ring for cattle. The infraorbital nerve is the continuation of the maxillary branch of the fifth cranial nerve after it enters the infraorbital canal. The infraorbital nerve has only sensory function and emerges on the face as a flat band through the infraorbital foramen where it is covered by the levator nasolabialis muscle.[2] The infraorbital nerve is blocked as it emerges from the infraorbital canal. The nerve is difficult to palpate but is located rostral to the facial tuberosity on a line extending from the nasomaxillary notch to the second upper premolar. A total of 20 to 30 mL of local anesthetic agent is injected deep into the levator nasolabialis muscle with an 18-gauge 3.8-cm needle (**Fig. 2**). The injection should be repeated on the opposite side.

ANESTHESIA OF THE EYE AND EYELID AND RELAXATION OF THE ORBIT

The globe, conjunctiva, nictitating membrane, and most of the eyelids are supplied by the ophthalmic branch of the trigeminal nerve. The extraocular muscles of the eye are innervated by the trochlear nerve, the abducens nerve, and the oculomotor nerve. The eyelids are innervated by the auriculopalpebral nerve. Topical and regional analgesia techniques are necessary for surgery of the eye and its associated structures, most commonly for squamous cell carcinoma, removal of foreign bodies from the cornea, and subconjunctival injections.[1]

Anesthesia of the Eyelid

Anesthesia of the eyelid is accomplished by performing a line block of the eyelid or by blocking the auriculopalpebral branch of the facial nerve. A line block is performed by using a 20- or 22-gauge 2.5-cm needle to inject 10 mL of a local anesthetic at multiple

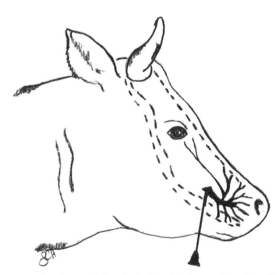

Fig. 2. Needle placement for desensitizing the infraorbital nerve in cattle. (*From* Edmondson M. Local and regional anesthesia in cattle. Vet Clin North Am Food Anim Pract 2008;24:211–26; with permission.)

sites 0.5 cm apart on a line approximately 0.5 cm from the margin of the lid.[1] This dose may be reduced to 5 mL for small ruminants. The auriculopalpebral nerve block is performed by using an 18- or 20-gauge 2.5-cm needle placed subcutaneously approximately 5 to 7.5 cm lateral to the zygomatic arch. A total of 5 to 10 mL of local anesthetic is then injected (**Fig. 3**).[2] Again, the dose of local anesthetic may be reduced to 2 to 5 mL for small ruminant patients. Because the auriculopalpebral nerve block only blocks the lower eyelid, if the surgical procedure to be performed also requires desensitization of the upper eyelid, a line block may be performed.

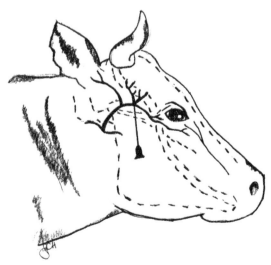

Fig. 3. Needle placement for desensitizing the auriculopalpebral nerve in cattle. (*From* Edmondson M. Local and regional anesthesia in cattle. Vet Clin North Am Food Anim Pract 2008;24:211–26; with permission.)

Anesthesia of the Eye and Orbit and Immobilization of the Globe

Anesthesia of the eye and orbit and immobilization of the globe that is necessary for such procedures as enucleation may be accomplished by performing a retrobulbar block or Peterson block.

Retrobulbar Block

The retrobulbar block is used for enucleation of the eye or for surgery of the cornea, and when properly performed, causes analgesia of the cornea, mydriasis, and proptosis. Adequate restraint of the head is necessary when performing this procedure. The sites for needle placement for retrobulbar injection are the medial and lateral canthus or the upper and lower eyelids.[3] An 18-gauge 15-cm needle is used and may be bent slightly to facilitate passage around the globe once it has been introduced through the eyelid or canthus at the orbital rim. The surgeon's finger is used to deflect the globe to protect it from the point of the needle (**Fig. 4**). Approximately 15 mL of local anesthetic is injected in small increments as the needle is advanced slowly toward the back of the orbit. The advantage of the retrobulbar block is that it is generally regarded as an easier technique to perform compared with the Peterson eye block. Some possible adverse effects of retrobulbar injections include penetration of the globe, orbital hemorrhage, damage to the optic nerve, dysrhythmias caused by initiation of the oculocardiac reflex, and injection into the optic nerve meninges.[2]

Peterson Eye Block

The Peterson eye block requires more skill to perform than the retrobulbar block, but it is safer and more effective if performed correctly. There is also less edema and inflammation associated with this block than with infiltration of local anesthetics into the eyelids and orbit. The Peterson eye block desensitizes the nerves (oculomotor, trochlear, abducent, and trigeminal) responsible for sensory and motor function of all structures of the eye except the eyelid.[2] An auriculopalpebral nerve block can be performed to

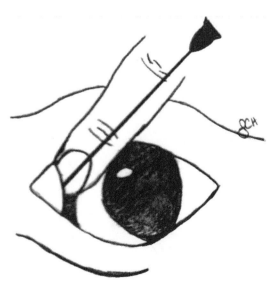

Fig. 4. Retrobulbar needle placement through the medial canthus of the eye in cattle. (*From* Edmondson M. Local and regional anesthesia in cattle. Vet Clin North Am Food Anim Pract 2008;24:211–26; with permission.)

anesthetize the eyelid. The landmark for needle placement for the Peterson eye block is the notch that is created by the supraorbital process cranially, the zygomatic arch ventrally, and the coronoid process of the mandible caudally. Approximately 5 mL of local anesthetic is injected subcutaneously at this site using a 22-gauge 2.5-cm needle. A 14-gauge 2.5-cm needle serves as a cannula and is placed through the anesthetized area as far anterior and ventral as possible in the notch. A straight or slightly curved 18-gauge, 10- to 12-cm needle is inserted into the cannula and directed horizontally and slightly caudally until it comes into contact with the coronoid process of the mandible at approximately 2.5 cm deep. The needle is then gently manipulated rostrally until its point passes medially around the coronoid process. It is then advanced to the pterygopalatine fossa rostral to the solid bony plate that is in close proximity to the orbital foramen at a depth of 7.5 to 10 cm (**Fig. 5**). Penetration of the nasopharynx and turbinates should be avoided. Aspiration ensures that the ventral maxillary artery has not been penetrated.[1,2] Approximately 15 mL of local anesthetic is then injected. Both the retrobulbar block and the Peterson eye block prevent blinking for several hours.[1] The cornea must be kept moist if these blocks are used for procedures other than enucleation. Caution must also be used with animals that are transported immediately following these procedures. A lubricating agent can be applied to the cornea, or the eyelids may be sutured together until motor function of the eyelids returns.

ANESTHESIA FOR LAPAROTOMY

Anesthesia of the paralumbar fossa and abdominal wall can be achieved by several techniques. These techniques include the proximal paravertebral nerve block, the distal paravertebral nerve block, the inverted L block, and infusion of the incision or line block. These anesthetic techniques are commonly used for abdominal procedures such as omentopexy, abomasopexy, rumenotomy, cesarean section, or other surgical procedures using a paralumbar fossa approach. Although these techniques can be theoretically performed in all ruminant species, they are most commonly used in cattle. The description of the techniques will be made using a bovine example. Please be aware that slight modifications will need to be made, especially a reduction in the dose of local anesthetic used if this procedure is to be performed in small ruminants.

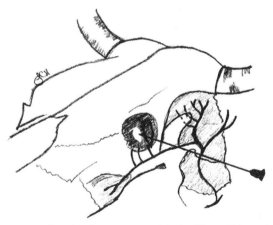

Fig. 5. Needle placement for the Peterson eye block. (*From* Edmondson M. Local and regional anesthesia in cattle. Vet Clin North Am Food Anim Pract 2008;24:211–26; with permission.)

Proximal Paravertebral Nerve Block

The proximal paravertebral nerve block desensitizes the dorsal and ventral nerve roots of the last thoracic (T13) and first and second lumbar (L1 and L2) spinal nerves as they emerge from the intervertebral foramina. To facilitate proper needle placement of anesthetic, the skin at the cranial edges of the transverse processes of L1, L2, and L3, and at a point 2.5 to 5 cm off the dorsal midline can be desensitized by injecting 2 to 3 mL of local anesthetic using an 18-gauge 2.5-cm needle. A 14-gauge 2.5-cm needle is used as a cannula or guide needle to minimize skin resistance during insertion of an 18-gauge 10- to 15-cm spinal needle. Approximately 5 mL of local anesthetic may be placed through the cannula to anesthetize further the tract for needle placement.

To desensitize T13, the cannula needle is placed through the skin at the cranial edge of the transverse process of L1 at approximately 4 to 5 cm lateral to the dorsal midline. The 18-gauge 10- to 15-cm spinal needle is passed ventrally until it contacts the transverse process of L1. The needle is then walked off of the cranial edge of the transverse process of L1 and advanced approximately 1 cm to pass slightly ventral to the process and into the intertransverse ligament. A total of 6 to 8 mL of local anesthetic is injected with little resistance to desensitize the ventral branch of T13. The needle is then withdrawn 1 to 2.5 cm above the fascia or just dorsal to the transverse process and 6 to 8 mL of local anesthetic is infused to desensitize the dorsal branch of the nerve.

To desensitize L1 and L2, the needle is inserted just caudal to the transverse processes of L1 and L2. The needle is walked off of the caudal edges of the transverse processes of L1 and L2, at a depth similar to the injection site for T13, and advanced approximately 1 cm to pass slightly ventral to the process and into the intertransverse ligament. A total of 6 to 8 mL of local anesthetic is injected with little resistance to desensitize the ventral branches of the nerves. The needle is then withdrawn 1 to 2.5 cm above the fascia or just dorsal to the transverse processes, and 6 to 8 mL of local anesthetic is infused to desensitize the dorsal branch of the nerves (**Fig. 6**). Evidence of a successful

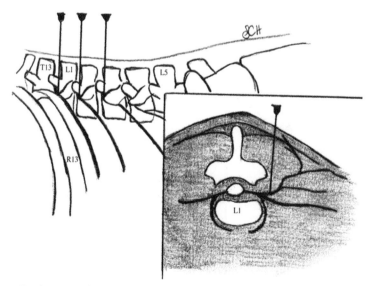

Fig. 6. Needle placement for the proximal paravertebral nerve block in cattle. Left lateral view and cranial view at the thoracolumbar junction. L1, first lumbar vertebra; L5, fifth lumbar vertebra; R13, last rib; T13, last thoracic vertebra. (*From* Edmondson M. Local and regional anesthesia in cattle. Vet Clin North Am Food Anim Pract 2008;24:211–26; with permission.)

proximal paravertebral nerve block includes increased temperature of the skin; analgesia of the skin, muscles, and peritoneum of the abdominal wall of the paralumbar fossa; and scoliosis of the spine toward the desensitized side. Advantages of the proximal paravertebral nerve block include small doses of anesthetic required, wide and uniform area of analgesia and muscle relaxation, decreased intra-abdominal pressure, and absence of local anesthetic at the margins of the surgical site. Disadvantages of the proximal paravertebral nerve block include scoliosis of the spine, which may make closure of the incision more difficult, difficulty in identifying landmarks in obese and heavily muscled animals, and more skill or practice required for consistent results.[2,3,8]

Distal Paravertebral Nerve Block

The distal paravertebral nerve block desensitizes the dorsal and ventral rami of the spinal nerves T13, L1, and L2 at the distal ends of the transverse processes of L1, L2, and L4, respectively. An 18-gauge 3.5- to 5.5-cm needle is inserted ventral to the transverse process, and 10 mL of local anesthetic is infused in a fan-shaped pattern. The needle can then be removed completely and reinserted or redirected dorsally, in a caudal direction, where 10 mL of local anesthetic is again infused in a fan-shaped pattern. This procedure is repeated for the transverse processes of the second and fourth lumbar vertebrae (**Fig. 7**). Advantages of the distal paravertebral nerve block compared with the proximal paravertebral nerve block include that it has a lack of scoliosis, it is easier to perform, and it offers more consistent results. Disadvantages of the distal paravertebral nerve block compared with the proximal paravertebral nerve block include larger doses of anesthetic required and variations in efficiency caused by variation in anatomic pathways of the nerves.[2,3,8]

Inverted L Block

The inverted L block is a nonspecific regional block that locally blocks the tissue bordering the caudal aspect of the thirteenth rib and the ventral aspect of the transverse processes of the lumbar vertebrae.[8] An 18-gauge 3.8-cm needle is used to inject up to a total of 100 mL of local anesthetic solution in multiple small injection sites into

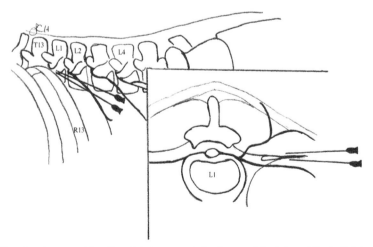

Fig. 7. Needle placement for the distal paravertebral nerve block in cattle. Left lateral view and cranial view at the thoracolumbar junction. L2, second lumbar vertebra; L4, fourth lumbar vertebra. (*From* Edmondson M. Local and regional anesthesia in cattle. Vet Clin North Am Food Anim Pract 2008;24:211–26; with permission.)

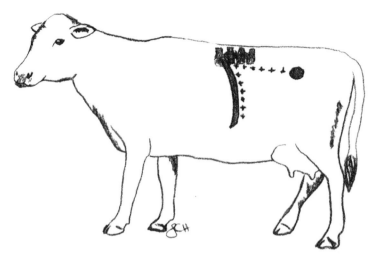

Fig. 8. Inverted L block for paralumbar anesthesia, showing multiple infusion sites (*asterisks*), the last rib, the lumbar vertebra, and tuber coxae. (*From* Edmondson M. Local and regional anesthesia in cattle. Vet Clin North Am Food Anim Pract 2008;24:211–26; with permission.)

the tissues bordering the dorsocaudal aspect of the thirteenth rib and ventrolateral aspect of the transverse processes of the lumbar vertebrae (**Fig. 8**), creating an area of anesthesia ventrocaudal to the block. Advantages of the inverted L block include that the block is simple to perform, it does not interfere with ambulation, and deposition of anesthetic away from the incision site minimizes incisional edema and hematoma.[3] Disadvantages include incomplete analgesia and muscle relaxation of the deeper layers of the abdominal wall (particularly in obese animals); possible toxicity after larger doses of anesthetic; and increased cost because larger doses of local anesthetic are required.[3]

Line Block

Infusion of local anesthetic into the incision site or a line block may also be used to desensitize a selected area of the paralumbar fossa. An 18-gauge 3.8-cm needle is used to infuse multiple, small injections of 10 mL of local anesthetic solution subcutaneously and into the deep muscle layers and peritoneum. Pain of successive injections may be alleviated by placing the edge of the needle into the edge of the previously desensitized area at an approximately 20° angle.[1] In heavily muscled or overweight cattle, it may be necessary to use an 18-gauge 7.5-cm needle to penetrate through the large amount of subcutaneous fat to reach the deep muscle layers. The amount of local anesthetic needed to acquire adequate anesthesia depends on the size of the area to be desensitized. Adult cattle weighing 450 kg can safely tolerate 250 mL of a 2% lidocaine hydrochloride solution.[1] Delayed healing of the incision site is a possible complication of infiltration of local anesthetic at the surgical site.

ANESTHESIA FOR REPRODUCTIVE PROCEDURES

Several anesthetic techniques have been used for obstetric manipulations and surgical procedures involving the tail, perineum, anus, rectum, vulva, vagina, prepuce, and scrotum. These techniques include caudal epidural anesthesia, continuous caudal epidural anesthesia, and internal pudendal nerve block. These techniques can also be used to relieve pain and control straining in cattle.

Caudal Epidural

Caudal epidural anesthesia is an easy and inexpensive method of analgesia that is commonly used in cattle. A high caudal epidural at the sacrococcygeal space (S5–Co1) desensitizes sacral nerves S2, S3, S4, and S5. The low caudal epidural at first coccygeal space (Co1–Co2) desensitizes sacral nerves S3, S4, and S5; as the anesthetic dose increases, nerves cranial to S2 may also become affected.[9] If possible the hair should be clipped and the skin scrubbed and disinfected. Standing alongside the cow, the tail should be moved up and down to locate the fossa between the last sacral vertebra and the first coccygeal vertebra or between the first and second coccygeal vertebrae. An 18-gauge 3.8-cm needle (with no syringe attached) is inserted on dorsal midline and directed perpendicular to the skin surface. Sometimes directing the needle slightly cranial will facilitate passage through the sacrococcygeal space. Once the skin is penetrated, place a drop of local anesthetic solution in the hub of the needle (hanging drop technique). The needle should then be advanced slowly until the anesthetic solution is drawn into the epidural space by negative pressure. The syringe may then be attached to the needle, and anesthetic solution is slowly injected with no resistance (**Fig. 9**). The dose of local anesthetic to be used is 0.5 mL per 45 kg of body weight. Animals that have had multiple epidurals may have abundant scar tissue dorsal to the sacrococcygeal space, which may impede spontaneous aspiration of the local anesthetic.

Sheep with severely docked tails can be difficult to achieve a caudal epidural. Thus, a lumbosacral epidural may be the only option in these animals. In goats, the tail should be pumped up and down to identify the cranial-most moveable space into which the needle is inserted at a 45° angle to the vertebrae. The hanging drop technique, which was previously described, is used to ensure correct placement of anesthetic into the epidural space. In small ruminants, the dose of 2% lidocaine hydrochloride ranges from 1 mL/50 kg to 1 mL/15 kg.[7] For tail docking of sheep, an epidural or local ring block just proximal to the site of docking may be used, although it appears that the local ring block was more beneficial than an epidural.[7]

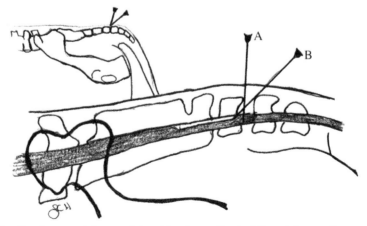

Fig. 9. Needle placement for caudal epidural anesthesia (A) and for continuous caudal epidural anesthesia (B) located between the first and second coccygeal vertebrae. (*From* Edmondson M. Local and regional anesthesia in cattle. Vet Clin North Am Food Anim Pract 2008;24:211–26; with permission.)

Continuous Caudal Epidural

Continuous caudal epidural anesthesia is used in cattle with chronic rectal and vaginal prolapse that experience continuous straining after the initial epidural. This procedure is performed by placing a catheter into the epidural space for intermittent administration of local anesthetic. A 17-gauge 5-cm spinal needle (Tuohy needle) with stylet in place is inserted into the epidural space at Co1 to Co2 with the bevel directed craniad. The stylet is removed, and 2 mL of local anesthetic is injected to determine if the needle is in the epidural space. A catheter is inserted into the needle and advanced cranially for 2 to 4 cm beyond the needle tip. The needle is then withdrawn while the catheter remains in place (see **Fig. 9**). An adapter is placed on the end of the catheter, and the catheter is secured to the skin on the dorsum. Local anesthetic solution may then be administered as needed.[1]

More recently, α_2-agonists and opioids either alone or in combination with local anesthetic solutions have been used for epidural anesthesia. Epidural administration of the $\alpha2$-agonist xylazine hydrochloride (0.05 mg/kg) diluted in 5 to 12 mL of sterile saline or xylazine hydrochloride (0.3 mg/kg) added to 5 mL of 2% lidocaine hydrochloride combinations offer similar anesthesia to lidocaine. Although the duration of anesthesia is prolonged (4–5 hours) using these combinations, systemic effects (sedation, salivation, ataxia) may also occur.[3] Epidural administration of opioids, such as morphine (0.1 mg/kg) diluted in 20 mL of sterile saline, is used to provide analgesia for a prolonged period (approximately 12 hours) without interfering with motor function. Disadvantages of using opioids for epidural anesthesia are that the analgesia is not as potent as lidocaine and the maximum effect of a morphine epidural may not occur for 2 to 3 hours. Caudal epidural administration of morphine may be used to help alleviate pain in the perineal area and straining.[6]

Lumbosacral Epidural

The lumbosacral epidural is a relatively easy and commonly used technique in sedated pigs for cesarean section, repair of hernias (umbilical, inguinal), prolapses (rectal, vaginal, uterine), and surgery of the rear limbs, penis, and prepuce. It is important to remember that epidural anesthesia is contraindicated in pigs with cardiovascular disease, bleeding disorders, or toxemic shock due to sympathetic blockade and resulting reduction in blood pressure. The 14-gauge needle can be used to guide and stabilize the spinal needle. The spinal needle needed varies according to the size of the pig with a 20-gauge, 6- to 8-cm needle appropriate for pigs weighing 10 to 20 kg and an 18-gauge, 10- to 16-cm needle for pigs weighing more than 100 kg. The site for needle placement is on the midline immediately caudal to the spinous process of the last lumbar (L6) vertebra. The injection site is felt as a palpable depression slightly caudal to a transverse line between the cranial prominences of the wings of the ilium on either side (0.5–1.5 cm in pigs weighing 10–50 kg and 1.5–2.5 cm in pigs weighing 50 kg or more). If the wings of the ilium are not palpable in larger pigs, a vertical line through the patella may be used as a guide to locate the lumbosacral space 2.0 to 3.0 cm caudal to the vertical line.[3] The spinal needle and stylet with the bevel of the needle directed cranially are inserted into the lumbosacral space using a 20° caudovertical angle. The depth of penetration of the needle depends on the size and condition of the pig. The depth may be up to 2 to 4 cm in pigs weighing between 10 and 20 kg and 4 to 10 cm in pigs weighing between 20 and 100 kg. The needle will meet resistance as it encounters the interarcuate ligament. Penetration through the ligament often feels like a slight pop and is associated with sudden movements indicating entrance into the vertebral canal. The lumbosacral aperture in the pig is relatively large (1.5 × 2.5 cm) and allows for some margin of error (Skarda3). The dose of anesthetic needed to provide anesthesia caudal to the umbilicus is 1.0 mL of 2% lidocaine hydrochloride per 4.5 kg of body weight at a rate of 1.0 mL per 2 to 3 seconds. Anesthesia should occur within 10 minutes and recovery within 2 hours. A smaller dose has been used with similar results by using 1.0 mL per 7.5 kg for pigs weighing up to 50 kg and an additional 1.0 mL for every 10 kg increase in body weight. A maximum dose of 20 mL of 2% lidocaine hydrochloride is suggested as the upper limit: for standing castrations, 4 mL per 100 kg, 6 mL per 200 kg, and 8 mL per 300 kg of body weight; for cesarean sections, 10 mL per 100 kg, 15 mL per 200 kg, and 20 mL 300 kg of body weight.[10]

The lumbosacral space in small ruminants can be accessed by palpating the space caudal to the dorsal vertebral process of the sixth lumbar vertebrae between the wings of the ilium. Typically, an 18- or 20-gauge, 3.8-cm needle is sufficient. Llamas and animals that are overconditioned may require an 8.4-cm spinal needle for the lumbosacral space. The needle is advanced on the midline of the animal perpendicular to the vertebrae until a pop is felt. A drop of 2% lidocaine hydrochloride placed into the hub of the needle should be drawn into the needle once the epidural space is entered. Injection of the anesthetic should not encounter any resistance. The injection should be given slowly over 60 to 90 seconds to prevent rapid cranial migration of the anesthetic.[7]

Sacral paravertebral nerve block

Sacral paravertebral anesthesia is used to relieve rectal tenesmus associated with rectal prolapse without affecting the sciatic nerve and the animal's ability to stand or tail function. The sacral paravertebral nerve block is used to provide analgesia to the pudendal nerve (pudic nerve), medial hemorrhoidal nerve (pelvic splanchnic nerve), and caudal hemorrhoidal nerve (caudal rectal nerve) by blocking S3, S4, and S5 as they branch off of the spinal cord. This block provides analgesia to the anus, vulva, and vagina.[10,11] In bulls, S3 supplies motor function to the retractor penis muscles. Physical restraint in a squeeze chute and/or sedation may be beneficial as to prevent lateral movement of the animal during the procedure. In addition, a caudal epidural may be helpful if the animal is fractious. The skin over the dorsal sacrum should be clipped of hair and surgically prepared for the procedure. The paired S5 foramina are 1 to 2 cm lateral to the sacral coccygeal joint. The S4 foramina are about 3 to 4 cm cranial and more lateral to the S5 foramina. The S3 foramina are an additional 3 to 4 cm cranial to the S4 foramina. A stab incision can be made dorsal to each foramen to aid in the introduction of a 5- to 7-cm, 18-gauge needle. The foramina can be palpated rectally with a finger placed in or over the ring, which allows for identification of the foramen and ensures correct needle placement. Once the needle has entered the osseous ring, inject 2 to 3 cc of lidocaine hydrochloride; this should be repeated for each foramen.[11] The use of a lidocaine/alcohol mixture has also been described to manage tenesmus following chronic cervicovaginal prolapse or rectal prolapse. A mixture of 1 cc of 2% lidocaine hydrochloride and 2 cc of 95% ethyl alcohol has been used effectively.[11]

The sacral paravertebral nerve block can also be used in sheep and goats by using an 18-gauge 7.5-cm needle. This block in small ruminants uses the same technique described for cattle with a reduced volume of 1 to 2 mL of 2% lidocaine hydrochloride per injection site.[10]

Internal Pudendal Nerve Block

The procedure for bilateral internal pudendal (pudic) nerve block was first described by Larson[12] to facilitate relaxation of the bull's penis without causing locomotor impairment. The internal pudendal nerve block can be used in the standing bull for penile relaxation and analgesia distal to the sigmoid flexure and examination of the penis. In the standing female, the internal pudendal nerve block can be used to relieve straining caused by chronic vaginal prolapse. This technique may also be used for surgical procedures of the penis, such as repair of prolapses, removal of perianal tumors, removal of penile papillomas or warts, and other minor surgeries of the penis and prepuce. This procedure involves desensitizing the internal pudendal nerve and the anastomotic branch of the middle hemorrhoidal nerve using an ischiorectal approach. The internal pudendal nerve consists of fibers originating from the ventral branches of the third and fourth sacral nerves (S3 and S4) and the pelvic splanchnic nerves. The skin at the ischiorectal fossa on either side of the spine is clipped, disinfected, and desensitized with approximately 2 mL of local anesthetic. A 14-gauge 1.25-cm needle is inserted through the desensitized skin at the ischiorectal fossa to serve as a cannula. An 18-gauge 10-cm spinal needle is then directed through the cannula to the pudendal nerve. The operator's left hand is placed into the rectum to the level of the wrist and the fingers directed laterally and ventrally to identify the lesser sacrosciatic foramen. The lesser sciatic foramen is first identified by rectal palpation as a soft depression in the sacrosciatic ligament. The internal pudendal nerve can be readily identified lying on the ligament immediately cranial and dorsal to the foramen and approximately one finger's width dorsal to the pudendal artery passing through the foramen. The internal pudendal artery can be readily palpated a finger's width ventral to the nerve. The spinal needle is held in the operator's right hand and introduced through the cannula in the ischiorectal fossa. The spinal needle is directed medial to the sacrosciatic ligament and directed cranioventrally (**Fig. 10**). The needle is not felt until it has been introduced approximately 5 to 7 cm and can then be repositioned to the nerve. Once at the pudendal nerve, 20 mL of local anesthetic is deposited at the nerve. The needle is then partially withdrawn and redirected 2 to 3 cm more caudodorsally, where an additional 10 mL of local anesthetic is deposited at the cranial aspect of the foramen to desensitize the muscular branches and the middle hemorrhoidal nerve. The needle is then removed, and the sites of deposition are massaged to aid in dispersal of the local anesthetic. This procedure is then repeated on the opposite side of the pelvis. Relaxation of the penis varies and may take as long as 30 to 40 minutes for full effect. The duration of the internal pudendal nerve block lasts from 2 to 4 hours.

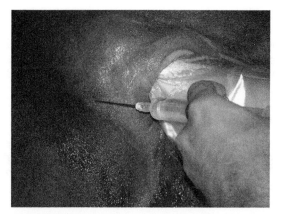

Fig. 10. Needle being inserted into the pararectal fossa of a bull for the purpose of blocking the pudendal nerve. Pudendal nerve block achieves paralysis of the retractor penis muscles and facilitates extension, manipulation, and surgery of the penis and prepuce.

Dorsal Penile Nerve Block

The dorsal nerve of the penis may be desensitized at a location just proximal to the surgical site. With the bull restrained, the penis should be manually extended and a towel clamp should then be placed under the dorsal apical ligament. Alternatively, a gauze tourniquet may be placed around the free portion of the penis to aid in penile extension. With the dorsal aspect of the penis thoroughly cleansed, 2 to 4 mL of 2% lidocaine hydrochloride should be infused subcutaneously across the dorsum of the penis proximal to the lesion.[13]

Alternatively, the dorsal nerve of the penis may also be desensitized as it passes over the ischial arch for penile anesthesia and relaxation. The skin associated with the penile body and located 10 cm ventral to the anus and 2.5 cm from midline is infiltrated with 2 to 4 mL of 2% lidocaine hydrochloride using a small-gauge needle (22–25 gauge). A 20-gauge, 4-cm needle is then inserted through the desensitized skin and advanced for 5 to 7 cm to contact the pelvic floor. Aspiration ensures that the needle is not in the dorsal artery of the penis. The needle is then withdrawn approximately 1 cm and the area infiltrated with 20 to 30 mL of 2% lidocaine hydrochloride. The procedure is then repeated on the opposite side of the penis. Analgesia and paralysis of the penis will occur within 20 minutes and should last for 1 to 2 hours.[10]

Local Anesthetic Procedures for Castration

Castration of bulls is a very common surgical procedure in general practice. Historically, castration was often performed with minimal or no anesthesia. However, anesthesia for castration is more commonly practiced because calves benefit from anesthesia with improved feed consumption and rate of gain. Depending on the age and size of the animal, the surgery is usually performed with chemical and/or regional anesthesia (scrotum and testicles). Depending on the size of the calf, the proposed line of incision for removal of the distal aspect of the scrotum should be subcutaneously infiltrated with 5 to 10 mL of 2% lidocaine hydrochloride. In bulls and boars, a 16- to 18-gauge, 3.8- to 7.5-cm needle is inserted at an angle (30° to 45°) into the center of the testicle and 10 to 15 mL of local anesthetic per 200 kg of body weight is injected into the parenchyma of each testicle. The anesthetic quickly enters the lymphatics and desensitizes the sensory fibers in the spermatic cord. For smaller animals or calves, a smaller needle (20 gauge, 2.5 cm) may be used to administer 2 to 10 mL of 2% lidocaine hydrochloride.[10]

Another method uses 10 mL of 2% lidocaine hydrochloride subcutaneously along the circumference of the neck of the scrotum followed by placement of 5 mL of 2% lidocaine hydrochloride into each spermatic cord.[14] In bull calves, rams, and bucks, a 20-gauge, 2.5- to 4-cm needle can be used to inject 2% lidocaine hydrochloride into the center of the testicle. The dose varies from 2 to 10 mL depending on the size of the animal.[10]

ANESTHESIA OF THE TEAT

Because most dairy cattle, sheep, and goats are accustomed to handling and restraint for milking, surgeries of the teat can often be performed with the animal standing and with minimal restraint. Because standing procedures are always preferred in cattle to prevent udder trauma, most surgical procedures of the teat are performed using local anesthesia.

Inverted V Block

The inverted V block is used primarily for specific lesions of the teat, such as a teat laceration or wart. Using a 25-gauge 1.5-cm needle, approximately 5 mL of local anesthetic is injected into the skin and musculature dorsal to the surgical site in an inverted V pattern (**Fig. 11**).[1,8]

Ring Block

The ring block is a commonly used procedure for teat surgeries. Using a 25-gauge 1.5-cm needle, approximately 5 mL of local anesthetic is injected into the skin and musculature encircling the entire base of the teat (see **Fig. 11**).[1,8]

Infusion of the Teat Cistern

The teat cistern may be infused with local anesthetic to assist in surgical conditions that only involve the mucous membranes (eg, removal of polyps). Before infusing the teat, the cistern should be milked out and the orifice thoroughly cleaned with alcohol. A tourniquet (rubber band) is then placed on the base of the teat with adequate tension to prevent leakage between the udder and teat cistern. A sterile teat cannula is introduced and approximately 10 mL of local anesthetic is infused to fill the teat (see **Fig. 11**). The teat cannula is removed, and the remaining anesthetic is milked out. Once the surgery is

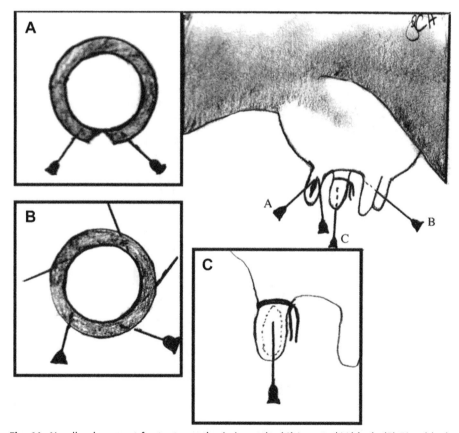

Fig. 11. Needle placement for teat anesthesia in cattle. (*A*) Inverted V block. (*B*) Ring block. (*C*) Placement of a tourniquet and teat cannula for infusion of local anesthetic into the teat cistern. (*From* Edmondson M. Local and regional anesthesia in cattle. Vet Clin North Am Food Anim Pract 2008;24:211–26; with permission.)

550

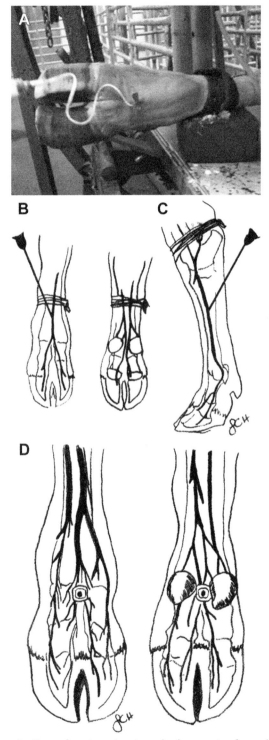

Fig. 12. Proper application of a tourniquet and placement of needle for intravenous administration of local anesthetic. (A) Intravenous regional anesthesia of the foot. Lidocaine 2% HCl (20 mL) is infused into the dorsal common digital vein distal to a rubber tourniquet. (B) Dorsal common digital vein III. (C) Cranial branch of lateral saphenous vein. (D) Axial dorsal proper digital vein III or IV. (From Edmondson M. Local and regional anesthesia in cattle. Vet Clin North Am Food Anim Pract 2008;24:211–26; with permission.)

performed, the tourniquet is removed. The musculature and skin are not desensitized using this technique.[1,8]

ANESTHESIA OF THE DISTAL LIMB

In many cases, intravenous regional anesthesia (Bier block) is the preferred technique for surgery of the foot. A tourniquet is placed proximal to the fetlock just before injection when the vein is maximally distended. In the thoracic limb, intravenous regional analgesia can be performed using the dorsal metacarpal vein, the plantar metacarpal vein, and the radial vein (**Fig. 12**). In the pelvic limb, the lateral saphenous vein or lateral plantar digital vein may be used for injection. Approximately 20 mL of local anesthetic is injected intravenously as close to the surgical site as possible using a 20-gauge 3.3-cm needle or 21-gauge butterfly catheter. It is only necessary to administer anesthetic into one vein to provide anesthesia to the entire area distal to the tourniquet. The tourniquet can be safely left on for up to 1 hour to provide hemostasis during surgical procedures of the foot. Anesthesia of the foot occurs within 5 to 10 minutes. Once the surgical procedure is complete, the tourniquet is released.

It is difficult to use the dorsal digital vein or the palmar (plantar) digital veins in small ruminants as is common in large ruminants. However, some have found the Bier block easier in small ruminants when the tourniquet was placed either above the elbow in the forelimb or below the tarsus in the hind limb. This placement allows use of the larger cephalic and recurrent tarsal veins, respectively. Using 3 to 4 mL in small goats typically results in limb anesthesia for as long as the tourniquet is in place.[7]

In cases of severe cellulitis, local intravenous anesthesia can be difficult to perform. In these cases, a simple ring block or 4-point nerve block may also be performed. A ring block is a simple method for regional anesthesia distal to the injection sites. Using a 22-gauge 2.5-cm needle, a total of 10 to 15 mL of local anesthetic is injected at multiple sites around the limb adjacent to the superficial and deep digital flexor tendons and medially and laterally to the extensor tendons. The ring block should be performed at the junction of the proximal and middle metacarpus or metatarsus. Although this is a simple technique to perform, multiple injection sites do increase the risk of infection. Problems achieving satisfactory or complete anesthesia of the digit may also be a concern when using a ring block.[1] The 4-point nerve block anesthetizes the area from the pastern distally. A 20-gauge 3.8-cm needle is inserted into the dorsal aspect of the pastern, in the groove between the proximal phalanges, just distal to the fetlock. Five milliliters of local anesthetic injected deep and another 5 mL of local anesthetic is injected superficially. This injection is then repeated on the palmar or plantar aspect of the pastern, just distal to the dewclaws. Five milliliters of local anesthetic is then used to block the digital nerve on both the medial and the lateral aspect of the fetlock, which lies approximately 2 cm dorsal and proximal to the dewclaw. The 2 interdigital injections performed in the 4-point block may also be used for removal of an interdigital fibroma.[6]

SUMMARY

Local, regional, and spinal anesthesia techniques are safe and effective methods for providing anesthesia for common surgical procedures and painful conditions in cattle and small ruminants. These techniques are inexpensive and easy to perform and offer a safe alternative to general anesthesia, in some cases.

REFERENCES

1. Skarda R. Techniques of local analgesia in ruminants and swine. Vet Clin North Am Food Anim Pract 1986;2:621–63.
2. Edwards B. Regional anaesthesia techniques in cattle. In Pract 2001;23:142–9.
3. Skarda R. Local and regional anesthesia in ruminants and swine. Vet Clin North Am Food Anim Pract 1996;12:579–626.
4. Anderson DE, Edmondson MA. Prevention and management of surgical pain in cattle. Vet Clin North Am Food Anim Pract 2013;29:157–84.
5. Elmore RG. Food animal regional anesthesia, bovine blocks: cornual. Vet Med Small Anim Clin 1980;75:1610–2.
6. Navarre C. Numbing: nose to tail. Proceedings from the 39th Annual Convention of AABP, vol. 39. Stillwater: Frontier Printers; 2006. p. 53–5.
7. Plummer PJ, Schleining JA. Assessment and management of pain in small ruminants and camelids. Vet Clin North Am Food Anim Pract 2013;29:185–208.
8. Noordsy J, Ames N. Local and regional anesthesia. In: Noordsy J, Ames N, editors. Food animal surgery. 4th edition. Yardley (PA): Veterinary Learning Systems; 2006. p. 21–42.
9. Noordsy J, Ames N. Epidural anesthesia. In: Noordsy JL, Ames NK, editors. Food animal surgery. 4th edition. Yardley (PA): Veterinary Learning Systems; 2006. p. 43–55.
10. Skarda R. Local and regional anesthetic techniques: ruminants and swine. In: Tranquilli, Thurmon, Grimm, editors. Lumb and Jones' veterinary anesthesia and analgesia. 4th edition. Oxford (United Kingdom): Blackwell Publishing Ltd.; 2007. p. 731–46.
11. Hopper R, King H, Walters K, et al. Management of urogenital surgery and disease in the bull: the scrotum and its contents. Clinical Theriogenology 2012; 4(3):332–8.
12. Larson LL. The internal pudendal (pudic) nerve block for anesthesia of the penis and relaxation of the retractor penis muscle. J Am Vet Med Assoc 1953;123: 18–27.
13. Wolfe D, Beckett S, Carson R. Acquired conditions of the penis and prepuce. In: Wolfe DF, Moll HA, editors. Large animal urogenital surgery. 2nd edition. Baltimore (MD): Williams and Wilkins; 1999. p. 237–72.
14. Rust R, Thomson D, Loneragan G, et al. Effect of different castration methods on growth performance and behavioral responses of postpubertal beef bulls. Bov Pract 2007;41(2):116–8.

Field Sedation and Anesthesia of Ruminants

Reza Seddighi, DVM, MS, PhD*, Thomas J. Doherty, MVB, MSc

KEYWORDS

- Bovine • Cattle • Ruminants • Field anesthesia • Sedation

KEY POINTS

- The general principles of anesthesia and monitoring should be applied to ruminants.
- Any change in the respiratory rate or tidal volume, subsequent to heavy sedation or general anesthesia, has a significant impact on respiratory function.
- Depending on the purpose of chemical restraint, different protocols and drug doses may be used; it is generally accepted that drug combinations are more effective for sedation and analgesia than any single drug.

INTRODUCTION

Dairy cows are generally tranquil and used to being handled; thus, many procedures can be performed using mild physical restraint with the aid of local or regional anesthesia while the animal is standing. This is fortunate, as recumbency and general anesthesia of ruminants have inherent risks. On the other hand, beef cattle are infrequently handled, and thus require more substantial forms of physical restraint and are more likely to require sedation. Additionally, beef cattle usually require larger doses of sedating and anesthetic drugs than do dairy cattle.

If recumbency is necessary for completion of a procedure, sedation can, in some cases, be used in association with a casting rope to induce recumbency. Surgical anesthesia is best performed with an endotracheal tube in place to protect the airway, but this may not always be feasible under field conditions.

Small ruminants, in contrast, are easier to handle, and many commonly performed procedures, such as cesarean section, can be done under local anesthesia, using mild physical restraint with the animal in lateral recumbency, and often without the need for sedation. Nevertheless, sedation has been shown to decrease the stress response and would be expected to improve the animal's comfort in some instances.

The authors have nothing to disclose.
Department of Large Animal Clinical Sciences, College of Veterinary Medicine, University of Tennessee, 2407 River Drive, Knoxville, TN 37996, USA
* Corresponding author.
E-mail address: mseddigh@utk.edu

CONSIDERATIONS FOR ANESTHESIA OF RUMINANTS

Sedatives and general anesthetics adversely alter cardiovascular and respiratory function; therefore, to improve patient safety, the general principles of anesthesia and monitoring should be applied to ruminants. In addition, ruminants have some unique features that distinguish them from monogastrics, and these must be considered in order to successfully manage the animal during the course of sedation and anesthesia.

Fasting

In adult cattle undergoing elective procedures, feed should be withheld for 24 to 48 hours, and water for 12 to 18 hours, depending on the size of the animal and the procedure to be performed. Small ruminants are generally not fasted longer than 24 hours, and water is not withheld for more than 12 hours. Excessive fasting should be avoided, as it may result in a change in ruminal flora and predispose the animal to ketosis.[1] In addition to decreasing the likelihood of regurgitation, fasting, by decreasing the mass of the ruminal contents, will ameliorate the effects of compression by the rumen on respiratory and cardiovascular function in the recumbent animal. Young ruminants on a milk diet are subject to developing hypoglycemia during episodes of fasting and anesthesia, as are all young animals; thus, they are not usually fasted. Additionally, it is prudent to periodically measure blood glucose in young animals under general anesthesia or, if that is not feasible, intravenous fluids should be supplemented with dextrose during the perioperative period. Older animals transitioning to solid feed are at a lower risk of developing hypoglycemia, and thus can be fasted for short periods.

Ruminal Tympany and Regurgitation

The volume of the rumen in the adult bovine can be up to 600 L, and because the rumen cannot be emptied by fasting prior to surgery, there is always a risk of bloating and regurgitation of ruminal contents. Distension of the rumen from gas accumulation and the loss of esophageal sphincter tone during a deep plane of anesthesia[2] can result in regurgitation of ruminal contents into the oropharynx.

Large volumes of gas, primarily carbon dioxide and methane, are produced in the rumen, and in the conscious animal, these gases are actively vented by eructation.[3] However, under general anesthesia or heavy sedation, ruminoreticular motility and eructation are reduced or absent, and this can result in accumulation of these gases, leading to ruminal tympany. Ruminal tympany also compounds drug-induced respiratory and cardiovascular compromise by compressing the lungs and vena cava, respectively (see further discussion in the cardiovascular section). Tympany usually resolves when the animal is placed in sternal recumbency during recovery from anesthesia.

Saliva Production

The volume of saliva produced in ruminants is considerable, and volumes up to 16 and 160 L/d have been reported for sheep and cattle, respectively.[3] The volume of saliva produced during anesthesia does not differ from the conscious state,[4] but due to the inability of the animal to swallow, it appears to be greater. In any case, this copious volume of salvia can cause obstruction of the unprotected airway. Anticholinergics, such as atropine and glycopyrrolate, are not used by the authors to decrease saliva production, because large doses of these drugs are necessary to achieve a decrease,

and there is a concomitant increase in the viscosity of saliva, thus making it more difficult to drain the pharyngeal area.

Airway Protection

Endotracheal intubation is the ideal way to protect the airway of an anesthetized animal, but it is not generally practical under field conditions. Although fasting decreases
the likelihood of regurgitation of ruminal contents, it is frequently necessary to anesthetize nonfasted ruminants for emergency procedures, and the risk of regurgitation
and aspiration can be decreased by attention to some details. If the animal is in lateral
recumbency, the risk of passive regurgitation can be decreased by elevating the proximal portion of the neck using padding and tilting the head downward to facilitate
drainage of saliva and regurgitated material from the oral cavity. It is more difficult
to drain the oral cavity with the animal in dorsal recumbency but, if possible, the animal's body should be placed on padding with the neck and head over the edge, and,
thus, at a lower level. This placement will allow the head and neck to be placed in a
more lateral position, and the head can also be tilted downward to facilitate drainage.

Endotracheal intubation poses some challenges in ruminants, and this is primarily
due to their narrow and long oral cavity and the rostro-dorsal angle of the laryngeal
entrance. It is also important that the animal be adequately anesthetized before
attempting endotracheal intubation, as attempting intubation on an inadequately
anesthetized animal may trigger regurgitation. In adult cattle, intubation is performed
most easily by initially placing a mouth gag and passing a suitably sized stomach tube
into the trachea using one's hand. The stomach tube serves as a guide over which the
endotracheal tube is passed; the cuff of the endotracheal tube is then inflated and the
stomach tube removed.

Endotracheal intubation in small ruminants and calves is commonly performed with
the aid of a laryngoscope and with the animal in sternal recumbency. It is also
possible, with practice, to pass a tube blindly, and this is facilitated by the use of a stylet to stiffen the tube. For this method, it is easiest if the animal is in lateral recumbency
with the neck extended; the mouth is held open by an attendant, and the larynx is
grasped gently in 1 hand to stabilize it. Then, the endotracheal tube is passed to
the oropharynx and gently manipulated into the larynx.

Nasotracheal intubation may be helpful in maintaining an airway if orotracheal intubation is not feasible.[5,6] The nasotracheal tube should be a few sizes smaller than the
corresponding tube used for orotracheal intubation. Passage of the nasotracheal tube
is facilitated by initially passing a smaller tube as a guide, and, depending on the size of
the animal, a stallion urinary catheter or small-bore stomach tube works well for this
purpose.

Respiratory and Cardiovascular Systems

Ruminants are sensitive to anesthetic-induced alterations in the respiratory system,
and, in comparison with many other mammals, disproportionately develop ventila-
tion/perfusion mismatch.[7] Unique features of the respiratory system in ruminants
include their smaller tidal volume and higher respiratory rate in comparison with
many other similarly sized mammals.[8] Therefore, any change in the respiratory rate
or tidal volume, subsequent to heavy sedation or general anesthesia, has a significant
impact on respiratory function. Hypercapnia and hypoxemia are common complications in anesthetized, spontaneously breathing ruminants, and these complications
occur more frequently and are of greater magnitude in nonfasted animals.[9] For these
reasons, oxygen supplementation is recommended, especially during prolonged
anesthesia.

To provide oxygen supplementation, the oxygen line should be passed into the trachea and the flow rate set to at least 15 L/min in adults. In the intubated large ruminant, it is possible to assist ventilation with the aid of a demand valve (eg, equine demand valve: JD Medical Dist. Co, Incorporated, Phoenix, Arizona) and an oxygen source. An E-type tank is suitable as an emergency source of oxygen but only lasts about 40 minutes at a flow of 15 L/min. In small ruminants, ventilation can be supported using a bag valve mask (eg, Ambu bag, Jorgensen Laboratories, Loveland, CO) to deliver air or supplemental oxygen from an E-type tank.

Anesthetic-related effects on the cardiovascular system result from the depressant effect of anesthetic drugs, and the effect of recumbency and compression by viscera on venous return and cardiac output. The latter effects are compounded in animals in dorsal recumbency and in nonfasted animals.

Musculoskeletal System

Myopathy and peripheral neuropathy are risks when large animals are immobilized. Muscle perfusion may be compromised during recumbency due to arterial hypotension, pressure on dependent muscles, poor positioning, noncompliant surfaces, and prolonged periods of recumbency. Maintaining adequate arterial blood pressure and providing padding are important preventive measures to decrease the risk of neuropathy and myopathy, particularly in large animals. A soft, grassy location or a well-bedded stall may be the best location for anesthetizing large ruminants under field conditions.

CHEMICAL RESTRAINT OF RUMINANTS

In the United States, lidocaine hydrochloride is the only modern anesthetic-related drug currently approved for use in cattle. Therefore, the administration of other sedatives and anesthetics is considered extralabel drug use.[10] On the other hand, the extralabel use of such drugs in cattle is increasing in order to improve veterinary care and welfare. In addition, withdrawal periods for commonly used drugs for animals used for milk and meat production, as recommended by the Food Animal Drug Residue Avoidance & Databank (FARAD), must be carefully followed (**Table 1**). Nevertheless, several different groups of sedative and analgesics, as sole agents or more commonly in combination, are used to provide restraint of small and large ruminants,

Table 1
Recommended withdrawal intervals for common anesthetic/analgesic agents in ruminants

Drug	Route of Administration	Withdrawal Intervals (d)	
		Meat	Milk
Acepromazine	IV or IM	7	2
Butorphanol	IV or IM	5 (2 for sheep)[35]	3 (2 for sheep)[35]
Detomidine	IV or IM	3	3
Guaifenesin	IV	3	2
Ketamine	IV or IM	3	3 (2 d)[34,35]
Lidocaine	SC (volume >20 mL)	4 (1 d)[35]	3 (1 d)[35]
Tolazoline	IV or IM	8	2
Xylazine	IV or IM	4 (5),[35] (5–10)[34]	1 (3),[35] (3–5)[34]
Yohimbine	IV	7	3

Abbreviations: IM, intramuscularly; IV, intravenously; SC, subcutaneously.
Data from Refs.[10,34,35]

either as premedication prior to general anesthesia, or for performing diagnostic or minor surgical procedures.

Route of Drug Administration

The intravenous route is the most effective method of administration in terms of bioavailability and onset of action. However, the intravenous route may not always be practical under field conditions, especially when dealing with unruly large bovines; in these animals, the intramuscular or subcutaneous route can be used initially to achieve sedation. The limitations of intramuscular and subcutaneous injection include incomplete bioavailability, delayed onset of action, and the limited volume that can be administered.

Intravenous administration of drugs

Depending on the animal in question and available facilities, intravenous drugs can be given into the jugular, auricular, or tail vein. The tail vein is commonly used for administration of small volumes when animals are restrained in a chute and when jugular injections are not practical due to an animal's disposition. It is advisable to place an intravenous catheter in a jugular vein if repeated drug administration is required or if tissue irritant solutions, such as guaifenesin, are to be administered. For large ruminants, a 14-gauge, 5.5-inch (approximately 14 cm) catheter is suitable for jugular vein cannulation, and an 18 to 20-gauge catheter is usually suitable for small ruminants or for auricular vein catheterization. Also, it is not prudent to administer guaifenesin and other potentially tissue irritant solutions into a small vein or an auricular vein, as thrombosis is likely to result, and, in the case of an auricular vein, this may result in sloughing of the pinna.

Drugs Commonly Used for Chemical Restraint of Ruminants

Alpha-2 adrenoceptor agonists

The main members of this group are xylazine, dexmedetomidine, romifidine, and detomidine. Xylazine is licensed for use in cattle in the United States and is the most commonly used sedative for chemical restraint of ruminants. An important aspect of alpha-2 adrenoceptor agonists is the availability of antagonists.

Generally, sedation induced by members of this group outlasts their analgesic effects, and xylazine administration results in the shortest duration of sedation and analgesia. Of interest, ruminants are much more sensitive to the sedating effects of xylazine than are horses; the dose of xylazine in ruminants is generally a tenth of the dose used in horses, and it also results in more profound sedation (**Table 2**).

Table 2
Doses of commonly used alpha-2 adrenoceptor agonists in ruminants

Drug	Route of Administration	Adult Cattle	Calf	Sheep	Goat
Xylazine (mg/kg)	IV	0.05–0.1	0.05–0.1	0.05–0.1	0.02–0.05
	IM	0.1–0.3	0.1–0.3	0.1–0.2	0.05–0.1
Dexmedetomidine (μg/kg)	IV	1–5	5–10	5–10	5–10
	IM	5–20	10–30	10–30	10–30
Detomidine (μg/kg)	IV	3–10	3–30	3–20	5–20
	IM	10–20	30–40	20–30	20–30
Romifidine (μg/kg)	IV	3–20	3–50	3–40	3–40
	IM	20–40	50–100	40–80	40–80

Abbreviations: IM, intramuscularly; IV, intravenously.

This is not the case for other alpha-2 agonists for which the drug dose is similar to that used in horses. It also seems that some breeds, particularly Brahman, are more sensitive than others to the sedating effects of xylazine. However, the response of an individual ruminant to xylazine can be quite variable, especially if the animal is excited or unruly. This topic is discussed further in the section on standing sedation.

Xylazine and other alpha-2 agonists have numerous dose-related adverse effects that necessitate special consideration. For example, small ruminants are particularly sensitive to the pulmonary effects of alpha-2 agonists.[11,12] Activation of pulmonary intravascular macrophages (PIMs) is the primary reason for the adverse effects of alpha-2 agonists on the pulmonary system. Once activated, PIMs release prostaglandins and other vasoactive substances; this can result in alveolar edema, an increase in transpulmonary pressure, a decrease in pulmonary compliance, and pulmonary congestion.[11,13] Although the cumulative clinical effect of these pulmonary changes can result in transient hypoxemia, these effects are well tolerated in healthy small ruminants.

Alpha-2 agonists, especially xylazine, increase the tone of the gravid uterus and constrict uterine vasculature, resulting in a decrease in uterine blood flow, and a decrease in fetal and maternal oxygen partial pressure.[14–17] Therefore, their use during the last trimester may result in premature labor or fetal hypoxemia.

Alpha-2 agonists decrease gastrointestinal motility, secondary to inhibiting the release of acetylcholine, and this can contribute to ruminal tympany. In cattle and sheep, detomidine and xylazine inhibited ruminal contractions, and this resulted in ruminal tympany.[18,19] The latter effect was eliminated by administration of the antagonist tolazoline, but not by yohimbine.

Phenothiazines

Acepromazine is the most commonly used agent in this group. Acepromazine has a delayed onset of action when compared with xylazine; maximum effect after intravenous administration may take 15 to 20 minutes, and its duration of action can be 4 to 6 hours. Acepromazine has minimal respiratory effects but may result in arterial hypotension, particularly at higher doses or in hypovolemic animals. Acepromazine lacks analgesic effects, and its sedative effect is less than xylazine. Therefore, as is discussed later, acepromazine is best used in combination with other drugs to achieve a clinically significant effect.

Benzodiazepines

Members of this family include midazolam, diazepam, and zolazepam. Zolazepam is commercially available only in combination with tiletamine in the product Telazol. These drugs act on gamma-aminobutyric acid receptors and, in the majority of animals, their administration results in sedation and muscle relaxation; however, when used alone in healthy animals, they can cause paradoxic excitation. It is recommended that diazepam be administered intravenously, as it is not water soluble, and intramuscular administration may be associated with tissue irritation and erratic absorption.

Benzodiazepines have minimal effects on the cardiovascular and respiratory systems and can be used for sedation in small ruminants and calves as the sole drug, but they are preferably used in combination with other agents. The use of benzodiazepines in cattle for standing sedation is not recommended, primarily because of the risk of inducing ataxia and recumbency; however, their muscle relaxant effects are beneficial when combined with ketamine for induction of anesthesia.[1]

Opioids

Opioid receptors are present in the peripheral and central nervous systems and are important components of the pain pathway. Although sedation and analgesia are the desired clinical effects of opioids, excitatory effects and behavioral changes have been associated with butorphanol administration to ruminants.[20,21] Nevertheless, excitatory effects are more likely to occur if opioids are administered at higher doses intravenously to nonsedated animals. Butorphanol has minimal analgesic effects, but, based on the authors' clinical impressions, it seems to potentiate the sedative and analgesic effects of other agents in ruminants. Morphine is a more efficacious analgesic agent and is recommended for more painful procedures. Morphine was not associated with behavioral changes in cows in 1 study,[22] but there have been anecdotal reports of morphine causing excitement in cattle (David Anderson, personal communication, 2015).

Standing Chemical Restraint of Adult Cattle

Depending on the purpose of chemical restraint, different protocols and drug doses may be used. It is generally accepted that drug combinations are more effective for sedation and analgesia than any single drug. Additionally, the response to a drug can be expected to vary greatly based on the animal's disposition and breed.

Various methods have been described to induce sedation in adult cattle. Regardless of the drug regimen used, it is important that the animal be left undisturbed for an adequate duration to get a clinically significant effect from the drug(s) before starting any manipulations. It is also important to keep in mind that the doses and combinations listed here are intended for use in healthy or minimally compromised animals, and doses should be adjusted in sick or debilitated animals.

Acepromazine

Although not a potent sedative when used alone, acepromazine combined with butorphanol or xylazine can be efficacious for sedation of tranquil bulls and dairy cows under certain circumstances. For example, in the authors' clinic, a mixture of acepromazine (10 mg) and xylazine (10 mg) is administered intravenously to sedate manageable bulls and cows for standing procedures, to facilitate placing animals on a tilt table, or to facilitate casting an animal using ropes (Sarel van Amstel, personal communication, 2016).

In a report on adult dairy cows undergoing standing cesarean section, intravenous acepromazine (7.5 mg) combined with butorphanol (10 mg) resulted in successful sedation.[5] In adult Jersey cows undergoing laryngoscopy, acepromazine (0.035 mg/kg, intravenously) did not profoundly change the laryngeal anatomic position and function, and, thus was deemed more appropriate than xylazine for sedation when evaluating laryngeal function.[23]

Alpha-2 agonists

Alpha-2 adrenoceptor agonists, particularly xylazine, are the mainstay of standing sedation, but it is important to give the appropriate dose to avoid inducing recumbency. On the other hand, if the animal is not adequately sedated with what seems to be an appropriate dose of an alpha-2 adrenoceptor agonist, it is best to add another drug from a different class rather than increasing the dose and causing recumbency or cardiorespiratory compromise.

Xylazine Xylazine is the most commonly used alpha-2 adrenoceptor agonist in cattle in North America. A simple and practical approach to achieving sedation in standing adult cattle is to administer xylazine (0.02–0.03 mg/kg, intravenously or 0.04–0.06 mg/kg, intramuscularly). These doses result in standing sedation in the majority of dairy cattle.

Detomidine Detomidine is licensed for intramuscular or intravenous use in cattle in Europe at doses of 0.01 to 0.04 mg/kg. In dairy cows, detomidine (0.01 mg/kg, intravenously) resulted in more profound sedation than did xylazine (0.02 mg/kg, intravenously), and the cows remained standing.[20]

Alpha-2 adrenoceptor agonists combined with opioids In dairy cows, xylazine (0.02 mg/kg, intravenously) or detomidine (0.01 mg/kg, intravenously) was combined with butorphanol (0.05 mg/kg, intravenously) to compare their sedative properties. Butorphanol did not increase the duration or intensity of the alpha-2 agonist induced-sedation in that study.[20] However, it has been reported that butorphanol (0.05 mg/kg, intravenously), when used in association with xylazine, seemed to create better analgesia of the body wall for laparotomies.[24] Although it is stated that the administration of xylazine and butorphanol eliminated the need for local anesthesia during laparotomy surgery in some cattle,[24] it is important to understand that these combinations do not induce a state of general anesthesia; thus local or regional anesthesia of the surgical site should be provided.

Combinations of alpha-2 adrenoceptor agonists ketamine and opioids (ketamine stun) The use of sedative combinations that include ketamine is known informally as the ketamine stun. The original technique was introduced for restraint of adult cattle,[25] but variations of these protocols have been used.[26] Using these combinations, sedation and some analgesia are achieved by administering subanesthetic doses of xylazine and ketamine. An opioid, butorphanol, or less commonly, morphine, is generally added to this combination to improve sedation and analgesia. An advantage of this technique is that a smaller dose of individual drugs is given, which helps decrease the adverse effects of each drug. In addition, there is an additive, or perhaps synergistic, effect when using more than 1 drug.

The ketamine stun, using xylazine (0.05 mg/kg, intravenously) with ketamine (0.1 mg/kg, intravenously), decreased distress behavior at the time of castration and attenuated the cortisol response for the initial 60 minutes in 4- to 6-month-old Angus calves, when used without local anesthesia.[26] Nevertheless, as was mentioned earlier, local or regional anesthesia is necessary to achieve complete sensory blockade of the surgical site.

5-10-20 combination Intravenously administered combinations of butorphanol (0.01 mg/kg), xylazine (0.02 mg/kg), and ketamine (0.05–0.1 mg/kg) result in effective standing sedation in most adult cattle.[25] This drug regimen is known colloquially as the 5-10-20 combination because it contains approximately 5 mg butorphanol, 10 mg xylazine, and 20 mg ketamine, and, when given intravenously, it is suitable for standing sedation of most adult cattle (500–600 kg). With this combination, animals may show a brief period of unsteadiness, and this can be minimized by administering the ketamine intravenously 10 minutes after the xylazine–opioid combination. Alternatively, the higher end of the ketamine (0.1 mg/kg) dose can be given intramuscularly concurrently with intravenous administration of xylazine–butorphanol to prolong the sedative effect for up to 20 minutes, and to prevent the risk of behavioral changes induced by intravenous administration of ketamine (David Anderson, personal communication, 2015).

10-20-40 and 20-40-80 combinations The ketamine stun combination can also be given intramuscularly or subcutaneously to prolong the duration of effect and to decrease the risk of ketamine-induced behavioral changes.[25] In the authors' practice, approximately twice the intravenous dose is used for intramuscular or subcutaneous administration. For cattle (500–600 kg), the combination is known colloquially as the 10-20-40 combination, because it includes 10 mg butorphanol (0.015–0.02 mg/kg), 20 mg xylazine (0.03–0.04 mg/kg), and 40 mg ketamine (0.06–0.08 mg/kg). The peak effect after intramuscular or subcutaneous administration is achieved in 15 to 20 minutes; thus, it is important not to disturb the animal in this time interval. Readministration of 25% to 50% of the initial doses of xylazine and ketamine can be performed to achieve the desired degree of cooperation and to prolong restraint.

For large bulls or more unruly animals, the 20-40-80 combination is used: 20 mg butorphanol, 40 mg xylazine, and 80 mg ketamine.

Table 3 contains a summary of the drugs administered for standing sedation in adult cattle.

Inducing Recumbency and General Anesthesia in Adult Cattle

Adequate sedation and analgesia are important to decrease distress and pain associated with immobilization and surgery. When recumbency is intended, particularly for general anesthesia, fasting the animal reduces the risk of regurgitation and ruminal tympany. As previously stated, adult cattle are fasted for 24 to 48 hours prior to general anesthesia for elective procedures. If repeated intravenous injections are planned or if a continuous infusion of drugs is contemplated, placement of a jugular catheter is

Table 3
Examples of drug(s) and drug combinations used for standing sedation in adult cattle

Drug(s)	Estimated Body Weight (kg)	Total mg of Each Drug	Route of Administration	Duration of Effect (min)	Comments
Xylazine	500–600	10–15	IV	10–20	Mild-to-moderate sedation
	500–600	20–30	IM	15–30	Mild-to-moderate sedation
Detomidine	500–600	5–20	IV, IM	40–50	Mild-to-moderate sedation; High end of dose range for IM administration
Acepromazine/ xylazine	500–600	10/10	IV	10–20	Mild-to-moderate sedation
Butorphanol/ xylazine/ ketamine	500–600	5/10/20	IV	10–15	Moderate sedation Alternatively, ketamine (50–60 mg) can be given IM instead of IV
	500–600	10/20/40	IM, SQ	20–40	More profound sedation To prolong effect, readminister 25%–50% of initial dose of xylazine and ketamine
	≥800	20/40/80	IM	20–40	For larger and/or unruly animals

Abbreviations: IM, intramuscularly; IV, intravenously; SC, subcutaneously.

recommended. It is important that the site chosen for induction of recumbency provides adequate footing and padding for the animal and, as mentioned previously, a soft, grassy area or a well-bedded stall are probably the best options.

A variety of drug regimens can be used to induce recumbency and general anesthesia, and the method used will depend on the intended purpose, type of patient, available drugs and facilities, and personal preference. Even if general anesthesia is induced, it is usually beneficial to also perform a local or regional block to anesthetize the surgical site to increase patient comfort in recovery, and help to prevent the animal from responding to surgical manipulation if the depth of anesthesia changes.

Xylazine

Use of xylazine as a sole agent can be a practical method of inducing recumbency for completion of nonpainful procedures, or it can be combined with local anesthesia for more invasive procedures. Most dairy cattle will become recumbent with xylazine doses of 0.05 to 0.10 mg/kg intravenously, and the dose is generally doubled for intramuscular administration. The administration of xylazine (0.05 mg/kg, intramuscularly) 15 minutes before positioning cows in lateral recumbency alleviated the stress response and pain-related behaviors associated with claw treatment and recumbency.[27] In general, beef cattle, and certainly boisterous cattle, require bigger doses of xylazine. Inducing recumbency in a xylazine-sedated animal is facilitated by the use of a casting rope.

Ketamine-xylazine-butorphanol

If the doses of individual drugs are increased over those used for standing restraint, the ketamine stun can also be used to induce recumbency and deep sedation, and, when combined with local or regional anesthesia, it is practical for performing some surgical procedures. To induce recumbency and deep sedation in an adult bovine (500–600 kg), using intravenous administration, 20 mg butorphanol, 25 mg xylazine, and 250 to 500 mg ketamine are used in the authors' practice. The duration of sedation and recumbency can be extended by administering half of the initial dose of ketamine alone or combined with 10 to 20 mg xylazine. Doses of xylazine and ketamine are doubled if the intramuscular route is chosen.

Xylazine-ketamine

A short duration (10–15 minutes) of surgical anesthesia can be achieved with the intravenous administration of xylazine (0.1 mg/kg) and a higher dose of ketamine (2 mg/kg). Alternatively, if the animal does not readily tolerate venipuncture, sedation can be induced with intramuscular xylazine (0.1–0.2 mg/kg), and anesthesia can be induced with intravenous ketamine (2 mg/kg) once the animal becomes sedated. Diazepam or midazolam (0.025–0.05 mg/kg) may be administered with ketamine to improve muscle relaxation, especially if endotracheal intubation is planned.

Another option is to administer xylazine (0.2 mg/kg) and ketamine (3–4 mg/kg) intramuscularly to provide a longer duration (15–30 minutes) of surgical anesthesia. The duration of surgical anesthesia can be further extended by administering ketamine (1–2 mg/kg) and xylazine (0.02–0.04 mg/kg) intravenously, as deemed necessary. Ideally the supplemental doses of xylazine and ketamine should be administered slowly to prevent apnea.

An opioid, butorphanol (0.02–0.04 mg/kg), or morphine (0.05–0.1 mg/kg) can be added to either of these drug protocols, with the lower end of the dose range being used intravenously.

Telazol–xylazine

Telazol has minimal muscle relaxing properties and is best combined with other drugs. At the authors' clinic, a combination of Telazol and xylazine is used predominantly to immobilize large bulls ($\geq$800 kg) for procedures such as foot trimming (Marc Caldwell, personal communication, 2016). Telazol is available as a powder, and each vial contains 250 mg each of tiletamine and zolazepam. In this case, the powder is reconstituted by adding 500 mg xylazine, and 3 to 5 mL of the mixture, depending on the size and demeanor of the animal, are given intramuscularly. This mixture will provide up to 45 minutes of immobilization, and the recovery is smooth. However, local anesthesia is necessary to perform surgical procedures on these animals. The main disadvantage of this protocol is the cost of Telazol. A variation of this method is to add 100 to 150 mg of xylazine to Telazol, and add ketamine to make the volume up to 5.0 mL (as described for capturing wild cattle).

Telazol can also be administered intravenously with xylazine to induce anesthesia in ruminants. In 1 study, a mixture of Telazol (4 mg/kg) and xylazine (0.1 mg/kg) was administered intravenously.[28] However, 4 mg/kg Telazol seems to be an excessive dose for intravenous administration in association with xylazine (0.1 mg/kg), and an initial dose of 1 to 2 mg/kg of Telazol is recommended for induction when used with this dose of xylazine, administering more Telazol, as needed.

Ketamine-xylazine-guaifenesin infusion (triple-drip)

This mixture is informally known as triple-drip, and it can be used to induce anesthesia or maintain a state of general anesthesia. Guaifenesin is used for its muscle-relaxing effects and does not appear to have clinically significant anesthetic actions. A caution with the use of triple-drip is that guaifenesin is an irritant to tissues; thus, perivascular leakage must be avoided.

Induction of anesthesia with triple-drip For induction of anesthesia with triple-drip in an adult bovine (500–700 kg), 50 mg xylazine and 1.0 to 1.5 g ketamine are added to 1 L of a 5% guaifenesin solution, and the mixture is given to effect. An advantage of inducing anesthesia with triple-drip is that the process is relatively gradual; thus, the animal is less likely to become apneic than when a bolus of induction drugs is administered. Also, the infusion rate can be changed depending on the desired effect.

Maintenance of anesthesia with triple-drip The triple-drip mixture can also be used for maintenance of anesthesia either after induction with triple-drip itself or 1 of the previously described methods. Triple-drip, as described previously, should maintain a surgical plane of anesthesia in an adult bovine (500–700 kg) for approximately 60 minutes, and the duration will be influenced by the drugs initially used for induction of anesthesia. If a large dose of xylazine was administered at induction, the amount of xylazine in the triple-drip should be decreased accordingly.

A constraint to the use of triple-drip is the lack of commercial availability and expense of guaifenesin; however, guaifenesin can be purchased in bulk as a powder, and it can be made into a 5% solution and autoclaved in preparation for clinical use.

Ketamine-Xylazine Infusion

Because of the aforementioned issues of cost and availability of guaifenesin, an alternative is to maintain anesthesia using an infusion of only xylazine and ketamine. To facilitate administration under field conditions, appropriate doses of xylazine and ketamine can be added to a 1 L bag of a balanced electrolyte solution, such as lactated Ringer solution, and administered to effect. As in the case of triple-drip, 50 mg xylazine and 1.0 to 1.5 g ketamine added to 1 L electrolyte solution should provide surgical anesthesia for approximately 60 minutes for an adult bovine (500–700 kg). Muscle relaxation should be satisfactory if an adequate dose of xylazine is used at induction, or it can be improved by administering 25 to 50 mg of midazolam or diazepam intravenously as a bolus or by increasing the infusion rate of xylazine and ketamine.

Capture of Wild and Aggressive Cattle

In certain instances, the behavior of an animal necessitates that sedative and anesthetic drugs be delivered remotely, and this may involve the use of a dart gun, a pole syringe, or a pistol or rifle. Under these circumstances, the volume of anesthetics that can be delivered and the distance of the animal from the delivery system are limiting factors. A pole syringe can be used at distances between 1 to 3 m (3–9 feet), and can deliver volumes up to 10 mL. Pole syringes can also be used to deliver drugs once the animal becomes recumbent but is still regarded as too dangerous to approach for hand injection. Blow pipes are useful in the range of 5 to 10 m (16–30 feet), and can deliver volumes of 3 to 5 mL. Also, blow pipes cause minimum tissue trauma due to the low-velocity injection. Pistols are generally effective within a range of 20 m (65 feet), and at distances of 20 to 40 m (65–130 feet); it is necessary to use a rifle to project the dart. In general, the maximum dart volume is 5 mL for a pistol and 10 mL for a rifle.

The volume limitation of remote capture devices restricts the drug options for capture of adult cattle. Thus, a practical option is to use a drug regimen based on Telazol, and to reconstitute 500 mg of the drug mixture with 1 mL xylazine (100 mg/mL) and add 3 to 4 mL ketamine (100 mg/mL) to bring the total volume up to 4.0 to 5.0 mL. This mixture should be sufficient to immobilize a 600 to 800-kg animal. Alternatively, the vial of Telazol powder can be reconstituted with 300 mg xylazine.

As is the case for all drug protocols, the response to these drug mixtures depends greatly on the animal's disposition. For smaller animals, the dose can be prorated. Xylazine can be reversed, if deemed necessary, at the end of the procedure.

A summary of the drugs administered for inducing recumbency and/or general anesthesia in adult cattle is included in **Table 4**.

Recovery from Recumbency and General Anesthesia in Cattle

In general, recovery from recumbency and general anesthesia in cattle is smooth, and the animals usually recover in a controlled manner. However, the site chosen for recovery should provide adequate footing and padding for the animal and be free of obstacles that could cause injury. Additionally, the animal should be placed and supported in sternal recumbency, and, if deemed appropriate, the alpha-2 portion of the drug combination can be antagonized (as will be discussed).

Alpha-2 adrenergic antagonists

A desirable property of alpha-2 adrenergic agonists is their ability to be reversed; however, the use of alpha-2 adrenergic antagonists must not be undertaken lightly. The available drugs in this category are yohimbine, tolazoline, and atipamezole. In the authors' experience, yohimbine is not an effective reversal agent in ruminants. Tolazoline is the most commonly used member of this group in ruminants and is efficacious at reversing the actions of commonly used alpha-2 adrenergic antagonists. Atipamezole is also effective in reversing the sedative (and analgesic) effects of alpha-2 agonists in ruminants,[29,30] but its use in cattle may be cost prohibitive.

Overdosage or rapid intravenous administration of alpha-2 adrenergic antagonists can lead to adverse effects on the cardiovascular, respiratory, and central nervous system, and these effects can result in death. Hypotension, due to vasodilation,

Table 4
Examples of drug(s) and drug combinations for inducing recumbency or general anesthesia in adult cattle

Drug(s)	Estimated Body Weight (kg)	Total mg of Each Drug	Route of Administration	Duration of Effect (min)	Comments
Xylazine	500–600	25–50	IV	10–15	Generally induces recumbency Facilitates casting with ropes, if necessary
	500–600	50–100	IM	10–20	
Xylazine/ketamine	500–600	50/1000	IV	10–15	Short period of general anesthesia Top-up doses of ketamine (1–2 mg/kg) with xylazine (0.02–0.04 mg/kg) slowly IV to prolong effect
	500–600	100/2000	IM	15–30	
Butorphanol/xylazine/ketamine	500–600	20/25/250	IV	20–30	Heavy sedation; Dose of ketamine can be increased to 500 mg to prolong recumbency
Telazol/xylazine	≥800	Reconstitute 500 mg Telazol with 500 mg xylazine and give 3–5 mL	IM	30–45	Heavy sedation with longer duration of recumbency and immobilization
Telazol/xylazine/ketamine	Wild/aggressive cattle (600–800 kg)	500/100/400	IM	30–45	Heavy sedation/general anesthesia, depending on animal's demeanor

Abbreviations: IM, intramuscularly; IV, intravenously; SC, subcutaneously.

seems to be the main adverse cardiovascular effect at clinical doses. Higher doses of alpha-2 adrenergic antagonists have an amphetamine-like effect that can result in central nervous system stimulation and tachycardia. Although these compounds can be administered intravenously, the authors generally recommend intramuscular administration to decrease the likelihood of causing adverse effects. If it is determined that the reversal is best given intravenously in a particular circumstance, the dose should be decreased and administered slowly.

Chemical Restraint of Small Ruminants

In comparison with cattle, small ruminants, especially sheep, are generally docile, are easier to handle, and can be physically restrained for intravenous or intramuscular injection. On the other hand, small ruminants are likely to become recumbent once sedated, so it is unusual to perform surgeries on sedated standing small ruminants. The same concerns regarding regurgitation, bloating, and protection of the airway described previously for large ruminants apply to small ruminants. Various drugs and drug combinations are used to induce sedation and general anesthesia, and some examples will be discussed.

Acepromazine

Acepromazine provides mild sedation but is rarely used alone for this purpose. In the authors' practice, acepromazine is sometimes used as a premedication prior to induction of general anesthesia with midazolam and ketamine. In small ruminants, acepromazine is often combined with opioids to augment its sedative effects.

Benzodiazepines

When used alone, benzodiazepines have limited application, but they can be used to induce mild sedation for nonpainful procedures (eg, radiography, ultrasonography) in tranquil animals. Midazolam (0.1–0.5 mg/kg, intravenously or intramuscularly) or diazepam (0.1–0.5 intravenously) can cause paradoxic excitation, especially if administered rapidly intravenously to healthy adult ruminants.

Benzodiazepines and butorphanol

In the authors' clinic, midazolam and butorphanol are sometimes administered intravenously or intramuscularly to induce a more profound state of sedation, compared with benzodiazepines alone. For example, this combination can be used to provide mild sedation in sheep or goats undergoing cesarean section in lateral recumbency in conjunction with local analgesia and mild physical restraint. Midazolam (0.1–0.5 mg/kg, intravenously or intramuscularly) or diazepam (0.1–0.5, intravenously) is combined with butorphanol (0.1–0.2 mg/kg, intravenously or 0.2–0.4 mg/kg, intramuscularly). An advantage of this method is that the effects of the benzodiazepines on the newborn can be reversed with the administration of flumazenil (0.01–0.02 mg/kg, intravenously), a benzodiazepine antagonist. The umbilical vein can be used for intravenous injections in the newborn.

Opioids

Opioids are mainly used in conjunction with other agents such as acepromazine, a benzodiazepine, or an alpha-2 adrenoceptor agonist for sedation and analgesia. Butorphanol (0.1–0.2 mg/kg, intravenously or 0.2–0.4 mg/kg, intramuscularly) is the most commonly used opioid, but morphine (0.05–0.1 mg/kg, intravenously or 0.25–0.5 mg/kg, intramuscularly) provides more profound analgesia. The authors have not observed adverse effects when using morphine at these doses in small ruminants.

Alpha-2 adrenoceptor agonists

Xylazine is the most commonly used drug in this group, and it produces reliable sedation; however, small ruminants are sensitive to the effects of these drugs. Xylazine doses of 0.03 to 0.05 mg/kg intramuscularly produce mild sedation, and a dose of 0.1 to 0.2 mg/kg intramuscularly produces deep sedation. However, the response depends greatly on the disposition of the animal. Nevertheless, deeply sedated animals can still be aroused and will respond to noxious stimuli. As was discussed earlier, alpha-2 agonists, particularly at higher doses and when administered intravenously, may result in significant ventilation–perfusion mismatch and hypoxemia; thus, it is best to limit the dose of these drugs and add a drug from a different group to augment sedation and analgesia.

Xylazine and butorphanol

The authors have used this combination to induce mild-to-moderate sedation at doses of 0.02 to 0.05 mg/kg intravenously for each drug, or intramuscularly at 0.05 mg/kg for xylazine and 0.1 to 0.2 mg/kg for butorphanol.

Xylazine and ketamine

This combination, at the appropriate doses, can be used to induce deep sedation in small ruminants. Administration of xylazine (0.1–0.2 mg/kg, intramuscularly) and ketamine (2–3 mg/kg, intramuscularly) produces deep sedation, but not surgical anesthesia, for about 30 minutes. For intravenous administration, the dose of each drug should be reduced; to prevent apnea, xylazine (0.02–0.05 mg/kg) can be administered initially to induce sedation, and ketamine (0.5–2.0 mg/kg) can then be administered to effect. Alternatively, the mixture can be given slowly intravenously.

Xylazine and Telazol

Telazol can be substituted for ketamine for administration with xylazine, and the dose of each can be varied to attain the desired degree of sedation. Administration of xylazine (0.1–0.2 mg/kg, intramuscularly) and Telazol (0.5–1.0 mg/kg, intramuscularly) will produce profound sedation for 30 to 45 minutes, and smaller doses of each can be given intravenously to induce a lesser degree of sedation.

General Anesthesia of Small Ruminants

Depending on the circumstances and the disposition of the animal, premedication may or may not be administered. Under field conditions, most drug regimens are based on ketamine. Although ketamine has been used as the sole anesthetic agent in small ruminants, the authors do not recommend this, because ketamine alone does not provide a complete state of general anesthesia. Ketamine is primarily used in combination with xylazine, but several other combinations have also been described.

Propofol could be used for induction and maintenance of anesthesia, but it is not practical under field conditions, as it has to be administered as an infusion to maintain anesthesia. Additionally, propofol is likely to cause apnea, which would have serious consequences if the animal was not endotracheally intubated and there was no means to supply positive pressure ventilation.

Ketamine and xylazine

For intramuscular administration, xylazine can be administered at 0.1 to 0.2 mg/kg, depending on the animal's health and disposition, in association with ketamine at 5 to 15 mg/kg. Surgical anesthesia usually lasts 20 to 30 minutes, depending on the dose of ketamine administered. The authors use this drug regimen for disbudding of kids, and the animals are usually standing within 45 minutes after xylazine (0.1 mg/kg) and ketamine (10–15 mg/kg) administered intramuscularly. The duration of anesthesia can be extended by readministering ketamine (3–5 mg/kg, intramuscularly) or 1 to 2 mg/kg intravenously as needed.

Animals may also be sedated with xylazine (0.1–0.2 mg/kg, intramuscularly), and anesthesia may be induced with ketamine administered IV to effect, but care must be taken to avoid causing apnea. In sheep, ketamine has been administered at a dose of 7.5 mg/kg intravenously in association with xylazine (0.1 mg/kg), and the combination induced a state of surgical anesthesia for 25 minutes.[31]

Ketamine and benzodiazepines

Anesthesia can be induced in nonsedated animals with ketamine (5–7 mg/kg) and a benzodiazepine (eg, midazolam or diazepam 0.25–0.5 mg/kg) administered intravenously. The dose of ketamine needed to allow endotracheal intubation depends greatly on the speed of administration. However, the duration of anesthesia is short (5–10 minutes), and premedication with xylazine (0.1–0.2 mg/kg, intramuscularly) will prolong anesthesia and decrease the dose of ketamine needed for induction of anesthesia.

Telazol and xylazine

In 1 study, Telazol (13.2 mg/kg) was administered intravenously to sheep either alone or in association with 0.11 mg/kg xylazine.[32] The duration of analgesia was approximately 40 minutes in the Telazol group and 100 minutes in the Telazol and xylazine group; however, this dose was associated with apnea in some animals. As mentioned previously, this dose of Telazol is excessive for most small ruminants, and it would be best to induce anesthesia with a much smaller dose (1–3 mg/kg) and supplement as needed.

Ketamine-xylazine-guaifenesin infusion (triple-drip)

This method can be used to induce and maintain anesthesia in small ruminants. In a study in sheep, a mixture of guaifenesin (50 mg/mL), ketamine (1 mg/mL), and xylazine (0.1 mg/mL) in 5% dextrose induced anesthesia at a mean dose of 1.2 mL/kg and maintained anesthesia at 2.6 mL/kg/h. Significant hypoxemia and hypercarbia were observed throughout the course of the study; however, administration of 100% oxygen via an endotracheal tube reduced the magnitude of hypoxemia. After 1 hour of anesthesia, the sheep stood at a mean time of 96 minutes, but recovery was prolonged another 50 minutes in others.[33] Administration of lower doses and titration of the infusion to effect would presumably reduce the severity of the adverse effects.

REFERENCES

1. Valverde A, Doherty TJ. Anesthesia and analgesia of ruminants. In: Fish RE, Brown MJ, Danneman PJ, et al, editors. Anesthesia and analgesia in laboratory animals. London: Academic Press Elsevier; 2008. p. 385–412.

2. Steffey EP. Some characteristics of ruminants and swine that complicate management of general anesthesia. Vet Clin North Am Food Anim Pract 1986;2:507–16.

3. Leek BF. Digestion in the ruminant stomach. In: Swenson MJ, Reece WO, editors. Dukes' physiology of domestic animals. 11th edition. Ithaca (NY): Comstock Publishing Associates; 1993. p. 387–416.

4. Kay RN. The rate of flow and composition of various salivary secretions in sheep and calves. J Physiol 1960;150:515–37.

5. Newman KD, Anderson DE. Cesarean section in cows. Vet Clin North Am Food Anim Pract 2005;21:73–100.
6. Quandt JE, Robinson EP. Nasotracheal intubation in calves. J Am Vet Med Assoc 1996;209:967–8.
7. Erhardt W, Kostlin R, Seiler R, et al. Respiratory functional hypoxia in ruminants under general anesthesia. Tierarztl Prax Suppl 1985;1:45–9 [in German].
8. Mortola JP, Lanthier C. Breathing frequency in ruminants: a comparative analysis with non-ruminant mammals. Respir Physiol Neurobiol 2005;145:265–77.
9. Blaze CA, LeBlanc PH, Robinson NE. Effect of withholding feed on ventilation and the incidence of regurgitation during halothane anesthesia of adult cattle. Am J Vet Res 1988;49:2126–9.
10. Smith GW, Davis JL, Tell LA, et al. Extralabel use of nonsteroidal anti-inflammatory drugs in cattle. J Am Vet Med Assoc 2008;232:697–701.
11. Celly CS, Atwal OS, McDonell WN, et al. Histopathologic alterations induced in the lungs of sheep by use of alpha2-adrenergic receptor agonists. Am J Vet Res 1999;60:154–61.
12. Celly CS, McDonell WN, Black WD, et al. Cardiopulmonary effects of clonidine, diazepam and the peripheral alpha 2 adrenoceptor agonist ST-91 in conscious sheep. J Vet Pharmacol Ther 1997;20:472–8.
13. Kastner SB. A2-agonists in sheep: a review. Vet Anaesth Analg 2006;33:79–96.
14. Hodgson DS, Dunlop CI, Chapman PL, et al. Cardiopulmonary effects of xylazine and acepromazine in pregnant cows in late gestation. Am J Vet Res 2002;63: 1695–9.
15. Jansen CA, Lowe KC, Nathanielsz PW. The effects of xylazine on uterine activity, fetal and maternal oxygenation, cardiovascular function, and fetal breathing. Am J Obstet Gynecol 1984;148:386–90.
16. Leblanc MM, Hubbell JA, Smith HC. The effects of xylazine hydrochloride on intrauterine pressure in the cow. Theriogenology 1984;21:681–90.
17. Sakamoto H, Misumi K, Nakama M, et al. The effects of xylazine on intrauterine pressure, uterine blood flow, maternal and fetal cardiovascular and pulmonary function in pregnant goats. J Vet Med Sci 1996;58:211–7.
18. Ruckebusch Y, Allal C. Depression of reticulo-ruminal motor functions through the stimulation of alpha 2-adrenoceptors. J Vet Pharmacol Ther 1987;10:1–10.
19. Sinclair MD. A review of the physiological effects of alpha2-agonists related to the clinical use of medetomidine in small animal practice. Can Vet J 2003;44:885–97.
20. Lin HC, Riddell MG. Preliminary study of the effects of xylazine or detomidine with or without butorphanol for standing sedation in dairy cattle. Vet Ther 2003;4: 285–91.
21. Waterman AE, Livingston A, Amin A. Analgesic activity and respiratory effects of butorphanol in sheep. Res Vet Sci 1991;51:19–23.
22. Machado Filho LC, Hurnik JF, Ewing KK. A thermal threshold assay to measure the nociceptive response to morphine sulphate in cattle. Can J Vet Res 1998; 62:218–23.
23. Anderson DE, Gaughan EM, DeBowes RM, et al. Effects of chemical restraint on the endoscopic appearance of laryngeal and pharyngeal anatomy and sensation in adult cattle. Am J Vet Res 1994;55:1196–200.
24. Levine HD, Dodman NH, Court NH, et al. Evaluation of a xylazine–butorphanol combination for use during standing laparotomy in dairy cattle. Agri Pract 1992;13:19–23.
25. Abrahamsen EJ. Ruminant field anesthesia. Vet Clin North Am Food Anim Pract 2008;24:429–41.

26. Coetzee JF, Gehring R, Tarus-Sang J, et al. Effect of sub-anesthetic xylazine and ketamine ("ketamine stun") administered to calves immediately prior to castration. Vet Anaesth Analg 2010;37:566–78.

27. Rizk A, Herdtweck S, Offinger J, et al. The use of xylazine hydrochloride in an analgesic protocol for claw treatment of lame dairy cows in lateral recumbency on a surgical tipping table. Vet J 2012;192:193–8.

28. Lin HC, Thurmon JC, Tranquilli WJ, et al. Hemodynamic response of calves to tiletamine-zolazepam-xylazine anesthesia. Am J Vet Res 1991;52:1606–10.

29. Rioja E, Kerr CL, Enouri SS, et al. Sedative and cardiopulmonary effects of medetomidine hydrochloride and xylazine hydrochloride and their reversal with atipamezole hydrochloride in calves. Am J Vet Res 2008;69:319–29.

30. Re M, Blanco-Murcia FJ, San Miguel JM, et al. Reversible chemical restraint of free-range cattle with a concentrated combination of tiletamine-zolazepam, ketamine, and detomidine. Can J Vet Res 2013;77:288–92.

31. Coulson NM, Januszkiewicz AJ, Dodd KT, et al. The cardiorespiratory effects of diazepam-ketamine and xylazine-ketamine anesthetic combinations in sheep. Lab Anim Sci 1989;39:591–7.

32. Lin HC, Tyler JW, Wallace SS, et al. Telazol and xylazine anesthesia in sheep. Cornell Vet 1993;83:117–24.

33. Lin HC, Tyler JW, Welles EG, et al. Effects of anesthesia induced and maintained by continuous intravenous administration of guaifenesin, ketamine, and xylazine in spontaneously breathing sheep. Am J Vet Res 1993;54:1913–6.

34. Craigmill AL, Rangel-Lugo M, Damian P, et al. Extralabel use of tranquilizers and general anesthetics. J Am Vet Med Assoc 1997;211:302–4.

35. Pascoe PJ, Pypendop BH. Comparative anesthesia and analgesia of dogs and cats. In: Grimm KA, Lemont LA, Tranquilli WJ, et al, editors. Veterinary anesthesia and analgesia. 5th edition. Ames (IA): John Wiley & Sons Inc; 2015. p. 721–1062.

Surgery of the Sinuses and Eyes

Jennifer A. Schleining, DVM, MS

KEYWORDS

- Sinusitis • Sinusotomy • Enucleation • Ocular squamous cell carcinoma
- Eye surgery

KEY POINTS

- Sinus lavage for the treatment of frontal and maxillary sinusitis can be very effective and is not difficult when the appropriate landmarks are identified.
- Conditions of the eye and eyelids necessitating surgery are common.
- When early intervention is performed, the outcome is generally favorable.
- Temporary tarsorrhaphy can be an effective means of supporting eyelid laceration repair and corneal preservation during periods of facial nerve paralysis.

Conditions of the head requiring surgery in cattle are not uncommon when considering the incidence of conditions such as ocular squamous cell carcinoma and requests for surgical dehorning. Surgery involving the eyes in cattle is relatively common, whereas surgery of the paranasal sinuses is less common. Generally speaking, however, surgery for conditions of the head tend to have a more favorable prognosis when there is early intervention.

PARANASAL SINUSES

Cattle have 6 paranasal sinuses: the frontal, maxillary, palatine, lacrimal, sphenoid, and conchal.[1] Even though disease can affect any of these sinuses, practically and clinically, only the frontal and the maxillary gain attention of the clinician. Similar to the horse, the frontal sinus is very large. However, in cattle, the frontal sinus is separated into multiple compartments with the caudal frontal sinus being the most expansive, extending into the horn (if present) of mature animals. This extension is often referred to as the cornual diverticulum. A second diverticulum is located behind the orbit and is identified as the postorbital diverticulum.[2] The further compartmentalization of the caudal frontal sinus by irregular osseous and membranous partitions can

The author has nothing to disclose.
Lloyd Veterinary Medical Center, Department of Veterinary Diagnostic and Production Animal Medicine, Iowa State University, 1809 South Riverside Drive, Ames, IA 50011-3169, USA
E-mail address: jschlein@iastate.edu

make successful treatment of purulent sinusitis a challenge due to the inability to thoroughly and completely lavage the sinus. The frontal sinus communicates with the nasal passage via multiple fenestrations into the ethmoid meatuses.[1] In longstanding or chronic cases, effective lavage may be achieved only with a frontal sinus flap. Within the maxillary sinus are contained the tooth roots of the upper premolar and molar teeth. Hence, in immature animals, the sinus is relatively small, whereas in older cattle, it becomes larger as the cheek teeth are extruded. The maxillary sinus communicates with the nasal passage through the nasomaxillary opening. However, this communication lies high on the medial wall of the sinus allowing fluid to accumulate below this opening in the rostral maxillary sinuses and palatine sinuses rather than draining out the nasal passages.[1]

CONDITIONS OF THE PARANASAL SINUSES
Sinusitis

Frontal sinusitis in cattle is frequently seen as a sequela to dehorning procedures in which the frontal sinus was entered via the horn base following horn removal. It also can be seen following traumatic fracture of the horn, tipping of horns (**Figs. 1** and **2**), sequestration of bone secondary to dehorning, and frontal bone fractures. Environmental and skin contaminants gain access to the caudal frontal sinus through these openings, causing inflammation, and in some cases, results in bacterial infection leading to accumulation of purulent material within the sinuses. Clinical signs of sinusitis can include lethargy, inappetance, purulent nasal discharge, head pressing, head tilt, and in chronic cases, distortion of the bones overlying the affected sinuses. There

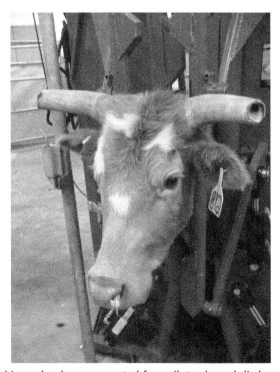

Fig. 1. A 5-year-old crossbred cow presented for unilateral nasal discharge and recent history of tipping the end of the horns.

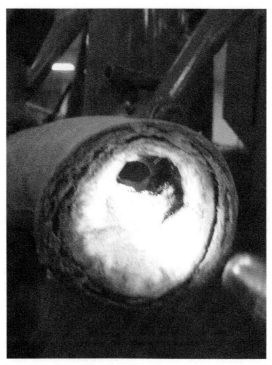

Fig. 2. Close up of the tip of the left horn showing communication of the horn with the caudal frontal sinus.

may be a history of recent dehorning, but in a study involving 12 cases of chronic sinusitis, only 8 of the affected animals had been dehorned within the 12 months before hospital admission for sinusitis.[3] Three cattle who did not have a history of dehorning had a history of recent respiratory disease. Physical examination may identify fever, foul odor to the breath or nasal secretions, draining tracts overlying a previous dehorning site or site of trauma, and a dull sound, and perhaps pain, on percussion of the affected sinus. Radiography confirms the presence of fluid within the affected sinus. Usually, lateral and dorsoventral projections are enough to confirm the diagnosis; however, oblique views, including a rostrocaudal oblique view to set off the caudal frontal sinuses, can be helpful in delineating the extent of the fluid and structures affected (**Fig. 3**). Culture of the fluid with subsequent sensitivity of bacterial isolates to common antimicrobials will help direct antibiotic treatment. *Truperella pyogenes* is the most common isolate from sinusitis following dehorning, whereas *Pasteurella multocida* is the most common isolate in cases without a history of dehorning.[3,4] As such, penicillin is a reasonable choice for therapy while awaiting sensitivity results. Antimicrobial therapy should be instituted along with sinus lavage. In acute cases of sinusitis, lavage can be performed through a small hole created in the caudal frontal sinus using a 4-mm Steinman pin inserted into a hand chuck. This hole will accommodate the male end of a fluid administration set or Simplex outfit providing for daily or twice daily lavage. In a study of 60 cattle with sinusitis, 4 different lavage solutions were compared. Cattle underwent sinus lavage with an unreported volume of fluid every 48 hours for 10 days. In that study, of the 15 cattle randomly assigned to each treatment group, 13 cases lavaged with 5% diluted povidone-iodine solution

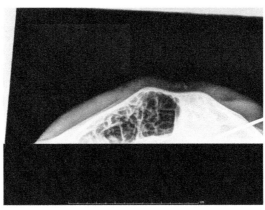

Fig. 3. A rostrocaudal oblique view of the caudal frontal sinuses showing a fluid-filled left frontal sinus. The metallic probe is placed into a draining tract communicating with the sinus.

achieved resolution compared with only 3 in the 0.9% sodium chloride group indicating povidone-iodine solution diluted to 5% resulted in a statistically better clinical outcome than using saline alone.[5] Chronic cases of sinusitis, however, usually require more invasive approaches to the sinus, which could include trephination or osteotomy (bone flap).

Maxillary sinusitis is uncommon and most commonly occurs secondary to an infected or fractured tooth root. Clinical signs include facial deformation (**Fig. 4**),

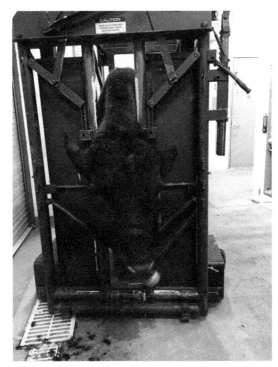

Fig. 4. Bilateral maxillary sinus swelling in a 4-year-old Wagyu bull.

unilateral mucopurulent nasal discharge, altered head carriage, and sometimes decreased appetite secondary to pain during mastication. Radiography should be performed to rule out dental disease as a cause of sinus swelling. If tooth root infection is diagnosed, sinusotomy with tooth repulsion and lavage should be performed and is curative. Differentials for maxillary swelling should also include neoplasia and other bacterial infection, such as *Actinobacillosis lignieresii* (**Fig. 5**).

Sinus Cyst

Cysts of the paranasal sinuses have been described in the literature. These include maxillary sinus cyst, sinonasal cysts, and conchal cysts.[6–8] Clinical signs include mucopurulent nasal discharge, increased respiratory effort, or noise due to partial or complete nasal obstruction, and/or facial deformity. Radiography will often identify a well-demarcated soft tissue opacity within the affected sinus with deviation of normal structures. Computed tomography can be a very useful adjunct to radiography when the full extent of the cyst is not able to be determined and/or to identify multiple cysts. Additionally, endoscopy should be considered for masses that enter the nasal passage. Treatment of sinus cysts will be predicated by the location of the cyst, but can include removal via the nasal passage under endoscopic guidance or via a maxillary or frontonasal bone flap technique. Complete removal of the cyst lining appears to be curative in cattle. In a study of 10 cattle undergoing surgical removal of paranasal and conchal sinus cysts, 9 returned to production and had no recurrence.[9] Not all well-demarcated soft tissue opacities in the sinuses or nasal passages should be assumed to be sinonasal cysts, however. Neoplasia can present very similarly and should be included in the differential list for paranasal sinus disease (**Fig. 6**).

Fracture

Depression fracture of the frontal bone, nasal bone, and orbit can occur resulting acutely in increased respiratory effort due to swelling, hemorrhagic nasal discharge (**Fig. 7**), abnormal head carriage, and inappetance depending on the severity and

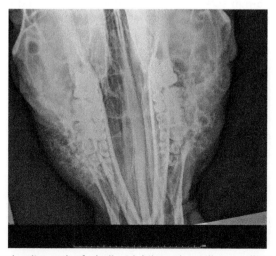

Fig. 5. Caudoventral radiograph of a bull with bilateral maxillary swelling diagnosed with *A lignieresii* sinusitis. Note the severe bone destruction and remodeling.

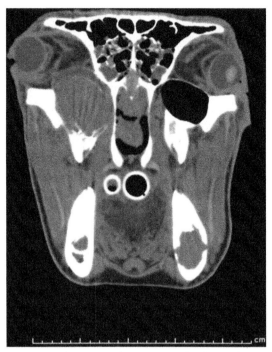

Fig. 6. Frontal plane computed tomography image at the level of the eyes in a 2-year-old Angus cow with lymphosarcoma believed to have been a sinonasal cyst. Note the right maxillary sinus is filled with fluid with a thick lining.

location of the fracture. The incidence of fracture is less than that reported in horses likely because of differences in behavior and animal use.[10] In cases of depression fracture, surgical repair can be performed under general anesthesia using bone reduction instruments or a 3.5-mm screw inserted proud into the fractured fragment to aid in reducing the fragment back into alignment. Cerclage wire may or may not be

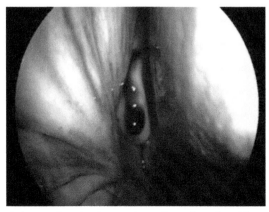

Fig. 7. An endoscopic image showing hemorrhage from the ethmoid meatus in a 5-year-old Simmental bull with a frontal bone fracture.

necessary to keep the fragment(s) in position. Orbital fractures can be repaired with various orthopedic techniques including string-of-pearls plates, dynamic compression plates, or cerclage wire depending on the configuration of the fracture. Minor closed fractures with minimal displacement may not require repair.

TREPHINATION
Preoperative Planning

Trephination can be completed using either a Galt or Michele trephine (**Fig. 8**). The advantage of the Galt trephine is that it results in a larger access portal to the sinus. The appropriate site should be chosen to best access the affected sinus (**Fig. 9**). **Box 1** lists the supplies needed for trephination of the paranasal sinuses.

Preparation and Patient Positioning

The patient should be restrained in a hydraulic chute or manual head catch. A halter should be used to further restrain the head to minimize movement during the procedure. The trephine site should be clipped allowing for at least 2-inch margins around the proposed site of trephination. A rough preparation of the site should be conducted with chlorhexidine scrub followed with alcohol. Ensure that these solutions do not contact the eyes, as they will cause severe chemical keratitis. A large bleb of lidocaine should be placed subcutaneously at the trephination site followed by a more thorough cleansing of the site with scrub and alcohol.

SURGICAL APPROACH AND PROCEDURE

Using a scalpel blade, a full-thickness circular area of skin should be removed corresponding to the size of the trephine extending to the periosteum of the frontal or maxillary bone. The trephine should then be used in a clockwise rotation to remove a section of bone allowing access into the sinus. At this time, a sample of the fluid within the sinus should be collected for culture and sensitivity. The sinus may now be lavaged and/or investigated further using flexible endoscopy if necessary.

IMMEDIATE POSTOPERATIVE CARE

The trephine sites should be left open to heal by second intention. Covering the trephination sites is recommended to keep debris and further contaminants from entering

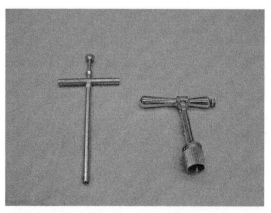

Fig. 8. A Michele trephine on the left and a Galt trephine on the right.

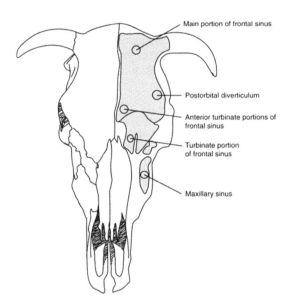

Main portion of frontal sinus

Postorbital diverticulum

Anterior turbinate portions of
frontal sinus

Turbinate portion
of frontal sinus

Maxillary sinus

Fig. 9. The circles indicate the site(s) of trephination for each sinus, and shaded areas are the frontal and maxillary sinuses. (*From* Gaughn EM, Provo-Klimek J, Ducharme NG. Surgery of the bovine respiratory and cardiovascular systems. In: Fubini S, Ducharme N, editors. Farm animal surgery. St Louis (MO): Saunders; 2004. p. 148; with permission.)

the sinus. A stent bandage using #2 polymerized caprolactam (Braunamid; Braun) (or other nonabsorbable suture material) is easily made by placing 2 loose interrupted sutures through the skin perpendicular to the surgical site, one above and one below the incision. A 12-inch segment of umbilical tape should be passed through each suture. A roll of 4 × 4 gauze sponges or a 4-inch roll gauze can then be placed over the incision and secured in place by the umbilical tape. The bandage may then be removed and replaced for subsequent sinus lavage procedures or alternatively left in place until the sinusotomy has been obscured by granulation tissue. Postoperative care also should include the use of anti-inflammatory medications such as meloxicam

---

Box 1
Supplies needed for sinus trephination

- Clippers with a #40 blade
- Lidocaine
- Chlorhexidine scrub and alcohol for site preparation
- Sterile trephine (Galt or Michele)
- Sterile surgical gloves
- #10 or #15 scalpel blade and handle
- Gauze sponges
- Culturette or sterile syringe
- #2 Braunamid suture
- One-half–inch Braunamid suture

(0.5–1.0 mg/kg by mouth once a day or every other day) or flunixin meglumine (1.1–2.2 mg/kg intravenously (IV) as needed).

OSTEOTOMY (BONE FLAP)
Preoperative Planning

List of supplies and instruments needed to perform a sinus osteotomy (**Box 2**).

Preparation and Patient Positioning

Although a frontal sinus bone flap procedure could be done in the standing animal, it is generally recommended to perform this procedure in the anesthetized animal. Maxillary bone flaps should be performed under general anesthesia. General anesthesia should be maintained with inhalant anesthesia with an appropriately inflated endotracheal tube cuff given the propensity of significant bleeding into the nasal cavity if the nasal concha are required to be punctured for creation of drainage. The patient should be placed in lateral recumbency with the affected sinus(es) up. The surgical site should be clipped and aseptically prepared as for any other surgical site.

SURGICAL APPROACH AND PROCEDURE: FRONTAL SINUS

Using a scalpel blade, a 3-sided, rectangular incision should be made extending to the bone and including the periosteum. The location for the incision should be as follows: the caudal margin should be a line extending from midline to a point bisecting the supraorbital foramen and poll, the lateral margin should extend from the caudal margin to the level of the center of the orbit approximately 3.5 to 4.0 cm medial to the medial canthus of the eye taking care to avoid the supraorbital foramen, and the rostral margin extends from midline to the rostral extent of the lateral margin. The periosteum should be gently reflected with a blunt periosteal elevator along with the skin and subcutaneous tissue. An oscillating bone saw or mallet and osteotome should then be used to create osteotomy incisions following the margins of the skin incision. The osteotomy incisions should be created at an approximately 45° oblique angle through the bone (**Fig. 10**). The rostral and caudal incisions at midline should be notched to facilitate "hinging" the flap axially. The flap may then be elevated and hinged.

Box 2
Supplies needed to perform an osteotomy

- Clippers with a #40 blade
- Chlorhexidine scrub and alcohol for site preparation
- Sterile surgical gloves
- #10 or #15 scalpel blade and handle
- Basic surgical pack
- Oscillating bone saw or mallet and chisels/osteotome set
- Gauze sponges
- Culturette or sterile syringe
- 6-inch roll gauze with fine weave
- 0 or 2-0 absorbable suture material
- 0 absorbable or nonabsorbable suture material or stainless steel staples for skin closure

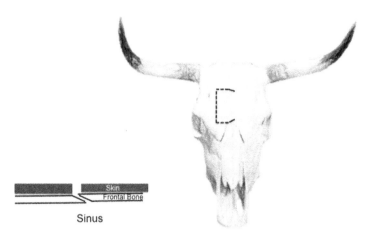

Sinus

Fig. 10. Location for the skin and osteotomy incisions for a frontal sinus bone flap. Note the angled notches at the axial border to facilitate flap hinging. The osteotomy angle is illustrated in the inset.

Depending on the chronicity of the condition and location of osseous structures within the sinuses, an osteotome may be necessary to manually dissect attachments of the flap to the sinus cavity. Fluid should now be collected for cytology and/or culture and sensitivity. Copious lavage and debridement of the sinus should be undertaken paying special attention to the postorbital diverticulum and other deep structures within the sinus. If drainage is not well established, a fenestration into the nasal passage may be made through the wall of the conchal sinuses using a probe, large hemostats, or other blunt instrument. This usually results in profuse hemorrhage and packaging of the sinus with fine-weave roll gauze should be performed. The front tail of the gauze should be exited the fenestration and secured to the nasal fold with a simple interrupted or mattress suture. A single, small tight knot should be placed at the back tail so that when the packing is removed, the visualization of the knot confirms that the entire packing was removed. A second option for packing the sinus includes exiting the gauze packing out a corner of the osteotomy site after removing a corner of the bone flap. If this option is chosen, a knot should not be used at the end of the gauze. This method of packing, however, will result in an open incision that will require further aftercare after the packing is removed. Following packing of the sinus cavity, the bone flap should be replaced. It is not necessary to suture the bone flap. The periosteum and subcutaneous tissues should be closed separately using 2 to 0 absorbable suture material. The skin can then be closed either with stainless steel staples or nonabsorbable suture material.

SURGICAL APPROACH AND PROCEDURE: MAXILLARY SINUS

Using a scalpel blade, a 3-sided, rectangular incision should be made extending to the bone and including the periosteum. The location for the incision should be as follows: the caudal margin should begin at the approximate level of the medial canthus of the eye 4 to 5 cm distal to the orbit extending distally to the level of the facial tuberosity, the ventral margin should begin at this point and extend rostrally 5 to 7 cm following a line drawn from the zygomatic arch to the facial tuberosity, the rostral margin then extends from this point dorsally 5 cm parallel with the caudal margin.[2] Care should be exercised during the incision so as to not incise the facial vein as it courses across the maxillary sinus. The osteotomy should then proceed as described previously with the bone flap hinged on its dorsal margin (**Fig. 11**). In young animals, the tooth roots will occupy much of the sinus and care should be taken not to disrupt normal roots. If a tooth is removed, the void should be filled with a temporary plug. The socket of the missing tooth should be packed with either a methylmethacrylate plug or rolled gauze secured to umbilical tape, which exits the sinusotomy site at a small removed corner. Following tooth removal and/or sinus lavage, closure of the osteotomy site should be performed as described previously. Methylmethacrylate plugs are left to fall out on their own, whereas gauze plugs should be changed every 5 to 7 days until there is no longer communication between the oral cavity and the sinus. The gauze packing should be secured with very long pieces of umbilical tape to allow the packing to be removed from the oral cavity through the mouth, a new packing secured to the umbilical tape, and then the umbilical tape again pulled taut from the sinusotomy site until the new packing is again secure within the socket. The tails are tied in a bow around a second roll gauze to keep the plug in place. An oral speculum is required for this packing change. The disadvantage of the methylmethacrylate plug is that if it falls out prematurely, feed material may become impacted into the sinus through the fistula requiring further intervention.

IMMEDIATE POSTOPERATIVE CARE

The surgical sites should be kept clean. Any sinus packing should be removed in 24 to 48 hours and sinus lavage instituted if needed at that time. Postoperative care also should

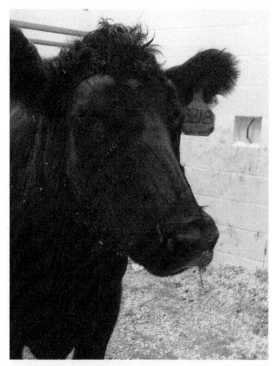

Fig. 11. Location for a maxillary bone flap. Note the nasal packing secured to the right nares.

include the use of anti-inflammatory medications, such as meloxicam (0.5–1.0 mg/kg by mouth SID – EOD) or flunixin meglumine (1.1–2.2 mg/kg IV as needed) and antimicrobial therapy as indicated. The skin sutures or staples should be removed in 14 days.

EYES

Surgery involving the periorbital structures and eyes is relatively common in ruminants. Conditions requiring surgery are varied and range from trauma to neoplasia to congenital.[10]

SURGICAL CONDITIONS OF THE EYE
Neoplasia

Ocular squamous cell carcinoma

Squamous cell carcinoma of the eye and associated structures is common in cattle and can affect the eyelids, the nictatans (third eyelid), the conjunctiva, and cornea (**Fig. 12**).[10,11] Although the complete etiology of ocular squamous cell carcinoma (OSCC) is not totally understood, cattle lacking pigment of the area around the eyes and exposed to high levels of UV sunlight have a higher incidence. The size and location of the lesion will likely determine the treatment. Smaller, well-defined, lesions (<50 mm) lend themselves to successful treatment with cryotherapy, hyperthermia, or surgical excision. Larger lesions provide more challenges and may require enucleation, sometimes involving extensive removal of periorbital tissues, to completely

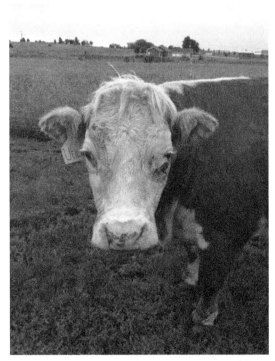

Fig. 12. An extensive OSCC of the periorbital tissues in a 6-year-old Hereford cow.

resolve the condition. When only the third eyelid is involved, the third eyelid may be removed without worry of further problems.

Lymphosarcoma

Neoplasia should always be included on a differential list for an animal presenting with exophthalmos. Lymphosarcoma is the most common neoplastic disease of the orbit in cattle and tends to be fairly invasive.[12] Digital palpation of the orbit should occur because foreign bodies can also cause retrobulbar or orbital abscesses resulting in clinical symptoms that may mimic lymphosarcoma. If lymphosarcoma is suspected, a fine-needle aspirate, biopsy, serology for bovine leukosis virus, and/or palpation of regional lymph nodes and abdominal lymph nodes via rectal palpation may assist in arriving at a final diagnosis. Cattle with lymphosarcoma can sometimes be salvaged long enough to birth or wean a calf, but quality of life should be taken into account when deciding on how to progress. Exenteration of the orbital contents may prolong the life of the animal, but in the author's experience the tumor tends to reoccur very rapidly and aggressively. Cattle with any outward signs of lymphosarcoma will be severely discounted at market and the carcass condemned at slaughter.

Trauma

Lacerations of the eyelids, although not common, do occur and may require surgical repair (**Fig. 13**). Depending on the location and extent of tissue trauma, this may be best done under general anesthesia in the interest of cosmesis, functionality of the lid, and integrity of the repair. It is important to perform a full ophthalmic examination when presented with an eyelid laceration to rule out globe trauma, corneal ulceration or laceration, and the presence of conjunctival foreign bodies that may have occurred during the traumatic event. The tissues often will be edematous and may contain mucous exudate. Practitioners should avoid the temptation to remove skin flaps, especially when the eyelid margins are involved in the laceration. The integrity of the margin is very important when considering the future functionality of the lid. Without the lid margin, entropion may occur resulting in chronic corneal irritation and ulceration from hair, or even worse, the eye may not be properly protected or able to maintain a tear film resulting in chronic exposure keratitis and discomfort. All efforts should be made to repair the eyelid.

Cryotherapy

List of supplies needed to perform cryotherapy of the eyelids or nictitating membrane (**Box 3**).

The patient should be restrained in a hydraulic chute with the head further restrained with a halter or hydraulic head restraint system. Topical ophthalmic anesthetic

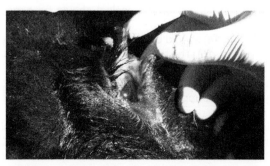

Fig. 13. Eyelid laceration in a yearling crossbred heifer. (Photograph courtesy of Dr Josh Ydstie.)

Box 3
Supplies needed for cryotherapy

Topical anesthetic (ie, Proparacaine)

Styrofoam coffee cup

Sterile lube

Cryotherapy unit (pen, gun, or other unit)

(proparacaine) should be generously applied to the eye. If the lesion is on the margin of the eyelid, the rim of the Styrofoam cup can be removed, lubricated, and inserted between the lid and the eye serving as a barrier to the liquid nitrogen.

Using either a contact probe or an open spray tip, a double freeze thaw cycle should be performed. The abnormal tissue should be frozen until either a thermocouple placed in the skin deep to the mass reads −25°C or until an ice ball is observed extending past the periphery of the mass. The second freeze cycle should occur immediately after the mass has thawed.

An antibacterial ointment should be placed in the eye following cryosurgery. Edema within the affected tissues will be evident within a few hours and is a normal sequela to cryosurgery. This edema gradually subsides within the next few days without further intervention. The eye should be relatively comfortable as cryotherapy results in death of nerve endings at the site of cryogen application.

Hyperthermia

Box 4
Supplies needed for hyperthermia to remove eyelid masses

- Topical anesthetic (ie, Proparacaine)
- Handheld radiofrequency unit
- Orbital retractor

The patient should be restrained in a hydraulic chute with the head further restrained with a halter or hydraulic head restraint system (**Box 4**). Alternatively, if a tilt table is available, the patient can be restrained in lateral recumbency with the affected eye up. Topical ophthalmic anesthetic (proparacaine) should be generously applied to the eye.

An orbital retractor (**Fig. 14**) should be gently placed behind the eye while avoiding the muscles of the eye (**Fig. 15**). The retractor will prevent the eye from moving during the procedure. The radiofrequency probes should then be placed in contact with the mass and the mass consequently heated to 50°C. Care should be taken not to overlap the direction of hyperthermia application on the cornea, as this may cause corneal perforation.

Antimicrobial ointment should be placed in the eye at the conclusion of the procedure. The use of anti-inflammatory medications, such as meloxicam (0.5–1.0 mg/kg by mouth SID – EOD) or flunixin meglumine (1.1–2.2 mg/kg IV as needed) also may be used as indicated.

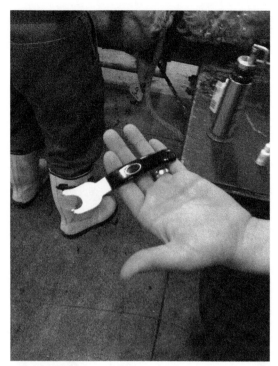

Fig. 14. A bovine orbital retractor.

Enucleation

Box 5
Supplies needed to perform enucleation
Clippers with a #40 blade
Chlorhexidine scrub and alcohol for site preparation
Sterile surgical gloves
#10 or #20 scalpel blade and handle
Basic surgical pack with towel clamps
Mixter forceps or other 90° forceps
Gauze sponges
0 absorbable suture material
#2 Braunamid or other nonabsorbable suture material

Three options exist for removal of the eye. They are enucleation, exenteration, and evisceration. Enucleation refers to the removal of the globe only. Exenteration refers to removal of the globe and all orbital contents including muscles, periorbital fat, and optic nerve and vessels. Evisceration is a procedure in which only the intraocular contents of the eye are removed, leaving the globe intact. Enucleation is by and far the most frequent surgical procedure used in bovine practice and is described here. The reader is directed to other texts for detailed descriptions of the other procedures.

The patient should be restrained in a hydraulic chute with the head further restrained with a halter or hydraulic head restraint system (**Box 5**). Alternatively if a tilt table is

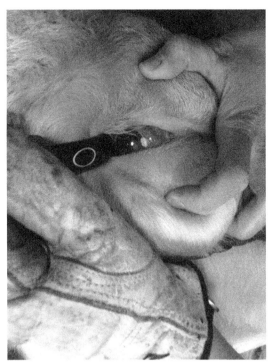

Fig. 15. The bovine orbital retractor placed behind the eye to prevent eye movement during hyperthermia.

available, the patient can be restrained in lateral recumbency with the affected eye up. If indicated, a broad-spectrum antibiotic can be administered at this time. The orbital area should be generously clipped and a rough scrub performed to remove surface debris. Care should be taken so as to not get scrub or alcohol into the eye. The eyelids and orbit should then be anesthetized (see Edmonson MA: Local, Regional, and Spinal Anesthesia in Ruminants, in this issue). Following tight apposition of the eyelids with a continuous suture pattern, a final surgical scrub should be performed. Another method of eyelid apposition is with the use of towel clamps rather than suturing the lids closed. An advantage of this technique is that the towel clamps may be used for traction of the globe during the surgical procedure.

An elliptical incision should be made 1 to 2 cm around the periphery of the eyelid margins. Using a combination of blunt and sharp dissection and using the orbit as a guide, the surgeon should proceed through the orbicularis oculi muscle and periorbital fascia while avoiding penetration of the conjunctiva. The ligaments at the medial and lateral canthi are substantial and will require sharp transection. After transection of the ligaments, the globe should be freely moveable. Dissection should proceed into the orbit transecting the oblique, rectus, and retractor bulbi muscles. When all the muscular attachments to the globe have been removed a Mixter forceps or other vascular clamp (such as a kidney clamp or large curved Kelly forceps) should be applied to the optic nerve and vessels at the base of the eye. The globe should then be sharply removed and, if possible, a ligature placed around the optic pedicle using an absorbable suture material. At this time, further debridement of the orbit can occur if necessary. The globe can then be lavaged before closure of the subcutaneous tissues with a 0 or 2 to 0 synthetic absorbable suture material capable of maintaining tension. Alternatively, if the pedicle is not able to be ligated effectively, the orbit can be packed with roll gauze to provide hemostasis while the incision is being closed. The gauze can then be removed just before placement of the final sutures in the subcutaneous layer. The lid margins should then be apposed using a continuous suture pattern of the surgeon's preference using #2 nonabsorbable suture (**Fig. 16**). If the animal is anticipated to rub at the surgical site postoperatively, a stent bandage can be placed over the surgical incision to protect the integrity of the sutures. This is accomplished by placing loose simple interrupted sutures with #2 nonabsorbable suture material at the rostral and caudal borders of the orbit through which umbilical tape passes in a "lacing" fashion. A rolled huck towel, laparotomy sponge, or rolled gauze can then be placed over the incision and under the laces. The laces are then tightened to secure the stent in place.

The surgical site should be monitored closely over the course of the next 3 to 5 days. Postoperative swelling usually subsides within the first week as the hematoma within the orbit resolves. The use of anti-inflammatory medications such as meloxicam (0.5–1.0 mg/kg by mouth SID – EOD) or flunixin meglumine (1.1–2.2 mg/kg IV as needed) should be considered. If present, the stent can be removed in 5 to 7 days and the skin sutures in 14 days.

Laceration repair

Box 6
Supplies needed to repair eyelid lacerations

- Dilute povidone-iodine solution (not scrub)
- Clippers
- Lidocaine
- Topical anesthetic (ie, Proparacaine)
- #15 scalpel blade and handle
- Brown Adson thumb forceps
- Gauze sponges
- 2-0 to 5-0 absorbable suture material
- Scissors

If the laceration is small, the patient may be restrained in a hydraulic chute with the head further restrained with a halter or hydraulic head restraint mechanism (**Box 6**). However, if the laceration is extensive or requires meticulous repair based on the location or configuration of the laceration, general anesthesia is recommended. The laceration margins should be locally anesthetized with subcutaneous injection of lidocaine and topical anesthetic liberally applied to the eye surface. The laceration should then be prepped for surgery using 5% dilute povidone-iodine solution. The use of scrub formulations and alcohol will result in chemical keratitis and should be avoided!

The margins of the laceration should be carefully and minimally debrided to preserve as much tissue as possible. This is important for proper eyelid function after the repair has healed. Flaps should not be removed and the tips of any flaps left in situ even if they look like they will not survive. Full-thickness lacerations should be repaired in 2 to 3 layers. The deep layer should include the fibrous tarsal plate, which is very important in the repair process.[10] The eyelid margins should be apposed meticulously and carefully. There are numerous suturing techniques for this type of

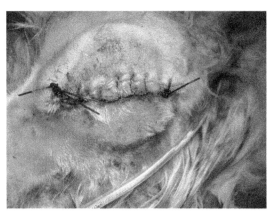

Fig. 16. A completed enucleation surgery showing skin closure.

repair depending on the configuration of the laceration and the reader is directed to ophthalmology texts for these specific suture patterns. The skin can be apposed in simple interrupted or mattress suture patterns. Extensive laceration repairs may require stenting after repair. This can occur in a number of different ways, including temporary tarsorrhaphy. If the eye requires medicating postoperatively, a subpalpebral lavage system is recommended to be placed before the tarsorrhaphy.

If the animal is amenable, the repair should be warm compressed 2 to 3 times a day to help reduce inflammation and pain. The use of anti-inflammatory medications, such as meloxicam (0.5–1.0 mg/kg by mouth SID – EOD) or flunixin meglumine (1.1–2.2 mg/kg IV as needed) should be considered. If indicated, the eye should be medicated through the subpalpebral lavage system with liquid medication or carefully at a site distant from the repair with ointment. If there was extensive tissue damage, broad-spectrum systemic antibiotics may be indicated. If a tarsorrhaphy was performed, it should be removed in 7 to 10 days.

Tarsorrhaphy

Box 7
Supplies needed to perform a tarsorrhaphy

- Lidocaine
- Topical anesthetic (ie, Proparacaine)
- 2-0 nonabsorbable suture material
- Rubber tubing (16 drops/s intravenous lines work well) cut into small pieces
- Needle holders
- Scissors

In cases such as described previously or when presented with an animal with facial nerve paralysis (such as sometimes seen in listeriosis) a temporary tarsorrhaphy can be a useful procedure to protect the laceration repair or the cornea from exposure keratitis (**Box 7**).

The animal should be restrained in a hydraulic chute with the head further restrained by a halter. A local injection of lidocaine should be performed subcutaneously at the site of each suture. The eye should be liberally dosed with a topical anesthetic.

The suture material should be placed through the rubber tubing. A partial-thickness bite through the upper lid exiting along the eyelid margin should then be performed. Next, the lower lid should be entered in the center of the eyelid margin opposite of the exiting suture of the upper lid and exited through the skin. The suture should then pass through a second piece of rubber tubing, the needle reversed, and the procedure repeated back through the lower lid and into the upper lid exiting near the upper rubber stent. The ends should then be tied together making a horizontal mattress suture pattern with the stents. A second and, possibly third if needed, stent suture can be placed to complete the procedure.

Postoperative care is minimal. The tarsorrhaphy sutures should be removed when no longer needed, preferably within 2 weeks. When the sutures are not removed in a timely fashion, large granulomas may form inhibiting normal lid function (**Fig. 17**).

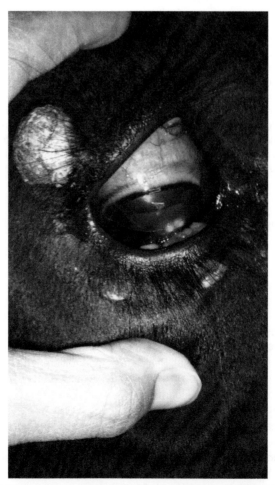

Fig. 17. Granuloma secondary to temporary tarsorrhaphy sutures left in place for 3 months. Note the corneal scar and conjunctivitis from improperly placed suture.

CLINICAL RESULTS

When used on appropriately sized OSCCs (demarcated lesions <50 mm), cryotherapy using a single freeze thaw cycle was curative in 66% of the lesions. When a double freeze thaw cycle was used, 97% of the lesions regressed completely.[13] Cryotherapy can also be used adjunctively following surgical debulking of the mass. However, because of the inability of the cryogen to effectively freeze deeper tissues, large tumors that invade deeper structures are not a candidate for cryotherapy. Hyperthermia has also been reported to have a favorable outcome on ocular squamous cell carcinoma.[14,15] In one study of 76 OSCCs, 60 tumors regressed completely after 1 hyperthermia treatment and another 9 regressed completely after a second treatment for an overall cure rate of 90.8%.[15] Tumors that are invasive or larger than 50 mm do not respond well to hyperthermia and other treatments should be considered. In a single-center retrospective study of 53 cattle undergoing enucleation, nearly 85% of eyes were removed consequent to OSCC. Despite nearly 20% of the cattle having surgical site infection in the 3 weeks postoperatively, cattle undergoing enucleation in this study largely were returned to production. The prognosis of the 22 cattle available for long-term follow-up was very good with a very low recurrence rate.[16]

SUMMARY

Although surgery of the paranasal sinuses may not be an everyday occurrence, familiarity with the anatomy can improve the veterinarian's comfort level and case outcome. The most common reason for sinus surgery is sinusitis secondary to previous dehorning or respiratory disease. Sinus lavage in early cases of sinusitis has a high success rate. Surgery of the eyes are more common given the incidence of OSCC and conditions requiring enucleation. Small lesions may be amenable to treatment with cryotherapy or hyperthermia, whereas larger lesions may require enucleation. Enucleation appears to have a good long-term outcome.

REFERENCES

1. Dyce KM, Sack WO, Wensing CJG. The head and ventral neck of the ruminants. In: Textbook of veterinary anatomy. Philadelphia: Saunders; 2002. p. 633–6.
2. deLahunta A, Habel RE. Paranasal sinuses. In: Applied veterinary anatomy. Philadelphia: Saunders; 1986. p. 51–3.
3. Ward J, Rebhun W. Chronic frontal sinusitis in dairy cattle: 12 cases (1978-1989). J Am Vet Med Assoc 1992;201:326–8.
4. Gaughn EM, Provo-Klimek J, Ducharme NG. Surgery of the bovine respiratory and cardiovascular systems. In: Fubini S, Ducharme N, editors. Farm animal surgery. St Louis (MO): Saunders; 2004. p. 146–8.
5. Silva L, Neto A, Campos S, et al. Evaluation of four different treatment protocols to sinusitis after plastic dehorning in cattle. Acta Scientiae Veterinariae 2010;38:25–30.
6. McPike Mundell L, Smith B, Hoffman R. Maxillary sinus cysts in two cattle. J Am Vet Med Assoc 1996;209:127–9.
7. Ross M, Richardson D, Hackett R, et al. Nasal obstruction caused by cystic nasal conchae in cattle. J Am Vet Med Assoc 1986;188:857–60.
8. Cohen N, Vacek J, Seahorn T, et al. Cystic nasal concha in a calf. J Am Vet Med Assoc 1991;198:1035–6.
9. Schmid T, Braun U, Hagen R, et al. Clinical signs, treatment, and outcome in 15 cattle with sinonasal cysts. Vet Surg 2014;43:190–8.

10. Irby N. Surgical diseases of the eye in farm animals. In: Fubini S, Ducharme N, editors. Farm animal surgery. St Louis (MO): Saunders; 2004. p. 429–59.
11. Tsujita H, Plummer C. Bovine ocular squamous cell carcinoma. Vet Clin North Am Food Anim Pract 2010;26:511–29.
12. Rebhun WC. Ocular manifestations of systemic diseases in cattle. Vet Clin North Am Large Anim Pract 1984;6:623–39.
13. Farris HE, Fraunhfelder FT. Cryosurgical treatment of ocular squamous cell carcinoma of cattle. J Am Vet Med Assoc 1976;168:213–6.
14. Grier RL, Brewer WG Jr, Paul SR, et al. Treatment of bovine and equine ocular squamous cell carcinoma by radiofrequency hyperthermia. J Am Vet Med Assoc 1980;177:55–61.
15. Kainer RA, Stringer JM, Lueker DC. Hyperthermia for treatment of ocular squamous cell tumor in cattle. J Am Vet Med Assoc 1980;176:356–60.
16. Schulz KL, Anderson DE. Bovine enucleation: a retrospective study of 53 cases (1998-2006). Can Vet J 2010;51:611–4.

Respiratory Surgery

 CrossMark

Sylvain Nichols, DMV, MS

KEYWORDS

• Surgery • Upper airway • Cattle • Larynx • Pharynx

KEY POINTS

- Inspiratory dyspnea is a common clinical sign of upper airway obstruction.
- Endoscopic evaluation of the upper airway helps localize the obstruction.
- Emergency drugs and a surgical kit to place a tracheostomy tube should be readily available when working on dyspneic animals.
- Pharyngeal trauma can cause severe head and neck cellulitis, causing dysphagia and dyspnea.
- Mandibular fractures are more frequent in calves and can be repaired with an intraoral splint when it involves the rostral mandible.

 Video content accompanies this article at http://www.vetfood.theclinics.com.

INTRODUCTION

Performing respiratory surgery in the field is an intimidating endeavor. Proper anesthesia of the head is challenging and sedation of an animal struggling to breathe is risky. However, with a good anesthesia protocol, surgical plan, and the right equipment, upper airway surgery can be successfully performed outside of a hospital setting. This article describes the different disorders affecting the upper airway. It highlights the clinical signs, the diagnostic approaches, and therapeutic options. Advanced surgeries, performed in referral centers, are briefly described to make readers aware of other possible treatment options to relieve upper airway obstruction.

CLINICAL SIGNS

Disorders affecting the upper airway can have an acute (eg, foreign body) or chronic (eg, cyst or neoplasia) evolution. They can potentially lead to obstruction causing various degrees of inspiratory dyspnea. The obstruction is accompanied by the characteristic inspiratory stridor (Video 1). Chronic cases may have secondary aspiration

Disclosure: The author has nothing to disclose.
Department of Clinical Sciences, Faculté de Médecine Vétérinaire, Université de Montréal, 3200 Rue Sicotte, St-Hyacinthe, Quebec J2S 2M2, Canada
E-mail address: sylvain.nichols@umontreal.ca

pneumonia. It is therefore important to carefully evaluate the chest through ausculta-tion and ideally an imaging technique before investing time and money in surgery. Portable radiography can be used in a field setup to evaluate the lungs in young calves.[1,2] However, ultrasonography is more readily available and was shown to be more efficient in detecting lung consolidation in calves and in older cattle (**Fig. 1**).[3–6] In referral centers, computed tomography (CT) can also be used to detect pneumonia in calves.[7,8]

Some conditions cause nasal discharge, asymmetric airflow through the nostril, skull deformation, chronic cough, and ocular discharge.[9] In some cases, swelling of the soft tissue surrounding the involved structure is present (eg, pharyngeal trauma).

DIAGNOSIS

Through the case history and a complete physical examination, a presumptive diag-nosis can usually be reached. A careful palpation of the head and neck can help localize the site of the obstruction. Oral palpation allows evaluation of the larynx and oropharynx. This evaluation can be performed by using the tongue of the animal as a speculum or any other type of mouth opener. The hand of the examiner is placed in a vertical orientation to pass between the cheek teeth. It is then placed in a horizon-tal position to palpate the larynx. This manipulation may exacerbate the respiratory distress. Therefore, it may need to be delayed after relieving the airway with the place-ment of a temporary tracheostomy tube.

The diagnosis is obtained by performing a nasal endoscopy. The technique has been described and is performed without sedation in most cattle.[10,11] A scope 9 mm in diameter and 1 m long is used and allows evaluation of the nasopharynx, lar-ynx, and proximal trachea. The structures seen are the nasal ventral meatus, the nasal septum, the pharyngeal septum, the opening of the eustachian tube, the epiglottis, the soft palate, the arytenoids, and the vocal cords (**Fig. 2**, Video 2). The opening of the

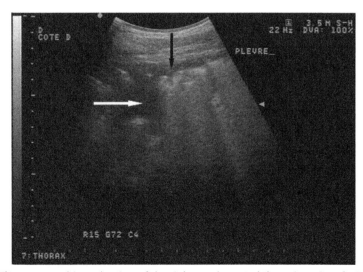

Fig. 1. Ultrasonographic evaluation of the right caudoventral thoracic cavity of a 2-year-old Holstein heifer with *Mannheimia haemolytica* bronchopleuropneumonia. A 3.5-mHz curvi-linear probe was used to obtained this picture. Fluids can be seen in the thoracic cavity (*black arrow*). The visceral pleura is irregular and an abscess is forming in the lungs (*white arrow*). (*Courtesy of* Dr Marie Babkine, University of Montréal, St-Hyacinthe, Québec, Canada.)

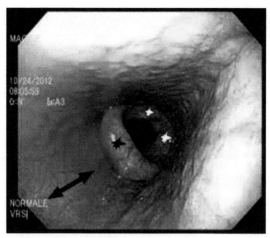

Fig. 2. Normal endoscopic evaluation of a 7-year-old Holstein cow. An endoscope 9 mm in diameter and a 1 m long was introduced through the left nostril of this cow. The nasopharynx, the soft palate (*black arrow*), the epiglottis (*black star*), and the arytenoids (*white stars*) are seen.

maxillary sinuses can be located in the middle meatus of the nasal cavity. During the endoscopy, the soft palate is frequently dorsally displaced without affecting the animal.[10] Black pigmentation is normally found in Jersey cattle.[10] The presence of discharge; asymmetry of the nasal cavity and the arytenoids; and, subjectively, the diameter of the nasopharynx and rima glottis are evaluated. Through the endoscope channel, a biopsy can be obtained. It is important to realize that the sample obtained is small and superficial and may not be diagnostically useful in cases of deeper disorder.

Radiography and tomodensitometry (CT scan) can be useful in finding disorders involving the sinuses, skull bone, and soft tissue surrounding the upper airway (**Fig. 3**).[12,13] It can also be used to find metallic foreign bodies that may be embedded in the soft tissue. The main advantage of the CT scan is the possibility to evaluate the head in cross section, thereby removing the superposition of the many structures forming the head. It can be performed under sedation in calves.

Ultrasonography has also been used to evaluate the soft tissue of the neck and larynx.[14–16] A description of the ultrasonic bovine larynx anatomy is lacking. The work done in horses is currently used as a guideline for bovine ultrasonography of the larynx.[17,18] The application of this diagnostic tool is to localize masses and to perform ultrasonography-guided aspiration of diseased tissue.

EMERGENCY PROCEDURES

In animals with severe inspiratory distress, emergency drugs to decrease swelling and edema should be given on presentation. Corticosteroids with or without a diuretic (eg, furosemide) can be given. The animal should be placed in a cool environment if possible. If the distress persists, a tracheotomy is performed and a temporary tracheostomy tube is inserted before the diagnostic work-up.

In animals with mild inspiratory distress, the diagnostic work-up is performed before attempting any procedure. It is important to realize that the condition of the animal may deteriorate rapidly during procedures like nasal endoscopy or if the animal has

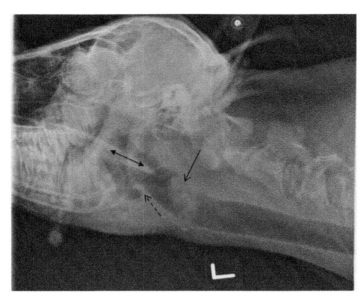

Fig. 3. Lateral radiograph of the head of a 6-week-old Holstein calf presented for dyspnea. A soft tissue opacity is located in the larynx (*black arrow*). Also shown are the epiglottis (*dotted arrow*) and soft palate (*double arrow*).

to be restrained during radiography or catheter placement. Emergency drugs and surgical instruments necessary to perform an emergency tracheotomy should always be available when working on a dyspneic animal.

Tracheotomy and Temporary Tracheostomy Tube Placement

The procedure is performed with the cow standing. It can be done in calves in dorsal recumbency. Preparation of the neck area varies according to the status of the animal. It is better to get the tube through a partially clean neck of a live animal than through the aseptically prepared neck of a dead calf. Therefore, if time permits, the neck is shaved, cleaned, and anesthetized. A line block using 10 to 20 mL of 2% lidocaine is performed on ventral midline at the junction of the cranial and middle third of the neck. At this location, the trachea is more superficial. The preoperative preparation is done with the head in normal anatomic position. At the time of surgery, the head is stretched up in the air or, if the procedure is to be performed in dorsal recumbency, the calf is turned on its back before the alcohol and chlorhexidine wipes are used. It is important to realize that those positions (head stretch or dorsal recumbency) may aggravate the respiratory distress of the animal. Therefore, it is crucial to be efficient.

With 1 hand, the trachea is mobilized while making a 10-cm ventral midline skin incision at the junction of the cranial and middle third of the neck (**Fig. 4**A). The paired sternohyoideus and sternothyroideus muscles are split on the midline using a combination of sharp and blunt dissection (**Fig. 4**B). Care should be taken to remain on the midline to avoid splitting the muscle fibers instead of separating the paired muscle. Using a Weitlaner retractor significantly helps to expose the tracheal rings (**Fig. 4**C). The annular ligament, between 2 tracheal rings, is sharply incised (**Fig. 4**D). The incision is extended making sure not to cut more than 50% of the diameter of the trachea. At this point, a hemostatic forceps is introduced in the trachea. The jaw is opened and the animal is allowed to breathe.

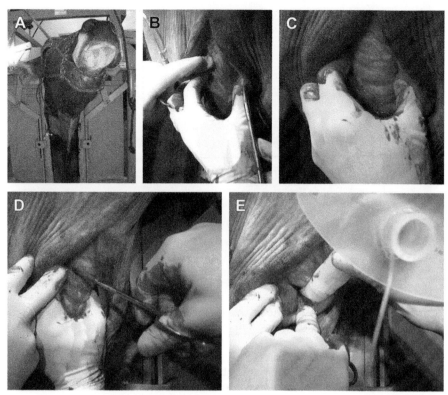

Fig. 4. Tracheotomy and insertion of a temporary tracheostomy tube. (*A*) Position of the head. (*B*) Incision on midline and exposure of the paired sternohyoideus and sternothyroideus muscles. (*C*) Mobilization of the trachea. (*D*) Incision of the annular ligament (no more than 50% of the circumference). (*E*) The tube is guided in the trachea with a curved Metzenbaum scissor.

The biggest tube fitting through the tracheotomy incision should be used. In calves, half the width of the rings surrounding the incised ligament can be excised with a curve Mayo scissor, which eases the insertion of the tracheostomy tube. A stylet, a forceps, or a finger is used to guide the tube within the trachea (**Fig. 4**E). With the tube in place, the skin incision is partially closed using nonabsorbable suture material in a cruciate pattern.

Silicone tracheostomy tubes of different sizes can be purchased. They can be cleaned and resterilized many times. However, they can be expensive especially because 1 size does not fit all. These tubes tend to get clogged by discharge if not cleaned frequently. Therefore, it is important not to inflate the cuff to allow the animal to breath around the tube if necessary. To avoid this complication, the tube has to be cleaned 2 to 4 times daily, which can be difficult to manage on the farm for an extended period of time.

An alternative to the silicone tube is the self-retaining stainless steel cannula (**Fig. 5**). They work well on cattle weighing more than 400 kg. Because they do not have an inner tube, they do not get clogged and therefore required less care than the silicone tubes. In heavily muscled cattle, they can be difficult to insert and may cause necrosis of the tracheal mucosa by compression.

Various items of everyday use can be used as a temporary tracheostomy tube. A popular item is the milk jug handle. The curve of the handle makes it easy to introduce

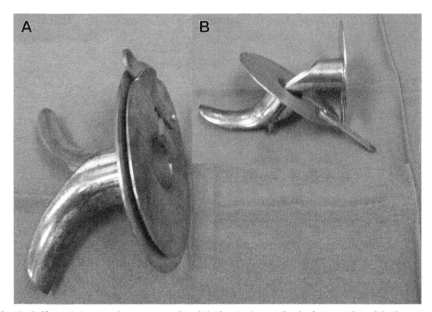

Fig. 5. Self-retaining tracheostomy tube. (*A*) The 2-piece tube locks together. (*B*) The pieces are apart to show how they are introduced in the trachea.

through the tracheotomy. It is readily available and inexpensive. The tube is sutured to the skin. This type of device works well in the short term but could be difficult to maintain for an extended period of time.

If the animal is not already on antibiotics, they are started and given for 3 to 5 days. Nonsteroidal antiinflammatory drugs (NSAIDs) are also indicated.

Complications associated with this procedure are cellulitis, tracheitis, bronchopneumonia, asphyxia, and death. It is important to monitor the surgery site for excessive swelling and foul discharge. A dyspneic animal has to have its tube removed to allow breathing through the tracheotomy site.

SEDATION, LOCAL ANESTHESIA, AND GENERAL ANESTHESIA

Sedation is usually not required for diagnostic procedures. However, if it is needed, the dose of drug used should be kept as low as possible. In ruminants, profuse salivation occurs with most of the sedative and anesthetic drugs, worsening the breathing of an already struggling animal.[19] Those drugs also cause a certain degree of pharyngeal collapse. In healthy cattle anesthetized with ketamine, it is common to hear snoring sounds caused by the soft palate vibrating when the animal breathes out.

Regional anesthesia is possible for the lips and the nares by blocking the infraorbital nerve (branch of the maxillary nerve) as it comes out of the infraorbital foramen.[20] To locate the foramen, a line is drawn from the nasoincisor notch to the first cheek tooth (**Fig. 6**). By palpation, the foramen is identified about 5 cm above the cheek tooth. Between 5 and 10 mL of 2% lidocaine are infiltrated into the canal.

The soft and hard palates and the nasal passage can be anesthetized using a Peterson block at the foramen orbitorotundum.[20] At this location, the maxillary nerve (branch of trigeminal nerve) can be blocked. The Peterson block is described in another article in this issue.

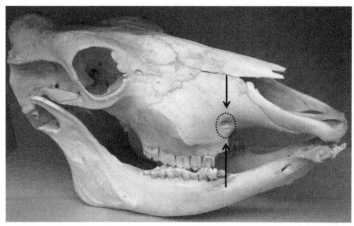

Fig. 6. An adult cow's skull. Lines are drawn from the nasoincisor notch (*black arrow* pointing ventrally) to the first cheek tooth (*black arrow* pointing dorsally) to locate the infraorbital foramen (*dotted black circle*). By infiltrating local anesthetic in this area, the infraorbital nerve is blocked. Surgery on the nares and upper lip can then be performed.

General anesthesia is frequently needed for more invasive upper airway surgery. It can be achieved by injection (double or triple drip) or by gas inhalation. In field practice, injectable anesthesia is used.

For laryngeal and pharyngeal surgery, it is not possible to perform an endotracheal intubation. Ideally, a temporary tracheostomy tube is placed before the surgery. At the time of the procedure, if the tube possesses a cuff, it is inflated to protect the airway from regurgitation. If it does not, it could be replaced by a regular endotracheal tube. If a tracheotomy has not been performed, it is important to realize that a respiratory collapse is more likely to occur. Therefore, the dosage of the anesthetic drug should be reduced and the approach of the airway should be performed quickly. When the trachea or the larynx is open, the breathing pattern improves significantly.

TRAUMA
Nasal Bone Fracture

Fractures of the skull, other than the mandible, are uncommon in cattle. They can involve the zygomatic, maxillary, or nasal bone. They rarely cause clinical signs other than a facial deformation. Therefore, they are fixed only for cosmetic purposes.

The procedure is delayed until the initial swelling has regressed. It is preferably done under injectable or gas inhalation general anesthesia. A local block is performed at the surgery site. Through a stab incision in the skin, a 5-mm hole is drilled through the fragment. A 90° bent 3.2-mm (0.125-inch) Steinmann pin is passed through the hole. The bent section is placed under the fragment before prying it in place. In most cases, no internal fixation is needed. The periosteum keeps the fragment in place. However, if the fracture remains unstable, sutures (monofilament stainless steel or polydioxanone) can be placed through small drill holes in the fragment and the intact bone. To easily place the sutures, the skin incision needs to be extended.[21]

All fractures involving the sinuses or the nasal cavity are considered open. Broad-spectrum antibiotics are indicated for the first weeks after the surgery. Chronic nasal discharge after the surgery may indicate the presence of a sequestrum that may need to be removed.

Mandibular Fracture

Mandibular fractures are more common in calves (**Fig. 7**). They are usually the result of improper use of chains around the mandible at calving.[22] The result is an open bilateral fracture at the diastema of both horizontal rami of the mandible. Many surgical techniques have been described to repair this type of fracture (pinless clamps, cerclage wires around the teeth, external coaptation, and oral splints).[23–27] Oral splint combined with cerclage wire seems to be the ideal way to repair this type of fracture because of the softness of the bone in young calves. It does not require expensive material and equipment and can be performed with the calf under deep sedation or general sedation.

Preoperative antibiotics and NSAIDs are given. The surgery site is cleaned before reduction of the fracture. A splint is created with dental acrylic or polymethyl methacrylate (PMMA). It is molded on the floor of the mouth, from the incisors to the premolars surrounding the base of the tongue (**Fig. 8**). An exothermic reaction occurs when the acrylic is prepared, so it must be allowed to cure out of the mouth to avoid burning the oral mucosa. Cerclage wires are used to attach the plate to the mandible. Skin stab incisions are done where the wires will be passed around the horizontal ramus of the mandible. Through a 14-gauge needle, the wires are passed from outside in (labial side) and inside out (lingual side). Ideally, 2 wires per side are passed caudal to the fracture. The rostral portion of the plate is attached by passing wires through holes drilled in the splint and the mandible (or around incisors if solid enough). When all

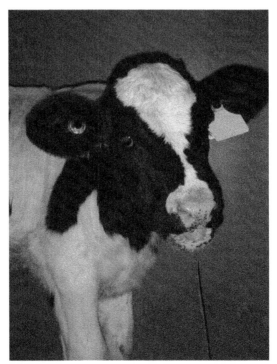

Fig. 7. A 2-day-old calf with a mandibular fracture sustained at calving. The rostral mandible cannot be closed, causing constant drooling. (*Courtesy of* Dr Hélène Lardé, Université de Montréal, St-Hyacinthe, Québec, Canada.)

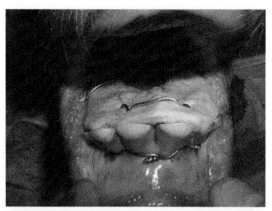

Fig. 8. Mandibular fracture repair of the calf pictured in **Fig. 7**. A PMMA splint was molded around the horizontal ramus and the symphysis of the mandible. The splint was attached with cerclage wire going around the horizontal ramus and between the incisor teeth. (*Courtesy of* Dr Hélène Lardé, Université de Montréal, St-Hyacinthe, Québec, Canada.)

the wires are passed, they are attached by twisting the ends together. The knots are located ventrally in the subcutaneous tissues for the caudal wires and on the labial side of the mandible just below the incisors for the rostral wires.

Antibiotics are given for 7 to 10 days. If possible, the calf is trained to drink from a bucket rather than a bottle. Discoloration of the gums is normal early after the surgery. The cerclage wires are cut and removed 4 weeks after the surgery.

Even if this type of fracture is open, the prognosis is excellent. This success is explained by the good blood supply and the low load that the mandible sustains compared with bones of the appendicular skeleton.

Mandibular fractures in older animals are more suitable to internal (plates and screws) or external skeletal fixators.[28,29] Therefore, they are usually sent to a referral center where the equipment is more readily available.

Pharyngeal Trauma

Pharyngeal traumas are common. They are frequently associated with the administration of Rumensin and calcium carbonate boluses.[30,31] The bolus gun used is often spring loaded. In the hands of an inexperienced manipulator, the bolus can be pushed through the oropharynx. The swelling that follows may cause dysphagia and dyspnea. If not treated rapidly with antibiotics and NSAIDs, cellulitis of the neck and mediastinitis can occur (**Fig. 9**).

The diagnosis is confirmed by oral palpation and endoscopy (**Fig. 10**, Video 3). A lateral radiograph is useful to evaluate the extent of cellulitis.[32]

The cavity is carefully explored and foreign material is removed. A tracheostomy tube is rarely necessary because of dyspnea. However, if there is dysphagia it may be necessary to create a rumen fistula in order to feed the animal during the healing phase.

In case of cellulitis of the neck, stab incisions are needed to drain and stop the progression of the infection. In more chronic cases, a pharyngeal or retropharyngeal abscess may be present.

Pharyngeal abscess can be drained orally, through a transcutaneous approach or through a pharyngotomy. The oral approach is favored more than the other techniques. However, because of limited access, this may not always be possible. The

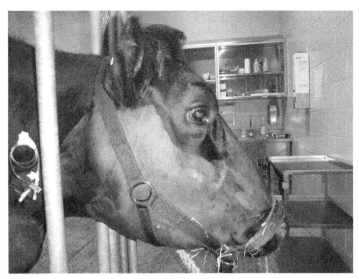

Fig. 9. A 3-year-old Holstein cow presented for severe swelling of the head and neck. The cow had a pharyngeal balling gun injury that caused dissecting cellulitis.

transcutaneous approach is evaluated with the help of the ultrasonography. Ideally, the access to the abscess should be superficial and ventrally located. It should not be over the linguofacial vein, the facial nerve, or the parotid gland. A small skin incision is created before inserting an appropriate-sized chest trocar in the abscess. The trocar is left in place for 5 days to allow daily lavage of the abscess.

If safe drainage cannot be achieved through either of those approaches, a pharyngotomy can be performed.[9]

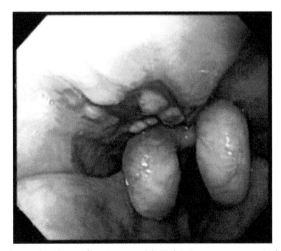

Fig. 10. Endoscopic evaluation of a 2-year-old Holstein cow presented for ptyalism. An endoscope 9 mm in diameter and 1 m long was introduced through the left nostril. The dorsal wall of the nasopharynx is granulating after sustaining a balling gun injury.

Pharyngotomy

Ideally, this procedure is performed with the animal under general anesthesia, intubated through a tracheotomy. The cow is placed in dorsal recumbency and the pharyngeal/laryngeal area is prepped for surgery. The skin incision begins at the thyroid cartilage caudally and travels rostrally, past the basihyoid bone, on ventral midline (**Fig. 11**). The oropharynx is approached by blunt dissection with a Metzenbaum scissor, between the paired sternohyoid muscles, until the oral mucosa is encountered and sharply incised. If needed, the basihyoid bone can be split using an osteotome. The tissues are retracted using a self-retaining retractor. The abscess is located, incised, drained, and flushed. The airways are protected by making sure the cuff of the endotracheal tube is inflated and by putting the animal in a Trendelenburg position during the flush. The surgical site is partially closed. First, the oral mucosa is closed with a simple continuous pattern with 2.0 absorbable suture materials. The basihyoid bone, if split, is repaired with steel sutures or polydioxanone. The sternohyoid muscles are sutured back together with a simple continuous pattern using 2.0 absorbable suture materials. The remainder of the incision is left to heal by second intention.

Fractured Ribs and Tracheal Collapse

Rib fractures occur at birth on calves with fetopelvic disproportion.[33] Most of the time, the fracture occurs at the costochondral junction. Pain-induced tachypnea may be present, especially if the fracture involves multiple ribs or if the diaphysis is involved. In this case, the sharp fragments can penetrate the pleural cavity and lacerate the lungs, causing a pneumothorax (**Fig. 12**). Depending on the rib involved, the sharp fragment can also traumatize the heart and cause an acute and fatal hemorrhage.

Fractures at the costochondral junction may not alter the general status of the calf and therefore rarely warrant repair. Fractures involving the diaphysis must be repaired to avoid further injury to the internal structures and to relieve the pain associated with the condition. Not all the fractured ribs have to be repaired. Because of the strong intercostal muscle, fixing every other rib is usually sufficient to stabilize the rib cage. Placing a small reconstruction plate, secured with screws and cerclage wire, is an efficient technique (**Fig. 13**).[34] It requires gas anesthesia and specific orthopedic material that may not be available in all clinics. A contoured Steinmann pin secured to each fragment with cerclage wire can replace the plate. The risk of using the pins is that

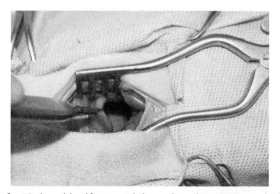

Fig. 11. Pharynx of a 10-day-old calf exposed through a pharyngotomy incision. The Adson-Brown forceps is holding the epiglottis. A Weitlaner is holding the skin, the muscles, and the oral mucosa. The soft palate can be seen past the epiglottis. This structure can be mobilized out of the incision.

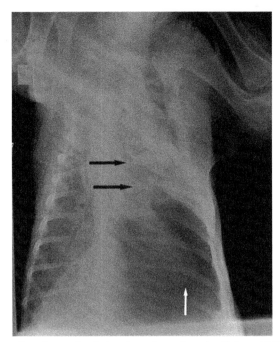

Fig. 12. Dorsoventral radiograph of the thoracic cavity of a 3-day-old Holstein calf. Fractured ribs can be seen (*black arrows*). The left lung is collapsed (*white arrow*), compatible with a pneumothorax.

it can migrate if a wire breaks or if not properly tied. Success has also been reported using the Securos canine cranial cruciate ligament repair system.[35]

If the fracture involves the first rib, it could go unnoticed early in the life of the calf. However, with time, a large callus will form and eventually compress the trachea, which will cause severe inspiratory distress.[36] Diagnosis is confirmed by performing a lateral radiograph (**Fig. 14**). Depending on the value of the calf, it could be referred

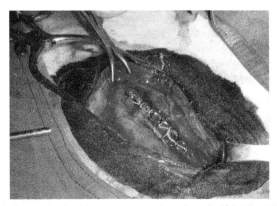

Fig. 13. Fractured rib repaired with a reconstructive plate (calf in **Fig. 12**). Two screws, on each side of the fracture, are holding the fragments together. Cerclage wires were added to reinforce the construct.

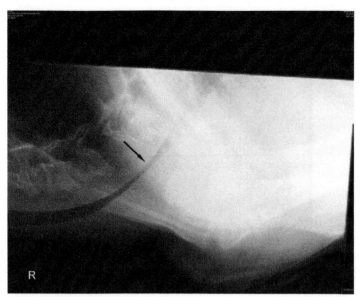

Fig. 14. Lateral radiograph of the lower cervical neck of a month-old Holstein calf. Tracheal collapse can be seen (*black arrow*). Fracture of the first ribs is difficult to appreciate on this radiograph. The fractures caused the tracheal collapse. (*Courtesy of* Dr André Desrochers, Université de Montréal, St-Hyacinthe, Québec, Canada.)

to a large animal hospital where the callus can be removed surgically and an extratracheal prosthesis placed around the trachea to resolve the collapse.[37]

INFECTIOUS DISEASES
Oral Necrobacillosis (Arytenoidal Chondritis)

Oral necrobacillosis is an infection caused by *Fusobacterium necrophorum*, affecting the larynx of young calves. If inappropriately managed in the early phase of the condition, it can cause death or permanent damage to the laryngeal cartilages.[38]

Calves with oral necrobacillosis have a decrease appetite, foul breath, and may have signs of inspiratory dyspnea. Antibiotics efficient against anaerobe bacteria are given in combination with corticosteroids. The treatment is continued until the clinical signs have resolved. If dyspnea persists after a week of treatment, further investigation is warranted. Endoscopy of the nasopharynx and larynx may reveal large immobile arytenoids or necrotic vocal cords (**Fig. 15**, Video 4). At this time, a temporary tracheostomy tube may be used to relieve dyspnea. Another week of broad-spectrum antibiotics may be given in combination with another dose of corticosteroids. Endoscopy is then repeated. If no improvement is noted, surgery is necessary to salvage the calf. Three procedures have been described: permanent tracheostomy,[39] tracheolaryngostomy,[40,41] and unilateral arytenoidectomy.[42] The latest is performed through a laryngotomy and necessitates a longer period of postoperative care. It is performed under general anesthesia in a referral center. The permanent tracheostomy and tracheolaryngostomy can be performed under sedation and local block in a field setting. The arytenoidectomy and tracheolaryngostomy surgery has a success rate of 60% and 58% respectively.[40,42]

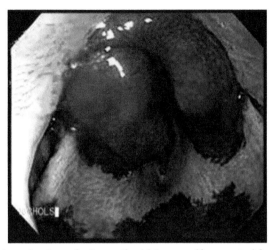

Fig. 15. Endoscopic evaluation of a 2-month-old Jersey calf presented for severe stridor. An endoscope 9 mm in diameter and a 1 m long was introduced through the right nostril of this calf. The right arytenoid is deformed and enlarged. Note the normal pigmentation of the Jersey mucosa.

Permanent tracheostomy

The surgery can be performed on a standing adult or in dorsal recumbency in calves. Preoperative antibiotics and NSAIDs are given. The tracheostomy is performed at the junction of the proximal and middle third of the neck. It may be difficult to do if a tracheostomy tube is in place. After infiltration of lidocaine and surgical preparation, a fusiform skin incision is created (**Fig. 16**A). The skin is removed and the paired sternohyoideus and sternothyroideus muscles are split. In beef cattle, part of those muscles can be excised to decrease tension on the tracheostomy. Three to 4 tracheal rings are selected. Their cartilages are incised on the midline and on each side of midline, to allow removal of approximatively one-third of the circumference of each ring. The incision does not implicate the tracheal mucosa. The cartilage is then carefully detached from the mucosa using a combination of sharp and blunt dissection. When the pieces of cartilage are all removed, the remaining mucosa is incised in a double Y pattern. In addition, the mucosa is sutured to the skin with an interrupted pattern using nonabsorbable monofilament suture material (**Fig. 16**B).

Antibiotics and NSAIDs are repeated for 5 and 2 days respectively. The surgery site is cleaned daily and the stitches are removed 14 days postoperatively.

In the early postoperative period, complete or partial dehiscence of the surgery site is the most likely complication. In the long term (more than 5 years), tracheal collapse at the surgery site has been seen by the author.

Tracheolaryngostomy

The surgery is performed with the calf in dorsal recumbency. Having a tracheostomy tube in place allows deeper sedation and anesthesia to be induced without causing respiratory collapse. Antibiotics and NSAIDs are given before the procedure. The approach is similar to the permanent tracheostomy surgery. The difference is the location of the incision. With the tracheolaryngostomy, the incision is centered on the first tracheal ring and the cricoid cartilage.

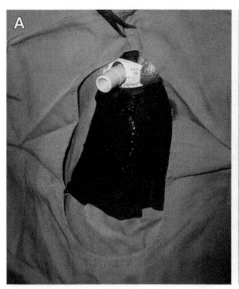
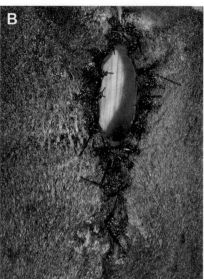

Fig. 16. Permanent tracheostomy performed on a 6-week-old Holstein calf. (*A*) The elliptical skin incision is performed just below the temporary tracheostomy tube. (*B*) Three tracheal rings have been partially removed, saving the mucosa. The mucosa was then sutured to the skin using nonabsorbable monofilament material with an interrupted pattern. (*Courtesy of* Dr André Desrochers, Université de Montréal, St-Hyacinthe, Québec, Canada.)

An oval or fusiform skin incision is made on the ventral midline (**Fig. 17**A). The skin is incised at an angle to facilitate closure. The paired sternohyoideus and sternothyroideus muscles are split by a combination of sharp and blunt dissection (**Fig. 17**B). In heavily muscled calves, these muscles have to be partially excised to decrease tension during creation of the tracheostomy. The cricoid cartilage and the first 2 tracheal rings are incised on the midline. The arytenoids and the vocal cord can be evaluated. Abscess can be drained and granuloma can be removed. However, if an arytenoidectomy is to be performed, the thyroid cartilage must be split in its center to expose the body and the corniculate process of the arytenoids. In young calves, the thyroid cartilage is easily split with a #21 scalpel blade. In older animals, a bone chisel and a mallet have to be used. At the end of the procedure, the cartilage is attached with simple interrupted suture pattern using an absorbable monofilament material.

After debridement of the larynx, the tracheolaryngostomy is realized. First, a wedge of the cricoid and tracheal cartilages is removed on each side of the midline incision (**Fig. 17**C). Ideally, the mucosa underneath the cartilage is saved. The cartilages are attached to the skin with horizontal mattress using polypropylene suture material. Then, the mucosa is attached to the skin with simple interrupted using USP2.0 polypropylene. The cranial and caudal parts of the skin incision are closed (**Fig. 17**B and D).

The tracheostomy tube, if present, is kept for 2 to 3 days postoperatively. The antibiotics are given for 5 to 7 days after the surgery. The surgery site is closely monitored for signs of infection or dehiscence. The skin sutures are removed 14 days after the procedure. Over time, the tracheostomy will reduce in size and may eventually close (3–4 months). Having performed an arytenoidectomy might allow the animal to breathe freely even with a stricture of the tracheolaryngostomy.

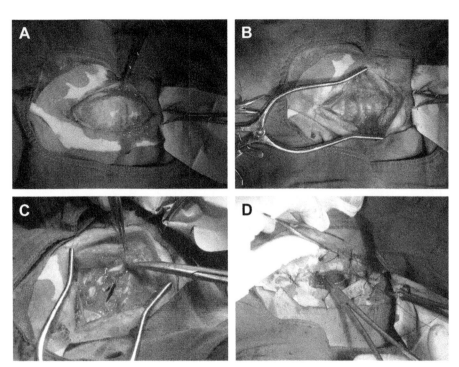

Fig. 17. Tracheolaryngostomy performed on a 4-week-old Charolais calf presented with chondritis of its arytenoidal cartilages. (A) Fusiform skin incision located above the cricoid cartilage and the first tracheal rings. (B) The paired sternohyoideus and sternothyroideus muscles were partially removed to decrease tension during closure. A Weitlaner is holding the soft tissue apart to expose the trachea and cricoid cartilage. (C) A third of the ventral cricoid cartilage and the first 2 tracheal rings were removed, saving the mucosa (incised in this picture). (D) The cartilages have been secured to the skin with horizontal mattress sutures. The mucosa is now secured to the skin using an interrupted suture pattern.

Early complications include dehiscence of the surgery site leading to acute upper airway reobstruction, ruminal bloat, and bronchopneumonia. Long-term complications include stricture of the surgery site leading to upper airway obstruction and chronic bronchopneumonia.

NEOPLASIA AND MASS
Lymphoma

The most common neoplasia involving the upper airway is lymphoma associated with the bovine leucosis virus. Some reports describe lymphoma infiltrating the nasal septum and the larynx.[43–45] Clinical signs are similar to any other upper airway obstruction. Endoscopic evaluation helps determine which structures are involved (**Fig. 18**, Video 5). A biopsy can be obtained through the endoscopic channel. It is frequently undiagnostic because only superficial mucosa is usually obtained. If the lymphoma involves the larynx, ultrasonography-guided fine-needle aspiration of the infiltrated tissue has a better chance to confirm the presumptive diagnosis. If the sample is again undiagnostic, ultrasonography evaluation of frequently involved structures in multicentric lymphoma has to be performed. The heart, the abomasum, and the uterus have to be evaluated.[46–49]

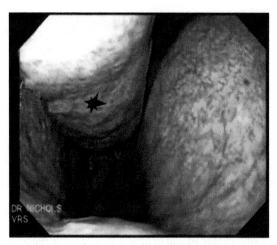

Fig. 18. Endoscopic evaluation of a 4-year-old Holstein cow presented for dyspnea. An endoscope 9 mm in diameter and 1 m long was introduced through the left nostril. The pharyngeal septum of this cow is 10 times the normal thickness (*black star*). After further investigation, it was determined that the enlargement was caused by a multicentric lymphoma.

Performing surgery on an upper airway neoplasia is unrewarding. If performed, the client has to understand that it may only provide temporary relief to allow the cow to carry its calf to term or to perform an embryo flush. In some cases, the stress of the surgery can speed up the proliferation of the cancer. Even if a nasal septum mass can be removed through nasal flaps, infiltrated arytenoid can be removed through a laryngotomy, and paralyzed arytenoid can be lateralized through a laryngoplasty, the use of a tracheostomy tube might be the ideal therapy in the short term.

Nasal Polyps

Polypoid masses can be found in the upper airway of cattle.[50] Their origin is unknown. They usually have broad attachments, making it difficult to dissect and control the bleeding (**Fig. 19**). Electrocautery or a laser can be used to decrease bleeding.

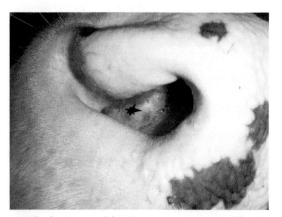

Fig. 19. The right nostril of a 3-year-old Holstein cow presented for dyspnea. Polyps were found in both nostrils obstructing the normal flow of air (*black star*).

However, the procedure is more rapidly done using sharp dissection with a blade or a scissor. The surgery site is then packed with a roll of gauze held together with umbilical tape and attached to the nares. The packing is removed the following day.

With a bilateral condition, the procedures are performed a day apart.

Nasal or Laryngeal Granuloma

Granuloma has been diagnosed most commonly in the nasal passages of cattle.[51,52] Sporadically, it has been diagnosed in the pharynx[53,54] and larynx.[55] It has been associated with chronic infection with *Nocardia* sp (nasal eosinophilic granuloma), with fungi such as *Bipolaris* sp and *Drechslera* sp (allergic granular rhinitis), and with bacteria such as *Actinobacillus lignieresii*.

Diffuse granulomatous lesions in the nasal passages can be difficult to remove and treat. A single mass in the pharynx has been successfully removed by using a chain écraseur, a laser, or a blade through an oral approach. All pharyngeal and laryngeal granulomas reported were caused by chronic infection with *A lignieresii*. Removal of the mass combined with systemic use of antibiotic efficiently resolved the obstruction.

CONGENITAL DEFECT
Cleft Palate

In cattle, cleft palates can be congenital or acquired. With the latter, a complete laceration of the palate may be caused by inappropriate delivery of oral medication. Congenital cleft palate is the result of incomplete fusion of the palatal folds following descent of the tongue in the mouth in the early embryonic state (**Fig. 20**). This condition could be inherited in Charolais and Hereford calves.[56] It is associated with other skeletal malformations such as arthrogryposis. It can also be caused by ingestion of teratogenic substances such as piperidine alkaloids, which are present in various plants.[57,58] It is thought that this substance decreases fetal movement (tongue and limb), leading to the formation of cleft palate and flexor tendon contracture.

In utero, the palate fuses from rostral to caudal. Therefore, the soft palate is always involved if the hard palate is not fused. In cattle, both the hard and soft palates are usually involved. The defect is usually large, which complicates surgical correction.

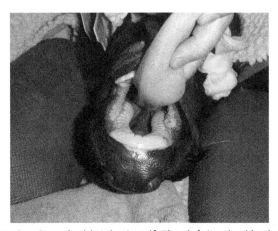

Fig. 20. Cleft palate in a 2-week-old Holstein calf. The cleft involved both the hard and soft palates.

Clinical signs include regurgitation of milk from the nose, aspiration pneumonia, and failure to thrive. The signs appear early in life and diagnosis is made at a very young age. It is obtained by oral examination or by nasopharyngeal endoscopy. It is important to evaluate the calf for any other congenital anomalies and to evaluate the severity of aspiration pneumonia.

Following diagnosis of cleft palate, 2 options are given to the owner: euthanasia or surgical correction.[59] Because of the frequent involvement of both palates, medical therapy alone will not allow the animal to grow and develop normally. With multiple congenital anomalies or with severe aspiration pneumonia, euthanasia should be the first option. If surgery is to be performed, the owner has to be informed of the high failure rate associated with repair of a large cleft palate, and the possible postoperative complications such as aspiration pneumonia, dysphagia, osteomyelitis, and cellulitis.[60] Some cases necessitate multiple surgeries to successfully close the defect, which involves a large investment from the owner. Before surgery, it is also important to discuss the possible hereditary nature of the disease and the risk of doing surgery for the genetic value of the animal. A large retrospective or prospective study about cleft palate repair in cattle is lacking. Our clinical impression is that 30% of calves have a positive outcome following surgical repair.

Because of the risk of aspiration pneumonia and the necessity of doing the surgery before the calf becomes a true ruminant, the procedure is not delayed as it might be in other species (horses). Multiple surgical approaches have been described: transoral, bilateral buccotomy, pharyngotomy, and mandibular symphysiotomy. Mandibular symphysiotomy is the only approach that allows correction of a cleft involving both the hard and soft palates. Therefore, it is the technique most frequently used in cattle. It is a procedure that has to be done under general anesthesia. It has a high morbidity rate that necessitates intensive postoperative treatments. It is therefore performed in referral centers.

Subepiglottic Cyst

Congenital subepiglottic cyst has been reported as a cause of intermittent upper airway obstruction in neonatal calves.[61] The obstruction is intermittent because the cyst can be swallowed to temporarily relieve the obstruction. Diagnosis is obtained by endoscopy. Most of the time, the cyst is pedunculated, allowing oral transection of the attachment. The procedure is done under general anesthesia, ideally with a tracheostomy tube in place. Laser ablation under endoscopic guidance is ideal. However, it can be done using a blade or a long curved scissor. No recurrence has been reported after surgical resection.

FUNCTIONAL OBSTRUCTION
Dorsal Displacement of the Soft Palate

Dorsal displacement of the soft palate causing clinical signs of exercise intolerance is uncommon in cattle. It has been reported as being a problem in breeding bulls.[62] In those bulls, strap muscle (sternohyoideus and sternothyroideus muscles) resection was performed successfully to resolve the displacement.

The surgery can be done with the animal standing or in dorsal recumbency under local or general anesthesia. The middle third of the ventral neck area is prepared for surgery and infiltrated with 2% lidocaine. A 15-cm ventral midline skin incision is made. The paired sternohyoideus and sternothyroideus muscles are exposed and isolated bluntly from the ventral trachea. Ten centimeters of each muscle are excised.

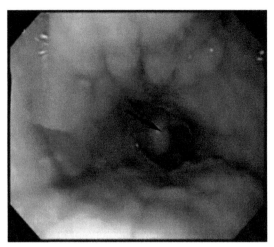

Fig. 21. Endoscopic evaluation of a 4-week-old Jersey calf presented for fever and labored breathing. An endoscope 9 mm in diameter and 1 m long was introduced through the right nostril of this calf. Severe collapse of the nasopharynx was found. The right arytenoid cartilage can be seen at the end of the collapsed pharynx (*black arrow*). This calf was diagnosed with bilateral middle ear infection and bronchopneumonia.

The subcutaneous tissue and the skin are closed separately. The clinical signs usually resolve within 24 hours after the surgery.

Pharyngeal Collapse

Neurologic pharyngeal collapse can be seen with disorders involving the brain stem or the cranial nerves. The author has seen it in cases of listeriosis or middle/inner ear infection. The glossopharyngeal and the vagal nerves innervate the muscle responsible for keeping the pharynx open during inspiration. Paralysis or paresis of these nerves can lead to pharyngeal collapse. When the condition is unilateral, no upper airway obstruction is present. However, with bilateral disorders (eg, bilateral middle/inner ear infection), a complete collapse of the pharynx may be seen (through endoscopy) to cause an upper airway obstruction (**Fig. 21**, Video 6).

Placing a temporary tracheostomy tube relieves the upper airway obstruction while the primary disease is being treated.

SUPPLEMENTARY DATA

Supplementary data related to this article can be found at http://dx.doi.org/10.1016/j.cvfa.2016.05.003.

REFERENCES

1. Farrow CS. Bovine pneumonia. Its radiographic appearance. Vet Clin North Am Food Anim Pract 1999;15:301–58.
2. Jones GF, Feeney DA, Mews C. Comparison of radiographic and necropsy findings of lung lesions in calves after challenge exposure with *Pasteurella multocida*. Am J Vet Res 1998;59:1108–12.
3. Babkine M, Blond L. Ultrasonography of the bovine respiratory system and its practical application. Vet Clin North Am Food Anim Pract 2009;25:633–49.

4. Abutarbush SM, Pollock CM, Wildman BK, et al. Evaluation of the diagnostic and prognostic utility of ultrasonography at first diagnosis of presumptive bovine respiratory disease. Can J Vet Res 2012;76:23–32.

5. Buczinski S, Forté G, Bélamger AM. Short communication: ultrasonographic assessment of the thorax as a fast technique to assess pulmonary lesions in dairy calves with bovine respiratory disease. J Dairy Sci 2013;96:4523–8.

6. Buczinski S, Forté G, Francoz D, et al. Comparison of thoracic auscultation, clinical score, and ultrasonography as indicators of bovine respiratory disease in preweaned dairy calves. J Vet Intern Med 2014;28:234–42.

7. Lubbers BV, Apley MD, Coetzee JF, et al. Use of computed tomography to evaluate pathologic changes in the lungs of calves with experimentally induced respiratory tract disease. Am J Vet Res 2007;68:1259–64.

8. Ohlerth S, Augsburger H, Abé M, et al. Computed tomography of the thorax in calves from birth to 105 days of age. Schweiz Arch Tierheilkd 2014;156:489–97.

9. Gaughan EM, Klimek-Provo J, Ducharme NG. Surgery of the bovine respiratory and cardiovascular systems. In: Ducharme NG, Fubini SL, editors. Farm animal surgery. 1st edition. St Louis (MO): Saunders; 2004. p. 141–9.

10. Anderson DE, DeBowes RM, Gaughan EM, et al. Endoscopic evaluation of the nasopharynx, pharynx, and larynx of Jersey cows. Am J Vet Res 1994;55:901–4.

11. Anderson DE, Gaughan EM, DeBowes RM, et al. Effects of chemical restraint on the endoscopic appearance of laryngeal and pharyngeal anatomy and sensation in adult cattle. Am J Vet Res 1994;55:1196–200.

12. Lee K, Yamada R, Tsuneda M, et al. Clinical experience of using multidetector row CT for the diagnosis of disorders in cattle. Vet Rec 2009;165:559–62.

13. Finnen A, Blond L, Francoz D, et al. Comparison of computed tomography and routine radiography of the tympanic bullae in the diagnosis of otitis media in the calf. J Vet Intern Med 2011;25:143–7.

14. Braun U, Föhn J, Pusterla N. Ultrasonographic examination of the ventral neck region in cows. Am J Vet Res 1994;55:14–21.

15. Braun U, Föhn J. Duplex ultrasonography of the common carotid artery and external jugular vein of cows. Am J Vet Res 2005;66:962–5.

16. Braun U, Lischer C, Koller U, et al. Imaging findings in a cow with a retropharyngeally displaced magnet. Vet Radiol Ultrasound 1999;40:162–3.

17. Chalmers HJ, Cheetham J, Yeager AE, et al. Ultrasonography of the equine larynx. Vet Radiol Ultrasound 2006;47:476–81.

18. Garrett KS, Embertson RM, Woodie JB, et al. Ultrasound features of arytenoid chondritis in thoroughbred horses. Equine Vet J 2012;45:598–603.

19. Lin HC. Comparative anesthesia and analgesia of ruminants and swine. In: Grimm KA, Lamont LA, Tranquilli WJ, et al, editors. Lumb and Jones veterinary anesthesia and analgesia. 5th edition. Ames (IA): Wiley-Blackwell; 2015. p. 743–53.

20. Valverde A, Sinclair M. Ruminant and swine local anesthetic and analgesic techniques. In: Grimm KA, Lamont LA, Tranquilli WJ, et al, editors. Lumb and Jones veterinary anesthesia and analgesia. 5th edition. Ames (IA): Wiley-Blackwell; 2015. p. 944–5.

21. Auer JA. Craniomaxillofacial disorders. In: Auer JA, Stick JA, editors. Equine surgery. 4th edition. St Louis (MO): Elsevier Saunders; 2012. p. 1469–73.

22. Aksoy O, Ozaydn I, Kilic E, et al. Evaluation of fractures in calves due to forced extraction during dystocia: 27 cases (2003-2008). Kafkas Univ Vet Fak Derg 2009;15:339–44.

23. Lischer CJ, Fluri E, Kaser-Hotz B, et al. Pinless external fixation of mandible fractures in cattle. Vet Surg 1997;26:14–9.
24. Purohit S, Malik V, Chaurasia MK, et al. Management of lower jaw fracture using interdental wiring (IDW) technique in adult bovine. Ruminant Sci 2013;2(1):99–101.
25. Rasekh M, Devaux D, Becker J, et al. Surgical fixation of symphyseal fracture of the mandible in a cow using cerclage wire. Vet Rec 2011;169:252.
26. Taguchi K, Hyakutake K. External coaptation of rostral mandibular fractures in calves. Vet Rec 2012;170:598.
27. Colahan PT, Pascoe JR. Stabilization of equine and bovine mandibular and maxillary fractures, using an acrylic splint. J Am Vet Med Assoc 1983;182:1117–9.
28. Pravettoni D, Fantinato E, Marconi S, et al. Transcortical fixation of a mandibular fracture in a heifer. Large Anim Rev 2010;16:158.
29. Wilson DG, Trent AM, Crawford WH. A surgical approach to the ramus of the mandible in cattle and horses. Vet Surg 1990;19:191–5.
30. Mann S, Nuss KA, Feist M, et al. Balling gun-induced trauma in cattle: clinical presentation, diagnosis and prevention. Vet Rec 2013;172:685.
31. Braun U, Salis F, Gerspach C, et al. Pharyngeal perforation in three cows caused by administration of a calcium bolus. Vet Rec 2004;154:240–2.
32. Farrow CS. Radiology of pharyngeal balling gun injuries. Vet Clin North Am Food Anim Pract 1999;15:391–5.
33. Schuijt G. Iatrogenic fractures of ribs and vertebrae during delivery in perinatally dying calves: 235 cases (1978-1988). J Am Vet Med Assoc 1990;197:1196–202.
34. Lugo J, Carr EA. Thoracic disorders. In: Auer JA, Stick JA, editors. Equine surgery. 4th edition. St Louis (MO): Elsevier Saunders; 2012. p. 655–7.
35. Ahern BJ, Levine DG. Multiple rib fracture repair in a neonatal Holstein calf. Vet Surg 2009;38:787–90.
36. Braun U, Ohlerth S, Sydler T, et al. Tracheal collapse with dyspnoea in 2 calves with multiple rib fractures. Schweiz Arch Tierheilkd 2009;151:83–5.
37. Fingland RB, Rings MD, Vestweber JG. The etiology and surgical management of tracheal collapse in calves. Vet Surg 1990;19:371–9.
38. Woolums AR. Disease of the pharynx, larynx and trachea. In: Smith BP, editor. Large animal internal medicine. 5th edition. St Louis (MO): Elsevier Saunders; 2015. p. 580–1.
39. Goulding R, Schumacher J, Barret DC, et al. Use of a permanent tracheostomy to treat laryngeal chondritis and stenosis in a heifer. Vet Rec 2003;152:809–11.
40. Gasthuys F, Verschooten F, Parmentier D, et al. Laryngotomy as a treatment for chronic laryngeal obstruction in cattle : a review of 130 cases. Vet Rec 1992;130:220–3.
41. West HJ. Tracheolaryngostomy as a treatment for laryngeal obstruction in cattle. Vet J 1997;153:81–6.
42. Nichols S, Anderson DE. Subtotal or partial unilateral arytenoidectomy for treatment of arytenoid chondritis in five calves. J Am Vet Med Assoc 2009;235:420–5.
43. Braun U, Brammertz C, Maischberger E, et al. T-cell lymphoma in the nasal cavity of a Brown Swiss heifer. Acta Vet Scand 2015;57:8.
44. Lardé H, Nichols S, Babkine B, et al. Laryngeal obstruction caused by lymphoma in an adult dairy cow. Cab Vet J 2014;55:136–40.
45. Crocker CB, Rings MD. Lymphosarcoma of the frontal sinus and nasal passages in a cow. J Am Vet Med Assoc 1998;213:1472–4.
46. Buczinski S, Bélanger AM, Francoz D. Ultrasonographic appearance of lymphomatous infiltration of the abomasum in cows with lymphoma. J Am Vet Med Assoc 2011;238:1044–7.

47. Campbell MW, Driskell EA, Tennent-Brown BS, et al. Vet med today: pathology in practice. J Am Vet Med Assoc 2011;238:47–9.
48. Malatestinic A. Bilateral exophthalmos in a Holstein cow with lymphosarcoma. Can Vet J 2003;44:664–6.
49. Angelos JA, Thurmond C. Bovine lymphoma. In: Smith BP, editor. Large animal internal medecine. 4th edition. St-Louis (MO): Elsevier; 2015. p. 1071–3.
50. Anderson DE, St Jean G. Surgery of the upper respiratory system. Vet Clin North Am Food Anim Pract 2008;24:319–34.
51. Shibahara T, Mitarai Y, Ishikawa Y, et al. Bovine nasal eosinophilic granuloma with blood eosinophilia caused by *Nocardia* species. Aust Vet J 2001;79:363–5.
52. Conti Diaz IA, Vargas R, Apopl A, et al. Mycotic bovine nasal granuloma. Rev Inst Med Trop Sao Paulo 2003;45:163–6.
53. Angelo P, Alessandro S, Noemi R, et al. An atypical case of respiratory actinobacillosis in a cow. J Vet Sci 2009;10:265–7.
54. Boileau MJ, Jann HW, Confer AW. Use of a chain écraseur for excision of a pharyngeal granuloma in a cow. J Am Vet Med Assoc 2009;234:935–7.
55. Gamboa JC, Angel KL, Shoemaker RS, et al. Laryngeal granuloma in a bull. J Am Vet Med Assoc 1992;201:460–2.
56. Russell RG, Doige CE, Oteruelo FT, et al. Variability in limb malformations and possible significance in the pathogenesis of an inherited congenital neuromuscular disease of Charolais cattle (syndrome of arthrogryposis and palatoschisis. Vet Pathol 1985;22:2–12.
57. Panter KE, James LF, Gardner DR. Lupines, poison-hemlock and nicotina spp: toxicity and teratogenicity in livestock. J Nat Toxins 1999;8:117–34.
58. Planter KE, Gardner DR, Molyneux RJ. Teratogenic and fetotoxic effects of two piperidine alkaloid containing lupines (*L. formosus* and *L. arbustus*) in cows. J Nat Toxins 1998;7:131–40.
59. Minter LJ, Karlin WM, Hickey MJ, et al. Surgical repair of a cleft palate in a American bison (*Bison bison*). J Zoo Wildl Med 2010;41:562–6.
60. Bowman KF, Tate LP Jr, Evans LH, et al. Complications of cleft palate repair in large animals. J Am Vet Med Assoc 1982;180:652–7.
61. Matton JS, Andrews D, Jones SL, et al. Subepiglottic cyst causing upper airway obstruction in a neonatal calf. J Am Vet Med Assoc 1991;199:747–9.
62. Anderson DE, St-Jean G, Gaughan EM, et al. Persistent dorsal displacement of the soft palate in two young bulls. J Am Vet Med Assoc 1994;204:1071–4.

Surgery of the Forestomach

Joseph W. Lozier, DVM*, Andrew J. Niehaus, DVM, MS

KEYWORDS

- Forestomach • Rumen • Rumenostomy • Rumenotomy • Vagal indigestion

KEY POINTS

- Forestomach surgery is usually performed in the left paralumbar fossa.
- Most forestomach surgery is either surgery on the rumen or using the rumen to gain access to other forestomach compartments (reticulum/omasum).
- The prognosis depends largely on the underlying problem, but timely surgical management can greatly influence outcome in certain disease situations.

SURGICAL ANATOMY AND PHYSIOLOGY

The forestomach, or proventriculus, in the ruminant consists of a rumen, reticulum, and omasum. All 3 are nonglandular and lined with stratified squamous epithelium, whereas glandular abomasum is the "true stomach." All are innervated almost entirely by the Vagus nerve which has both motor-parasympathetic and sensory fibers. It is divided into the ventral and dorsal vagi as it enters the abdomen. The ventral vagi innervates the cranial and medial parts of the reticulum, omasum, and abomasum. The dorsal branch innervates the rumen and parts of other segments of the stomach.[1] Blood supply comes from the celiac artery from the aorta and branches into the ruminal and splenic arteries. The left ruminal artery gives off a branch to the reticulum and the celiac continues to become the omasoabomasal artery.[2]

The reticulum is the smallest of the compartments and it lies just cranial to the rumen between the sixth and ninth intercostal spaces with equal parts on either side of midline. Ventrally it contacts the sternum and diaphragm. The left aspect contacts the spleen and costal diaphragm while the right is in contact with the left hepatic lobe, omasum, and abomasum.[2] The interior has a "honeycomb" appearance.[3]

The authors have nothing to disclose.
Farm Animal Surgery, Department of Veterinary Clinical Sciences, College of Veterinary Medicine, The Ohio State University, 601 Vernon L. Tharp Street, Columbus, OH 43210-1089, USA
* Corresponding author. Large Animal Surgery, Department of Veterinary Clinical Sciences, College of Veterinary Medicine, The Ohio State University, 601 Vernon L. Tharp Street, Columbus, OH 43210-1089.
E-mail address: lozier.29@osu.edu

Reticular contractions are biphasic with one partial contraction followed by a relaxation and another, full contraction just before ruminal contractions.[2]

The rumen lies on the left side of the abdomen extending from the pelvis to the seventh to eighth rib space. It is the largest of the compartments and grows in adult cattle from one-half of the size of the abomasum at birth[4] to holding roughly 100 to 150 L[2] and is the site of fermentation of cellulose. It has a dorsal and ventral sac divided by right and left longitudinal grooves. The left and right longitudinal grooves are also the attachment sites for the superficial and deep leaves of the greater omentum, respectively. The rumen has additional dorsal and ventral grooves demarcating the caudodorsal and caudoventral blind sacs. The ruminal recess refers to the blind end to the cranial most portion of the ventral sac of the rumen, whereas the atrium or cranial sac refers to the cranial most portion of the dorsal sac which opens into the reticulum. This lies between the cranial pillar and the ruminoreticular fold. The ruminoreticular fold is a septum that separates the rumen from the reticulum. The cardiac opening, the opening of the esophagus, is just dorsal to the reticulum at the eighth intercostal space. Internally, the ridges formed by the exterior grooves are referred to as pillars. The inside of the rumen is covered by ruminal papillae, which are roughly 1 cm long. Adequate forage and fiber mat in the rumen is required for appropriate ruminal papillae development.[3] Contractions of the rumen start just after a reticular contraction when the omasal orifice relaxes with a primary contraction. Primary contractions begin cranially and spread over the dorsal sac into the ventral sac. This contraction mixes and distributes ingesta and substrates. Following 2 primary contractions is 1 secondary contraction in which the ventral sac then contracts from caudal to cranial.[2] Secondary contractions push gas to the cardia and allow eructation to occur. There should be approximately 3 rumen contractions in 2 minutes.

The omasum is a spherical viscus that lies between ribs 7 to 11 just right of midline. It is sometimes called the "Butcher's Bible" as the muscular laminae covered with short papillae resemble pages of a book.[4] It has a capacity of 7 to 18 L. In the normal cow, 2 omasal contractions per minute can be auscultated at the ninth intercostal space at the level of the elbow.[2]

The gastric groove in suckling calves allows milk to bypass the forestomach and go straight to the abomasum. In the adult it is divided into the reticular groove, which leads to the reticulo-omasal opening and the omasal groove (as well as the abomasal groove).[3]

PATHOLOGY OF THE FORESTOMACH

Pathology of the forestomach often falls into a category of what is commonly referred to as "vagal indigestion." The syndrome was named after the clinical signs were produced experimentally by transecting different branches of the Vagus nerve by Hoflund.[1] This at times leads to confusion, as Vagus nerve damage or inflammation is rarely the cause of vagal indigestion. The classification scheme of vagal indigestion most used by the authors is the Ferrante and Whitlock classification and is as follows: 1, failure of eructation or free gas bloat; 2, omasal transport failure; 3, abomasal impaction; 4, partial obstruction of the stomach. Only types 1 and 2 are conditions of the forestomach, but all 4 types can result in similar presentation so physical examination findings and diagnostics must be used to appropriately diagnose the animal and the type of vagal indigestion.[1]

Type 1 Vagal Indigestion

Excessive free gas in the dorsal sac of the rumen is not a cause of a disease but a clinical sign. Fermentation in the rumen produces gas (methane and carbon dioxide) which must be eructated. Therefore, type 1 vagal indigestion does not occur as a result of overproduction of gas, but a failure to eructate the normally produced gas. This can occur for several reasons. One cause may be a physical obstruction of the esophagus, or choke. This most commonly occurs due to a foreign body but can also more rarely occur with myopathy or lymphadenopathy, as well as other tumors. Lesions may occur along the esophagus or at the cardia. Animals in right lateral recumbency may also occlude the esophageal groove due to ingesta falling onto and covering the cardia.[1]

Bloat may also occur in disorders of fermentation due to grain overload and acidosis. Weak ruminations due to rumen acidosis may not adequately move the gas layer and clear the cardia to allow for eructation. Gas trapped in a stable foam creating frothy bloat would also prevent gas eructation and can be diagnosed by failure to relieve the bloat on passing a tube to the rumen. This is usually attributed to consumption of legumes and rapidly fermented materials resulting in the production of froth and bubbles with high surface tension. The result is that gas is trapped in a foam that cannot be eructated. Severe hypocalcemia can also result in failure to eructate.[1,2]

Type 2 Vagal Indigestion

Type 2 vagal indigestion, or omasal transport failure, is most commonly a result of traumatic reticuloperitonitis (TRP). Adhesions, and peritonitis as well as masses, herniation of reticulum through the diaphragm, or foreign obstruction and impaction may also result in this condition. Inflammatory lesions of the ruminoreticulum may inhibit excitatory input to gastric centers from the Vagus nerve and result in paralysis of the omasum and reticulo-omasal orifice. Reticular adhesions after TRP might prevent delivery of ingesta to the reticulo-omasal orifice and the omasum.[1,4]

Damage to the Vagus nerve itself in the thorax or abdomen are rare, but could result in both Vagal trunks being affected and would result in forestomach atony as well as free gas bloat.[1]

CLINICAL FINDINGS

General signs of disease in cattle include decreased milk production, decreased feed intake, weight loss, and depression.

Free gas bloat results in left-sided distention, particularly dorsally, which progresses to generalized abdominal distention. If the cause is an esophageal obstruction, the head may be extended and the animal excessively salivating. In the case of carbohydrate overload, the rumen pH may be low and animals may have a metabolic acidosis.[4]

Type 2 vagal indigestion creates an "L" or "papple" shape, with left-sided distension accompanied by low, right-sided distention created by overdistention of the ventral sac of the rumen, which reaches across midline to the right side of the abdomen (**Fig. 1**). The rumen will be hypermotile, although some are amotile, and the animal will have a poor appetite along with decreased fecal production as contents accumulate in the forestomach. The feces often have increased fiber size and are pasty. The increased contractions are disordered primary and secondary contractions and result in a homogenously frothy material rather than the 3-layered stratification of the normal rumen. On rectal examination, the ventral sac of the rumen may be felt crossing midline and a full rumen on the left side of the abdomen will be palpated.[1]

Both types 1 and 2 vagal indigestion are often associated with a bradycardia due to stimulation of the Vagus nerve.[1] Types 3 and 4 are involved with outflow of the abomasum and will not be discussed further in this article. Forestomach and

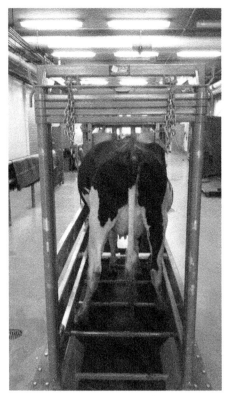

Fig. 1. Type 2 vagal indigestion. Note the bloated left and low distension on the right.

abomasal outflow conditions can be difficult to differentiate. A rumen chloride of greater than 30 meq/L would indicate abomasal reflux and suggest a pyloric outflow issue, as would a systemic hypochloremic, hypokalemic, metabolic alkalosis with hypocalcemia, and aciduria.[1]

If the underlying cause of disease is TRP, the animal may have fever and an elevated heart and respiratory rates. The animal may stand with a kyphotic posture, abducted elbows, and refuse to ventroflex when the withers are pinched due to cranial abdominal pain. In acute cases, bloodwork will reveal a neutrophilia with a left shift and elevated fibrinogen levels. In chronic cases total protein and serum globulin will be elevated.[4]

Imaging such as ultrasonography and radiography can be useful in the diagnosis and treatment of ruminal pathology. Ultrasound is useful in identifying areas of peritonitis or abscessation. Ultrasound can also be useful in guiding abdominocentesis. Radiographs can also be used to identify soft tissue–gas interface indicating an abscess or metallic foreign bodies.[4]

NONSURGICAL THERAPY

Some of the conditions affecting the forestomach may be amenable to nonsurgical management. In the case of esophageal obstruction, orogastric intubation can be performed in an attempt to push the obstruction into the rumen. Gentle water lavage may assist in this maneuver.

TRP prevention can be achieved by administering a magnet orally. Magnets first fall into the cranial sac of the rumen and are brought to the reticulum by normal rumen contractions. Although reticular magnets are very effective at preventing cases of TRP, an animal that is already experiencing disease likely will not be helped greatly by magnet administration. Affected animals often will have decreased rumen contractions and therefore magnets administered orally may not find their way into the reticulum. Also magnets likely are ineffective at pulling metallic foreign bodies back through the wall of the reticulum and do nothing to treat peritonitis, which is a large component to the pathology of the syndrome.

Impactions of the rumen, omasum, or abomasum may be alleviated by oral fluids and laxatives. Omasal or abomasal impactions may be more successfully treated by rumenotomy and direct administration of fluids and laxatives through the rumeno-omasal orifice.

Grain engorgement (rumen acidosis) is one of the most life-threatening conditions affecting the forestomach compartments. Affected animals may require rumenotomy to fully evacuate the rumen and thwart systemic side effects. If surgical management is not an option, rumen lavage may be accomplished with a Kingman tube. These animals will also benefit from a (possibly multiple) transfaunation to reestablish a healthy microbial population. Intravenous fluid therapy will also be beneficial.

Rumen tympany (bloat) typically is 1 of 2 forms, frothy and free gas. Frothy bloat may be treated medically with a detergent such as poloxalene. This surfactant functions to destabilize the foam and allow the small gas bubbles to coalesce and be eructated. Free gas bloat often will be relieved by orogastric intubation.

SURGICAL TECHNIQUES
Left Flank Celiotomy

After the flank is blocked and sterilely prepped, a 25-cm incision is made through the skin, external and internal abdominal oblique muscles, transversus abdominis, and peritoneum 4 cm caudal to the ribs. This facilitates exploration of the cranial abdomen without coming too close to the ribs, which makes closure much more difficult. If the surgeon reaches caudally behind the rumen, the bladder, uterus, left kidney, and intestinal mass can be palpated. Cranially the surgeon can feel the pylorus and abomasum, the omasum, and reticulum. Care is take if adhesions are found to not disrupt and spread possible contamination. If adhesions are found cranially they are likely due to TRP. Rumenotomy can be performed to gain access to the reticulum. If found ventrally they are likely due to abomasal ulcers. The area most suspected of pathology should be explored last to reduce the chances of carrying contamination to other parts of the abdomen.[4]

Rumenotomy

Indications for a rumenotomy include adhesions found cranially associated with the reticulum, hardware disease, foreign body ingestion, such as speculum or drenching tips, or ingestion of toxins or frothy bloat, which must be evacuated. The same approach through the left flank is made. A sufficient seal must be created so that when rumen contents escape the rumen through the incision, they will not contaminate the abdomen or layers of the body wall. The rumen is pulled out of the incision and sutured to the skin with a cutting needle in short runs of a Cushing pattern to create a seal between the rumen serosa and the skin. The mucosa of the rumen should not be penetrated. Interruptions within the continuous pattern should be used to avoid creating a purse-string affect. Blood clots from the incision may form at the ventral aspect of the incision (**Fig. 2**). These should be left in place, as they help provide

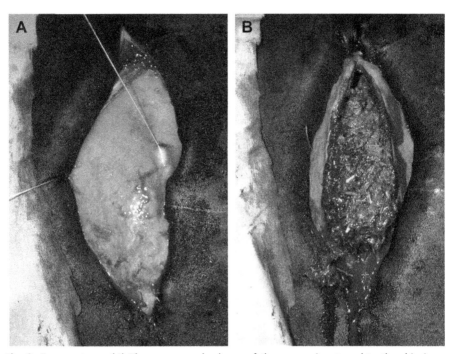

Fig. 2. Rumenotomy. (*A*) The seromuscular layer of the rumen is sutured to the skin in an inverting pattern to create a seal. Blood that has accumulated at the ventral aspect of the incision is left in place because it helps create a better seal. (*B*) The rumen has been opened to complete the rumenotomy. (*Courtesy of* Dr Bruce Hull, Columbus, Ohio.)

additional seal between the skin and rumen serosa. Once a seal has been created, the rumen wall is incised in a vertical direction, leaving at least 3 cm and the dorsal and ventral margins to avoid interfering with the sutures placed. Alternatively, a rumen board (**Fig. 3**) or Weingarth apparatus may be used. In this technique, the dorsal sac of the rumen is grasped dorsally and ventrally with large non-crushing forceps and exteriorized. The rumen is incised ventrally and hooks are placed in the cut edge and attached to the apparatus. As the incision is continued dorsally, more hooks are applied until the ventral forceps are reached. When closing this incision, a double-layer dorsal to ventral inverting pattern is used. Other methods include using only 4 stay sutures or simply clamping the rumen to the skin with 6 to 8 towel clamps spaced evenly around the incision. These 4 techniques were compared in a study by Dehghani and Ghadrdani[5] for time of procedure and postoperative body temperatures and white blood cell counts. Based on these variables, the rumenotomy with skin sutures took significantly longer than the other 3 methods. The stay suture method produced a significantly higher body temperature within its group for the first 4 days, and it had a statistically significantly higher white blood cell count and neutrophil-to-lymphocyte ratio on day 4 when compared with the other groups. Based on these results, the 4 stay suture technique was inferior at preventing abdominal contamination.[5] If available, a wound edge protector can serve as a shroud to protect the tissue edge from excess contamination. Commercial wound edge protectors (Steri-Drape 1076 Wound Edge Protector; 3M, St. Paul, MN) are plastic drapes that have an adhesive surface to adhere to the outside of the patient or the patient's drape. They also have an inner hole attached to a rubber ring that will collapse, allowing it to be inserted

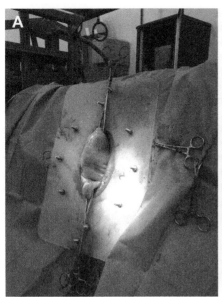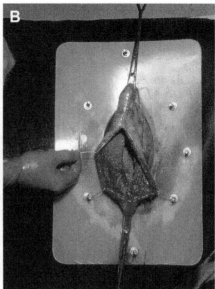

Fig. 3. Gabel rumen retractor (rumen board) is used to prevent rumen retraction and abdominal contamination during rumenotomy. (*A*) The rumen board is holding the rumen exterior to the body via 2 Vulsellum forceps placed on the dorsal and ventral aspects of the rumen. (*B*) The rumen is partially open and the leading edge of the rumen is being retracted by hooks placed around bolts in the periphery of the rumen board. (*Courtesy of* Dr Bruce Hull, Columbus, Ohio.)

through the rumenotomy. Once inside the rumen, it will expand and hold the drape in place. This will prevent rumen contents from touching the surgery site (**Fig. 4**).

The rumen may be evacuated by hand or by creating a syphon with a Kingman tube if it is filled with liquid. The reticulum, omasum, and abomasum may all be palpated transruminally. The ruminoreticular fold, esophageal orifice, and omasal orifice should all be palpated for lesions. The ventral sac of the rumen should be thoroughly explored for foreign bodies. The reticulum should then be explored for foreign bodies and

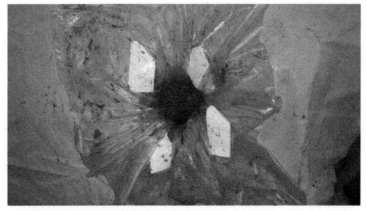

Fig. 4. A wound edge protector is a plastic drape that has an expandable rubber ring, holding the drape open on the interior of the rumen. The outside of the drape is adhered to the patient. This protects the surgical site from contamination from the rumen contents.

adhesions. More ruminal contents may need to be evacuated to reach the cranial portion of the reticulum. All foreign bodies should be removed whether they are penetrating or not. An ultrasound probe may also be used within the reticulum. If abscesses are identified, they can be lanced into the reticulum provided they are tightly adhered. Reticular abscesses are mostly commonly found on the medial wall of the reticulum. If an abscess is identified but not tightly adhered, a ventral midline celiotomy must be performed under general anesthesia to remove or drain the abscess. An ultrasound-guided drain can also be placed into the abscess and flushed daily in lieu of surgery.[4]

Once the ruminal explore is complete, the ruminal incision is closed in 2 layers. The first layer is closed while the rumen is still attached to the skin. Following thorough lavage, the rumen is released from the skin and oversewn with an inverting pattern using #2 absorbable suture. The second layer should be wide enough to oversew the suture holes that were created when the rumen was sutured to the skin. Once the rumen is closed, it is again thoroughly lavaged and cleaned of all debris before being released and allowed to return to the abdomen. The flank incision is closed in 3 layers using #2 or #3 absorbable suture closing the peritoneum and transversus abdominis together and the external and internal abdominal obliques together. The skin is closed with #3 nonabsorbable suture in a Ford-Interlocking pattern with 2 to 3 interrupted sutures at the bottom of the incision, which can be opened in the case of seroma or incisional abscess.[4]

Rumenostomy

Rumenostomy may be indicated in the case of bloat (**Fig. 5**) that is unable to be resolved by orogastric intubation or for enteral support of an animal unable to eat due to oral or pharyngeal trauma (**Fig. 6**). In emergency situations in which an animal is in respiratory distress and will not survive long enough to perform a rumenostomy, a rumen trocar may be used. A self-retaining rumen trocar is preferred if available. Peritonitis following rumen trocarization is very common, so this procedure should be avoided if possible. For rumenostomy, a similar approach is taken as that for a left flank laparotomy, except a small circle of skin is excised. Four stay sutures are placed at 12, 3, 6, and 9 o'clock before incising the rumen. Once incised, towel clamps can be used to secure the incised edges of the rumen to the skin to minimize contamination

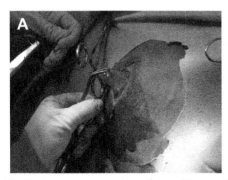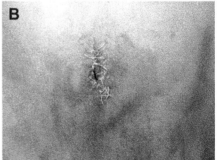

Fig. 5. A rumenostomy is performed in a calf with chronic rumen bloat. (*A*) The rumen is pulled through the gridded abdominal incision with the aid of towel clamps, and the seromuscular layer of the rumen wall is sutured to the body wall creating a seal. This prevents rumen contents from contaminating the peritoneal cavity. (*B*) The rumen is opened, and the leading edge is sutured to the skin creating a permanent stoma. As gas builds in the rumen it will open and allow gas to escape. This stoma will close when the rumen pressure is low, maintaining a favorable anaerobic rumen environment.

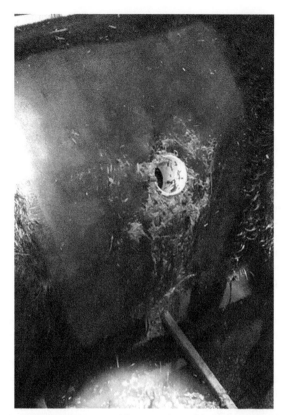

Fig. 6. A rumenostomy is created to provide enteral nutrition in a calf with listerosis. A small hard-plastic bottle is cut and used as a cannula to prevent the stoma from closing and to allow periodic feedings.

while the skin is apposed to the rumen. In the authors' experience, interrupted everting patterns with either vertical or horizontal mattress sutures result in the best rumen to skin seal while avoiding contamination of ruminal contents. If left open, the rumenostomy will granulate in on its own. If the surgeon wishes for the rumenostomy to be maintained, a commercial cannula or home-made stoma may be inserted into the rumenostomy (see **Fig. 6**). Chigerwe and colleagues[6] published successful enteral support for 3 cattle, 1 suffering from signs of listeriosis, 1 with mandibular fracture repair, and 1 with severe oral trauma, highlighting the importance of this procedure's potential therapeutic benefits for a variety of conditions.

Rumen Cannulation

Rumen cannulation is a commonly performed procedure typically for animals entering nutritional studies or to create animals to provide rumen contents for transfaunation of sick animals. Rumen cannulation has been described as a 1-stage and 2-stage technique.

One-stage rumen cannulation

After local or regional anesthesia, but before the sterile scrub has occurred, the cannula plug can be traced or scored into the left flank to mark the circular skin excision. Care should be taken to place the cannula in a location in which the edges of the cannula will not contact the transverse processes, ribs, or tuber coxa, as this may result in sores long term. Also rumenostomies placed on the flank fold may result in abnormal pull on the stoma by the internal abdominal oblique muscles and result in an oblong stoma. This effect may result in a loose fitting cannula.

Following the sterile scrub, a circular skin excision is made using the trace previously described, and the circumscribed skin removed. The external and internal abdominal oblique muscles should then be separated parallel with their fibers rather than sharply incised. This creates a grid that will close tightly around the cannula once the procedure is complete. The transversus abdominis and peritoneum are then incised. The serosa of the rumen is scarified with a sterile sponge or scored with a needle to encourage adhesion formation. The rumen is pulled through the incision laterally. The rumen should not be elevated dorsally as this will create excessive tension on the surgical site and the rumen may tear away. The same procedure as described in the rumenostomy section is performed, securing the edges of the rumen to the skin edge (**Fig. 7**). Once a tight seal has been created, the cannula is placed. The method of cannula insertion varies by cannula design. Most traditional cannulas are inserted by partially inverting the inner flange into the cannula's lumen and then allowing it to unfold once it is through the rumenostomy site. The cannula should fit tightly within the stoma created.

Two-stage rumen cannulation

In the 2-stage rumen cannulation, a physiologic seal is created between the skin, body wall, and rumen before the rumen is incised. In this manner, the risk of contamination of rumen contents into the peritoneal cavity or body wall is reduced. The rumen must be secured to the skin for 1 week. Historically, a metal rumen clamp has been described. The use of a wooden rumen clamp was described more recently by Martineau and colleagues[7] in 172 dairy cows. A vertical incision is made through the skin and the muscles gridded as previously described. Stay sutures with #3 nonabsorbable suture are placed on either side of the incision. The rumen serosa is scarified and pulled through the incision. The clamp is placed against the body wall and clamped to the rumen while the sutures are pulled through slots in the clamp. Mattress sutures are tied across the clamp. In this way, the clamp is secured to the flank of the cow and the rumen is held out. After 1 week, sufficient time for adhesions to form between the rumen and the skin, the clamp is removed. An incision is made into the rumen, and a cannula is placed. In the technique described by Martineau and

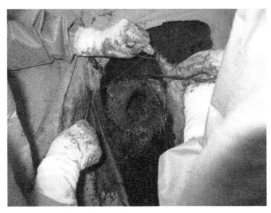

Fig. 7. Suturing the rumen to the skin in the 1-stage rumen cannulation technique.

colleagues,[7] a 7.5-cm cannula was initially placed and was a replaced with a 10-cm cannula after 1 more week. Complications were rare, but 2 cows experienced perioperative abortion, 3 had either the rumen slip from the clamp or the clamp slip off but were successfully replaced, and 2 developed peritonitis and died due to incomplete seal formation.

Omasal Impaction

The omasum can become impacted. In these cases, oral fluids, transfaunate, and laxatives may be beneficial. If this fails to work, a tube may be inserted into the omasum via a rumenotomy. By injecting fluid, mineral oil, and laxatives into the leaves of the omasum, along with manual massage, omasal impactions can be relieved.[2] The omasum can be found via ultrasound examination between the 6th and 11th intercostal spaces below the costal arches, although it is difficult to assess pathology in this manner.[8,9]

Omasal Dilatation and Displacement

A case series has been published on 4 cattle believed to have omasal dilatation and displacement. In all cases the animals presented due to right-sided abdominal distention and low milk production. Rectal examination on all animals revealed a large, doughy viscus on the right side of the abdomen. A ping was auscultated in 1 cow. Three of the cows underwent right flank laparotomy to decompress the omasum. Rumen, cecum, and abomasum were all identified and ruled out as the viscus in question. Three of the 4 were decompressed and found to have foam, fluid, and gas within them. None of the 3 returned to the normal anatomic position after decompression. One of the 4 was euthanized and the viscus in question was confirmed to be the omasum.[10]

PERIOPERATIVE CONSIDERATIONS

Despite the surgeon's best attempts at sterility, procedures involving the rumen are considered clean contaminated. Perioperative antibiotics are indicated. A study by Haven and colleagues[11] showed that a dose of penicillin at the time of surgery significantly decreased abscess formation after a rumenotomy. However, additional days of penicillin therapy postoperatively did not attribute to lower rates of abscess development.

Animals should be properly restrained and a regional block performed before surgery. Animals that are in shock should be hemodynamically stabilized. Efforts should be taken to prevent excessive movement or to prevent the animal from going down during the procedure. These scenarios increase the risk of abdominal contamination. Obviously, emergency rumenostomies may be life-saving and this risk must be weighed against the risk of immediate death. Recumbent animals should be appropriately restrained to prevent rolling to the opposite side, for example.

Common complications of rumen surgery include incisional abscess and peritonitis. The authors have also seen abscesses between the body wall and skin that were attributed to dehiscence of sutures placed between the body wall and rumen to provide additional security. If sutures are placed between body wall and rumen, it may be beneficial to remove these sutures after the rumen is attached to the skin to avoid sutures creating a hole in the rumen.

According to Hartnack and colleagues,[12] in which medical records of 95 cattle receiving rumenotomy (53 animals), rumenostomy (24 animals), or elective rumen cannula placement (18 animals) were examined, the complication rates were as follows: short-term (less than 30 days) follow-up for rumenotomy had a roughly 15% complication rate, including incisional infection, seroma, continuing regurgitation, and death/euthanasia/removal from the herd. Rumenostomy short-term follow-up showed a 13% complication rate with 1 animal developing an incisional infection and 2 either died or were removed from the herd. Finally, short-term follow-up for cannulated cattle had a 17% complication rate, with 1 animal developing an incisional infection and 2 experiencing cannula loosening.

SUMMARY

Most surgeries of the forestomach are safe and can be performed in the field with the appropriate restraint and equipment. Most surgical approaches to the forestomach compartments are performed in the left paralumbar fossa either on the rumen or using the rumen to gain access to other forestomach compartments (reticulum or omasum). Many surgical lesions cannot be corrected from a left flank laparotomy, so a thorough physical examination and appropriate diagnostics should be competed to determine the cause and the site of the lesion before performing surgery.

REFERENCES

1. Franklyn G, Craig M. Indigestion in ruminants. In: Jones, Smith SL, Bradford P, editors. Large animal internal medicine. 5th edition. St. Louis (MO): Elsevier; 2015. p. 777–99.
2. Hofmeyr CF. The gastrointestinal tract, surgical ruminant gastroenterology. In: Oehme FW, editor. Textbook of Large animal surgery. 2nd edition. Baltimore (MD): Williams & Wilkins; 1988. p. 435–72.
3. Pasquini C, Spurgeon TL, Pasquini S. Ruminant stomach. anatomy of domestic animals : systemic and regional approach. 7th edition. Pilot Point (TX): Sudz Pub; 1995. p. 270–3.
4. Ducharme NG, Fubini SL. Surgery of the ruminant forestomach compartments. In: Fubini SL, Ducharme NG, editors. Farm animal surgery. St Louis (MO): Saunders; 2004. p. 184–96.
5. Dehghani SN, Ghadrdani AM. Bovine rumenotomy: comparison of four surgical techniques. Can Vet J 1995;36(11):693–7.
6. Chigerwe M, Tyler JW, Dawes ME, et al. Enteral feeding of 3 mature cows by rumenostomy. J Vet Intern Med 2005;19(5):779–81.
7. Martineau R, Proulx JG, Cortes C, et al. Two-stage rumen cannulation technique in dairy cows. Vet Surg 2015;44(5):551–6.
8. Braun U, Blessing S, Lejeune B, et al. Ultrasonography of the omasum in cows with various gastrointestinal diseases. Vet Rec 2007;160(25):865–9.
9. Imran S, Tyagi SP, Kumar A, et al. Ultrasonographic imaging of normal and impacted omasum in Indian crossbred cows. Vet Med Int 2011;2011:485031.
10. Bicalho RC, Mayers HM, Cheong SH, et al. Omasal dilation and displacement in 4 Holstein dairy cows. Can Vet J 2009;50(4):393–6.
11. Haven ML, Wichtel JJ, Bristol DG, et al. Effects of antibiotic prophylaxis on postoperative complications after rumenotomy in cattle. J Am Vet Med Assoc 1992; 200(9):1332–5.
12. Hartnack AK, Niehaus AJ, Rousseau M, et al. Indications for and factors relating to outcome after rumenotomy or rumenostomy in cattle: 95 cases (1999-2011). J Am Vet Med Assoc 2015;247(6):659–64.

Surgical Management of Abomasal Disease

Andrew J. Niehaus, DVM, MS

KEYWORDS

- Abomasum • Abomasopexy • Laparotomy • Displaced abomasum
- Abomasal ulcers • Abomasotomy • Abomasal obstruction

KEY POINTS

- Abomasal disease is common in ruminants and frequently requires surgical intervention.
- The most common surgical abomasal disorder is abomasal displacements.
- Abomasal displacements can be corrected with conventional surgical techniques as well as minimally invasive techniques.
- Other abomasal diseases such as intraluminal abomasal obstruction and abomasal ulcers may be treated by surgery.

Conditions affecting the abomasum can result in a severe and potentially life-threatening situation for the affected animal. Some of these conditions may not be amenable to surgical therapy, whereas others may be exacerbated by surgical intervention. However, surgical management of abomasal disease remains a treatment option for several of these conditions. Surgical therapies for various abomasal conditions are reviewed herein. Abomasal disease can be divided broadly into disorders that result in altered abomasal outflow and those that result in loss of abomasal wall integrity. Abomasal outflow alterations include abomasal displacements, intraluminal abomasal obstruction, abomasal wall lesions that obstruct flow of abomasal ingesta, and extraluminal masses that obstruct the flow of ingesta. Conditions that result in the loss of abomasal wall integrity include abomasal ulceration and abomasal fistula formation (**Fig. 1**).

ABOMASAL DISPLACEMENTS

Surgery to correct abomasal displacements likely accounts for the majority of nonelective surgical procedures in cattle, but is uncommon in small ruminants.

The author has nothing to disclose.
Farm Animal Surgery, Department of Veterinary Clinical Sciences, College of Veterinary Medicine, The Ohio State University, 601 Vernon L. Tharp Street, Columbus, OH 43210, USA
E-mail address: niehaus.25@osu.edu

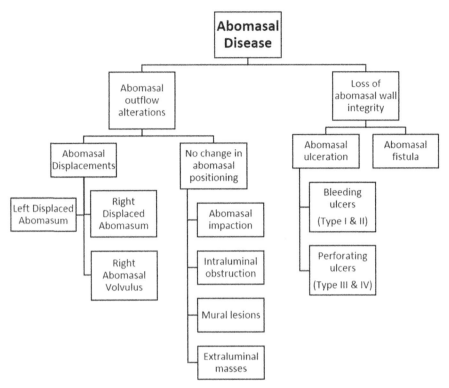

Fig. 1. Relationship between various conditions affecting the abomasum.

The most common surgical procedures performed on the abomasum in cattle are for correction of a left displaced abomasum followed by correction of other abomasal displacements (right abomasal dilatation/displacement and right abomasal volvulus [RAV]). Multiple surgical procedures have been advocated for repair of the displaced abomasum ranging from blind techniques (closed abdomen) to open laparotomy techniques to minimally invasive procedures. Most of the techniques are associated with a good outcome, depending mostly on the perioperative status of the patient.

PATHOGENESIS OF ABOMASAL DISPLACEMENTS

An abomasal displacement is an abnormal positioning of the abomasum within the abdominal cavity, and is divided into 3 broad categories: left abomasal displacement (LDA), right abomasal displacement (RDA), and RAV. In the healthy bovid, the abomasum lies to the right of the rumen against the ventral abdominal wall. Abomasal positioning changes during gestation. As the gravid uterus expands cranially, the abomasal length decreases and the length increases resulting in a more transverse oriented abomasum that gets pushed leftward on the ventral abdominal wall.[1]

The etiology of abomasal displacements is multifactorial. It is thought that the genesis of all abomasal displacements is abomasal atony. Abomasal atony leads to gas accumulating within the abomasum creating a gas-filled viscus. This gas-filled viscous is buoyant within the abdomen and floats dorsally. If it floats up on the left side of the rumen, an LDA is formed; if it remains on the right side, an RDA is formed. An RDA can twist again, creating a RAV or can involve the omasum forming a right abomasal omasal volvulus. The direction of the twist is counterclockwise as viewed from the hind (RDA), and counterclockwise as viewed from the top (RAV). It is thought that all cases of RAV begin as RDAs.

Any concurrent diseases or conditions that cause gastrointestinal (GI) atony can lead to formation of a displaced abomasum. Infectious diseases such as mastitis, metritis, enteritis, and peritonitis, as well as noninfectious causes such as hypocalcemia, hypokalemia, and ketosis, can lead to stasis of the GI tract and subsequent GI and abomasal atony. Abrupt changes in diet can also cause upsets that can cause GI atony. Cattle that have recently calved are at a much higher risk for developing a abomasal displacement. In addition to physically changing the position of the abomasum in late gestation, an abrupt void created within the abdomen after parturition has been speculated to predispose to displacements in the early postpartum period, but this is likely a minor contributing factor. Also, recently fresh cattle are at a much higher risk for development of other conditions such as metritis, mastitis, hypocalcemia, and ketosis. Eighty percent of LDAs occur within the first month after parturition and 57% within the first 2 weeks.[2] In the author's practice, the median number of days after calving for cases of LDA was 14 and the median age of cows was 4.2 years.[3]

An LDA occurs when the abomasum becomes displaced to the left of the rumen and floats up between the rumen and the left body wall, and owing to the buoyancy of the gas-filled abomasum, it becomes trapped on the left. An RDA occurs when the abomasum becomes gas distended and floats dorsally but remains along the right side of the rumen, sliding along the right body wall. If the RDA flips along its long axis, then an RAV occurs. The abomasal volvulus may include the omasum within the twist, becoming a right abomasal omasal volvulus.

An LDA and RDA create a partial outflow obstruction to abomasal contents. The abomasum is usually only mildly to moderately distended and the animal is typically not colicky. The animal will usually be depressed in feed intake and, if a lactating dairy cow, the animal will generally drop in milk production over the course of the disease. The signs of a RAV are generally more severe. The onset of clinical signs is more acute with an RAV. The abomasum is typically severely distended and the luminal pressures can reach upwards of 30 mm Hg.[4] Signs of colic are common with elevated heart and respiratory rates. As the luminal pressure increases, the abomasal perfusion decreases.[5] The abomasal tissue may be totally devitalized, resulting in necrosis of the abomasal wall. Signs of shock and endotoxemia may result. RAV is an emergency condition. If the omasum is involved within the twist, the condition is worsened with a poorer prognosis.[6]

PROGNOSIS

Much of the recent research in the realm of abomasal displacements investigates predicting outcome based on preoperative and postoperative factors. In general, cattle with abomasal volvulus have more hemodynamic compromise, leading to a poorer prognosis than cattle with simple displacements. One study found that prognosis to return to a productive life averaged 81.2% for RDAs and 67.3% for RAVs.[7]

Historically, poor prognosis of cattle with RAV have been associated with preoperative findings of tachycardia, poor hydration status, and a longer period of inappetence[8] than cattle without these findings. Intraoperative findings of omasal involvement, large abomasal fluid volume, venous thrombosis, and dark abomasal color before decompression were associated with a poor prognosis.[6] Anion gaps of 30 mEq/L or greater were a poor prognostic indicator for cattle with abomasal volvulus. This same study showed that anion gap measurements was a more accurate prognostic indicator then either serum chloride or base excess values.[9] Preoperative blood lactate concentrations are a better predictor of outcome in cows after right abomasal disorders (RDA and RAV) than heart rate; however, the best predictor of outcome has been shown to be the combination of blood lactate concentrations with heart rate together. More recent studies investigating the correlation between blood lactate and outcomes found that lactate concentrations of 2 mmol/L or greater were associated with a favorable outcome, whereas lactate concentrations of 6 mmol/L or greater were associated with a poor outcome.[10] Another study showed that postoperative blood lactate could be useful to predictor of outcome in cattle with RDA or RAV; however, the change in blood lactate (difference between preoperative and postoperative values) was not predictive of outcome.[11] In a review of 106 cases of right-sided abomasal displacements, 1 study found that a heart rate of 90 bpm or greater, blood urea nitrogen of 10 mmol/L or greater, potassium of 3.3 mmol/L or less, and a chloride of 85 mmol/L or less were associated with a nonproductive outcome. High γ-glutamyl transferase was a preoperative indicator that could be used to differentiate an abomasal volvulus from an RDA.[7] An early report looked at base excess as a predictor of outcome and as a biomarker to preoperatively differentiate RDA from RAV. This study found that the survival rate decreased as the base excess decreased and the lowest survival rate was found in cattle with base excess of −0.1 mEq/L or greater.[12]

In general, cows with LDAs have a good prognosis for returning to a productive life after surgical replacement. It has been shown that, in cows that have fatty liver disease with LDA, the prognosis after surgical correction of the LDA was related inversely to the severity of the fatty liver. Therefore, it is useful to be able to predict the severity of the hepatocellular damage. One study found that there was a strong correlation between serum levels of ornithine carbamoyl transferase and hepatocellular damage during cases of fatty liver disease. These results support the use of these compounds use as clinical anylates in cases of cattle with abomasal displacements and fatty liver.[13] Dermal carotenoids (a reflection of the animal's antioxidant status) were investigated in a more recent study. In a group of cattle that had an LDA surgically repaired, it was found that cattle with a favorable outcome had an increase in dermal carotenoids over time, whereas the dermal carotenoids decreased over time in cattle with a poor outcome. Although dermal carotenoids are not routinely used clinically as a prognostic indicator in cattle suffering from LDA, these may prove to be useful to prognosticate cattle with LDA.[14] Higher magnesium levels and, counterintuitively, higher β-hydroxybutyrate levels, have been found to be protective for herd survival in cattle with LDA. No association between surgical procedure and longevity in herd was found. Dystocia before LDA and β-hydroxybutyrate of less than 1.2 mmol/L were associated with decreased herd survival.[15] Although abomasal displacements in beef cattle are rare, 1 study looking at beef cattle with LDA showed increased serum glucose and decreased serum insulin concentrations compared with cattle without abomasal displacements, suggesting that cattle with LDA had altered glucose metabolism. Beef cattle with LDA that did poorly postoperatively had significantly lower serum insulin concentrations compared with cattle that did well.[16]

Diagnosis

Diagnosis of abomasal displacements is made based on clinical signs and auscultation and percussion of the abdomen. Auscultation and percussion over the displaced abomasum reveals a hyperresonant "ping" either on the left (LDA) or right (RDA and RAV) abdomen over the gas-distended abomasum. The rectal examination is likely to be normal, but a distended abomasum may be felt in the right paralumbar fossa with large RDAs or RAVs or in the left paralumbar fossa with very distended LDAs. An LDA pushes the rumen away from the left body wall, which may be appreciated on routine rectal examination.

Although cattle having a simple right displacement generally are not regarded as having a surgical emergency, they should be operated on immediately given the difficulty in distinguishing preoperatively between cattle with RDA and RAV on physical examination. In a study investigating base excess in cattle with right-sided displacements, all cows that had a base excess of −5.0 mEq/L or less had an abomasal volvulus rather than a simple displacement.[12] Ultrasound examination of the abdomen is occasionally used to differentiate RDA and RAV. Cattle with an RAV have an abomasum that is more distended, and typically pushes the liver medially away from the right body. However, ultrasonographic visualization of the liver, omasum, and intestines has been shown to be more difficult in cattle with right abomasal disorders compared with cattle without, and the usefulness of ultrasonography in distinguishing between RDAs and RAV is questionable.[17]

MEDICAL THERAPY

Medical therapy is seldom used alone for treatment of abomasal displacements, but is combined frequently with surgical correction. Goals of medical therapy include correction of the underlying cause of the abomasal atony, promotion of GI motility, and correction of metabolic derangements. The restoration of abomasal motility should result in gas being expelled and allow it to return to its normal anatomic position.[2] Oral or systemic calcium to correct hypomotility owing to hypocalcemia may be useful. Promotility agents such as parasympathomimetic agents can help to stimulate GI motility. Dehydrated animals or animals that suffer from severe electrolyte imbalances may benefit from oral or systemic fluid therapy.

Postoperative ileus and abomasal hypomotility can be a complicating factor in cattle undergoing surgical correction of LDA. Preoperative erythromycin can increase the postoperative abomasal emptying rate in these cattle.[18] Preoperative erythromycin has been shown to be effective at ameliorating postoperative abomasal hypomotility in cattle undergoing RAV correction via right flank omentopexy.[19]

Cows are in a state of negative energy balance after freshening. If severe, ketosis can ensue and lead to appetite suppression as well as hypomotility and be a cause of GI atony predisposing to a displaced abomasum. An abomasal displacement can further exacerbate the negative energy balance by decreasing appetite and nutrient assimilation. Mild ketosis may resolve after correction of the abomasal displacement and an increase in appetite; however, severe cases of ketosis should be treated. Intravenous dextrose, insulin therapy, oral niacin, and oral propylene glycol can be used for treating ketosis.

Metabolic derangements are common in cattle with abomasal pathology. Hypochloremic, hypokalemic, metabolic alkalosis typifies the metabolic abnormalities in cattle with functional, proximal GI obstructions. Fluid therapy is beneficial in these animals to correct electrolyte and acid–base abnormalities. Cattle with abomasal volvulus suffer from severe hemodynamic compromise. Hypertonic saline administration has been shown to improve hemodynamic function in these patients.[20]

SURGICAL THERAPY

Surgical correction of abomasal displacements is one of the most commonly performed surgeries in cattle by food animal surgeons.[21–23] Several surgical techniques are available for correction of abomasal displacements (**Box 1**). The chosen technique depends largely on surgeon preference, available facilities and equipment, assistance available, value and purpose of the cow, direction of displacement, presence of adhesions, and prior displacement with surgical correction. Cattle having surgical correction of the uncomplicated abomasal displacements have a good to excellent prognosis for return to productivity.[3,24–27]

Many surgeons prefer right flank techniques because they can be done standing, allow versatility in working with different abdominal structures, and allow the surgeon to perform a thorough abdominal exploration. Right flank techniques are also preferred because they allow the surgeon to work alone.[21] The right flank omentopexy is a procedure by which the greater omentum attaching to the greater curvature of the abomasum is fixed to the right body wall holding the abomasum in near anatomic position.[1] It is critical that the correct positioning be achieved and that sutures are placed through the omentum in close proximity to the pylorus. If this is not achieved, the omentum can stretch and the abomasum can displace again.[5,23]

The pylorus usually serves as a landmark and is brought to the level of the flank incision to assure correct positioning of the abomasum (**Fig. 2**).[21] With this technique, no suture is placed in the abomasal wall decreasing the likelihood of developing leakage of abomasal contents, which can result in peritonitis or fistula formation.

Disadvantages of the right flank approach include inability to visualize and work with adhesions of the abomasum to the left body wall which may occur in cases of chronic or recurrent LDA or cases of LDA complicated by abomasal ulcers or peritonitis. Correcting an LDA in cattle in late gestation can be challenging. These conditions make a left flank approach (left flank abomasopexy) preferable. The greater omentum is friable and can stretch or break down allowing for redisplacement of the abomasum, after an omentopexy. Many surgeons advocate adding a "pyloropexy" to the omentopexy to increase the strength of the fixation. Owing to possible complications of pyloric stricture and secondary abomasal outflow problems, it is best not to pass suture through

---

Box 1
Techniques for correction of abomasal displacements

Right flank omentopexy

Right pyloricantropexy ("pyloropexy")

Left flank abomasopexy[a]

Right paramedian abomasopexy

Rolling[b]

"Roll and tack"[b]

"Roll and toggle"[b]

One-step laparoscopic abomasopexy[b]

Two-step laparoscopic abomasopexy[b]

   [a] Only an option for left abomasal displacements.
   [b] Minimally invasive techniques. Only advised to correct left abomasal displacements.

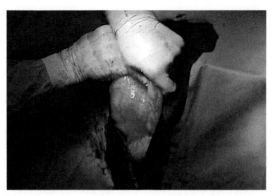

Fig. 2. Exposure of the greater omentum during a right flank omentopexy on a cow. Note the paler pink area at the bottom of the incision representing the pyloric area of the abomasum. Visualization of this landmark indicates to the surgeon that the abomasum has been replaced to its correct anatomic position. (*Courtesy of* Dr Jen Ewoldt, Eldridge, IA.)

the muscular pylorus, but rather through the pyloric antrum of the abomasum, approximately 3 to 5 cm orad to the pylorus (pyloricantropexy). It can be used as a standalone procedure, or it can be combined with an omentopexy to increase the security of the omentopexy. Although providing added security to the pexy, there is greater risk of abomasal perforation and fistula formation. Indications for performing a pyloricantropexy are those situations where the surgeon feels that an omentopexy may not provide enough security to hold the abomasum in place. In overconditioned cattle, the fatty omentum is friable and tears easily. Cases where omentum tears as the abomasum is being replaced has weakened omentum and is a candidate for omentopexy failure.[28] Although intuitively we feel that standalone omentopexies are a relatively weak method of abomasal fixation, studies have found that recurrence rates of LDAs are approximately equivocal[29,30] for correction via omentopexy (4.0%[30]) versus techniques like paramedian abomasopexy, which are thought to have a very secure fixation (2.4%,[31] 3.6%,[32] and 4.3%[33]). Another study comparing the right flank omentopexy, right flank omentoabomasopexy (pyloricantropexy), and the left flank abomasopexy found that all techniques could be successfully used for returning cattle to normal milk production after left displaced abomasum; however, a small but statistically significant poorer outcome (milk production) was noted in cattle with LDA corrected with an omentopexy combined with a pyloricantropexy. It is noted that this difference may be owing to case selection and the retrospective nature of the study.[3]

The left flank abomasopexy technique is performed by laparotomy incision in the left paralumbar fossa. Although there have been methods described preventing a left displaced abomasum via left flank approach,[34] in general, the left flank approach can only be used for the correction of left displaced abomasum, which is a clear disadvantage if the veterinarian is unsure of a diagnosis. Owing to blockage by the rumen, the left flank approach also limits the surgeon's ability to perform a complete exploratory of the peritoneal cavity. Another disadvantage of performing a left flank abomasopexy as compared with the right flank approaches is that the left flank abomasopexy requires an assistant to guide the needle through the ventral abdominal wall so as to achieve correct positioning of the pexy and to avoid vascular structures.[35] One indication for performing a left flank abomasopexy in cases of an LDA where adhesions are present between the abomasum and the left body wall. These adhesions can be visualized and subsequently broken down through a left flank approach. Other forms of abomasal pathology like gastric ulcers or perforations can be oversewn from the left flank approach.[21] Surgical correction of LDAs during late stage pregnancy may be difficult to perform from the right flank owing to the large gravid uterus preventing replacement of the abomasum; these cattle may be good candidates for a left flank abomasopexy.

A small, 10- to 15-cm square should be prepared on the ventral abdomen of the standing cow before left flank abomasopexy. The ideal location for fixation of the abomasum has been determined to be 20 cm caudal to the xyphoid and 5 to 10 cm to the right of midline.[1] These landmarks should be identified and a permanent marker can be used to mark the area so that an assistant can help to guide suture placement. Two paramedian marks, approximately 5 cm apart in a sagittal plane, should be identified centered over the previously described landmarks. Care should be taken to identify the milk veins so that they are not inadvertently punctured. A left flank laparotomy, approximately 15 cm in length, is made in the left paralumbar fossa. A left flank exploratory should reveal the left displaced abomasum lateral to the rumen (**Fig. 3**). The laparotomy should be started approximately 5 to 10 cm ventral to the transverse processes of the lumbar vertebrae. A long piece of continuous, nonabsorbable suture (#3 Braunamid) is required. The length of the suture should be approximately 2 times as long as the surgeons "wingspan." The left displaced abomasum is visualized, and multiple continuous bites of a nonabsorbable suture (#3 Braunamid) are placed in the greater curvature of the abomasum. The ends of the suture should protrude from the abomasum equally at the ends of the suture line. The ends of this suture are passed ventrally along the left body wall, cross the midline, and emerge through the right paramedian abdominal wall at the locations previously identified on the external abdomen. An assistant is needed to guide the surgeon. Both suture ends are passed thought the ventral body wall before the abomasum is replaced to normal positioning. The abomasum is pushed ventrally by the surgeon as the assistant pulls the excess suture tight. Deflation of the abomasum is useful during this step. Once the abomasum has been successfully replaced, the assistant ties the sutures externally to fix the abomasum in position.[21]

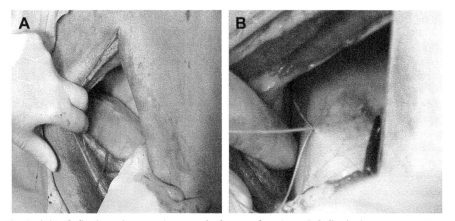

Fig. 3. (*A*) Left flank exploratory in a cow before performing a left flank abomasopexy. Note the left displaced abomasum in the foreground and the rumen medial to it. (*B*) A #3 Braunamid suture is placed through the greater curvature of the abomasum. This suture will be passed ventrally to perform the abomasopexy. (*Courtesy of* Dr Jen Ewoldt, Eldridge, IA.)

If nonabsorbable sutures are used, sutures must be removed after formation of an adhesion. It is recommended to remove the sutures at 14 days postoperatively. Failure to remove these sutures may result in abomasal fistula formation.

An abomasopexy can also be performed from a right paramedian approach. With this approach, the cow is placed in dorsal recumbency. An incision is created parallel to and 3 to 4 cm to the right of midline, extending caudally from a point 4 to 5 cm caudal to the xyphoid (**Fig. 4**). The incision should be approximately 15 to 20 cm in length (see **Fig. 4**).[2]

After repositioning of the abomasum, the seromuscular layer of the abomasum is sutured to the peritoneum and the internal rectus fascia. Some surgeons suture the abomasum with the incisional closure and others describe pexying the abomasum to the body wall remote from the incision. Potential advantages of this approach include achievement of a stronger adhesion as well as the ability to work with prior abomasal adhesions. Complications with this technique include complications with maintaining the cow in dorsal recumbency during surgery, abomasal fistula formation, and herniation of abomasal leaves.

Minimally Invasive Approaches

Minimally invasive approaches capitalize on the buoyancy of the distended, gas-filled, abomasum. When the cow is rolled on her back, the abomasum tends to float to the ventral abdomen. If the cow is tilted slightly onto her left side (putting the right abdomen in a nondependent position), the abomasum floats into a right paramedian location. In this manner, by laying a cow down on her right side and slowly rolling her through dorsal recumbency and slightly onto her left side, an uncomplicated left displaced abomasum can be replaced. Rolling should only be performed for cases of LDA because it is thought that an abomasal volvulus can result from rolling a cow with an RDA. Advantages of minimally invasive techniques include less expense on average compared with traditional open approaches. The procedures are generally faster, cattle have shown a decreased need for antimicrobials, and cattle have shown a faster recovery and return to milk production compared with traditional open approaches.[26,27,36,37] Even though all methods of abomasal displacement correction results in sterile inflammation within the abdominal cavity, minimally invasive techniques

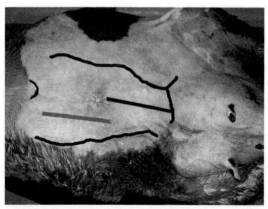

Fig. 4. Ventrum of a cow illustrating the correct placement of the paramedian incision (*red line*) for a paramedian abomasopexy. The xyphoid, milk veins, and midline are outlined in black. (*Courtesy of* Dr Bruce Hull, Columbus, OH.)

have been shown to result in less muscle damage compared with traditional surgical techniques.[38]

Multiple methods of abomasal fixation can be performed after rolling of the cow to replace the displaced abomasum. First described by Hull in 1972,[39] the "blind stitch" abomasopexy technique is the first and the simplest of the minimally invasive techniques and involves passing a large gauge, large diameter needle (and suture) through the skin, body wall and abomasal wall fixing the abomasum to the ventral abdomen. Although auscultation and percussion can and should be used to determine the relative location of the distended abomasum, the primary disadvantage of this technique is that the surgeon cannot be certain that the abomasum has been penetrated, decreased confidence in proper anatomic repositioning of the abomasum, and the possibility that other structures have been trapped between the abomasum and the body wall.[40] In 1982, Grymer and Sterner published a technique that replaced the "blind stitch" technique and has become the basis for percutaneous (minimally invasive) abomasopexy today.[41] The Grymer-Sterner method involves placing a pair of bar sutures (toggle sutures) into the lumen of the abomasum and the attached suture passes through the abdominal wall and is tied externally. The primary advantage of this technique is the verification of abomasal penetration by analysis (odor/pH) of the gas/fluid that is obtained after penetration of the viscus. This technique has remained popular through today and has been associated with equivocal outcomes compared with open techniques.[27,42]

Laparoscopy has been combined with the general principles of the Grymer-Sterner method and has been described as either a 2-step[42] method or as a 1-step[43] laparoscopic abomasopexy. Laparoscopic viewing of the abomasum ensures accurate penetration of the abomasum while avoiding other abdominal structures.

The 2-step laparoscopic abomasopexy was described by Janowitz[42] in 1998. This technique uses a specialized bar suture with two 80-cm-long sutures attached to its midpoint with a dyed present marker used to indicate that the abomasum has been pulled adjacent to the body wall. Placement of the toggle pin suture within the abomasal lumen and deflation of the abomasum is first accomplished with laparoscopic guidance via the left paralumbar area in a standing cow, followed by laparoscopic suture retrieval via the right paramedian area after the cow has been rolled into dorsal recumbency.[42,44] Similar to the sutures of the left flank abomasopexy, the suture is cut 2 to 3 weeks postoperatively. A retrospective study investigating the outcome of cows who underwent an LDA surgically repaired with a 2-stage laparoscopic repair technique found that the cows had a good outcome. There was no difference in 305-day milk yield between control cows and LDA cows after laparoscopic repair.[24]

The disadvantages of this procedure include the additional cost of the laparoscopic equipment, the necessity to reposition the cow during the procedure, and the need for 2 separate surgical preparations. The main advantages of the 2-step laparoscopic abomasopexy is the ability to confirm the diagnosis of the LDA and the ability to evaluate adhesions between the abomasum and body wall or rumen.

The main disadvantage of the 2-step laparoscopic abomasopexy is the need to reposition the cow during the surgical procedure. This has led to the evolution of the 1-step laparoscopic abomasopexy.

Multiple versions of the 1-step laparoscopic abomasopexy have been described and can be performed with cattle either standing[45] or in dorsal recumbency.[25,43] Advantages of the 1-step laparoscopic abomasopexy procedures compared with the 2-step include fewer surgical preparations, fewer incisions, and no need to reposition the cow midway through the procedure, resulting in less operative time.

The original 1-step technique developed by Christiansen[45] involves placement of a bar suture within the abomasal lumen under laparoscopic guidance via the left paralumbar area in a standing cow (similar to step 1 in the 2-step laparoscopic abomasopexy). The suture ends are then passed ventrally against the left body wall using a specialized tool ("spieker"; TR-78–766, Fritz LLC, Veterinary Endoscopy America, Louisville, KY). The spieker tip is a long instrument used to advance the suture ventrally to exit the right paramedian area. Excess suture material is withdrawn by an assistant (similar to the left flank abomasopexy). Advantages of this technique include confirmation of the LDA, ability to evaluate adhesions, and the ability to perform this surgery while the animal remains standing.

The 1-step procedure developed by Newman[43] involves placement and suture retrieval with laparoscopic guidance via the right paramedian area in a dorsally recumbent cow. Placement of the bar suture within the lumen of the abomasum is similar to the technique described by Grymer and Sterner.[41] A reported complication of this technique was accidental placement of the cannula for the viewing portal into the omental bursa before insufflation of the abdomen in one cow. This complication was immediately corrected and did not cause any long-term complications.[43]

Ventral laparoscopic abomasopexy utilizing intracorporeal suturing rather than the bar suture principle has been described.[25] This technique was used successfully in 17 LDA cases and 1 RDA case. Follow-up laparoscopy at 90 days postoperative indicated good adhesion formation of the abomasum and the body wall. Unlike the laparoscopic techniques using the bar-suture principle, this ventral laparoscopic abomasopexy technique requires more intraabdominal laparoscopic maneuvers and therefore is more technically challenging. It also requires the need for a surgical assistant and therefore its use may be limited to hospital settings.[25,46]

POSTOPERATIVE COMPLICATIONS OF ABOMASAL FIXATION

As with any surgical procedure, complications include incisional infections, abscessation, and dehiscence. Catastrophic complications are rare. Techniques that perforate the abomasal lumen could result in peritonitis from leakage of abomasal contents from the lumen. Abomasal fistulation is also possible and most commonly result from ventral abomasopexy procedures that penetrate the abomasal lumen. Failure to remove the abomasopexy suture in a timely manner is associated with the development of abomasal fistulation.

Duodenal sigmoid flexure volvulus has been reported in cattle. Affected cattle present with clinical signs similar to abomasal volvulus or duodenal obstruction: a dorsal right-sided ping, succussable fluid, and a severe hypochloremic, hypokalemic metabolic alkalosis with high bilirubin. Cattle that have had previous history of surgical fixation of the abomasum are overrepresented with 20 of 29 cattle having a previously performed omentopexy or pyloropexy. Timely surgical intervention generally yields a fair to good prognosis.[47]

ABOMASAL ULCERS

Abomasal ulcers, similar to gastric ulcers of other species, are erosions of the abomasal wall. Abomasal ulcers are divided into 4 categories based on the depth of the ulceration. Types I and II are nonperforating ulcers. Types III and IV are perforating ulcers with localized and diffuse peritonitis, respectively. Animals with type I ulcers present with vague clinical signs including decreased appetite, weight gain, and rumen motility. Fecal occult blood may be positive. Type II ulcers commonly bleed and cause melena from digested blood. If blood loss is great, the cow may be anemic with pale mucous membranes and very low packed cell volume. Surgical management of type I and II ulcers is not indicated and may be contraindicated in anemic patients. Type III ulcers are perforating ulcers that result in localized peritonitis because the omental sling contained the abomasal leakage. Type IV ulcers are perforating ulcers that result in diffuse peritonitis.

Although management of type I and II ulcers are generally focused on medical management, reduction of stress, treatment of concurrent diseases, and correction of metabolic disturbances, surgery may be indicated for perforating ulcers; however, the prognosis is often poor and depends on the location and size of the ulcer, as well as the extent of peritonitis.[48] One report indicates that surgical resection of perforating abomasal ulcers was successful in 4 out of 10 calves.[49]

Often ulcers or secondary changes (peritonitis, adhesions) are found on exploratory surgery performed for correction of a displaced abomasum. If encountered during surgery, or if performing surgery to correct a perforating abomasal ulcer, the ulcer can be resected or oversewn to close the defect. The low pH of abomasal contents confers a relative sterility to the contents of this viscus as compared with that of other parts of the GI tract. Therefore, leakage of abomasal contents into the abdomen causes a self-limiting chemical peritonitis rather than a septic peritonitis. This may explain the surprisingly good outcome experienced by cows with perforating abomasal ulcers. Most abomasal ulcers are thought to be predisposed by stress. Stressors include environmental stress (transport, heat stress, etc), stress from high metabolic demands (high milk production), or stress induced by concurrent diseases (mastitis, metritis, ketosis, etc). Abomasal lymphosarcoma can also cause abomasal ulcerations. The prognosis for abomasal lymphosarcoma is poor and treatment is generally not warranted, although exploratory laparotomy with abomasal biopsy may be needed to confirm the diagnosis. Ultrasound imaging has been shown to be useful in diagnosing cows affected with abomasal lymphosarcoma. Enlarged lymph nodes caudal to the reticulum[50] and a thickened pylorus were visualized by ultrasonography in cattle affected by abomasal lymphosarcoma.[50,51] In addition, transabdominal ultrasonography can be a useful diagnostic tool in cattle presenting with signs of pyloric outflow obstruction caused by abomasal lymphosarcoma to avoid the time and expense incurred by exploratory laparotomy.[51]

Other Abomasal Surgery

Abomasal impaction can be treated by abomasotomy, abomasal massage, or pyloromyotomy. This study showed that abomasal massage with mineral oil delivered orally can be an effective treatment of abomasal impaction.[52] A case report of an abomasotomy for removal of a bezoar in a 4.5-year-old standing Holstein cow indicated that the cow was doing well and had integrated well into the milking herd with a similar milk production as the herd average at 6 months postoperatively.[53]

Midline body wall defects occasionally entrap the abomasum. This is especially true in young ruminants, where the abomasum is the largest of the gastric compartments. Adhesions of the abomasum to the body wall or to omentum in these young ruminants may need to be broken down. Care should be taken to avoid accidental abomasal perforation. If adhesions are present, part of the abomasal wall may need to be resected and oversewn.

A Richter's hernia is a hernia where only the antimesenteric wall of a viscus protrudes through the hernia. Although it is unlikely that the entire abomasum will become herniated owing to the size of the viscus, it is possible that 1 wall of the abomasum can protrude through a ventral hernia and become strangulated. This may necessitate resection of the strangulated portion of the abomasum (**Fig. 5**).

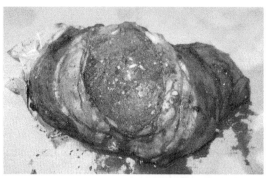

Fig. 5. Richter's hernia after resection from a 3-month-old calf. The open abomasal lumen can be visualized where it was resected from the rest of the body of the abomasum.

SUMMARY

The majority of abomasal surgeries are performed to correct abomasal displacements in cattle. Many different procedures for abomasal displacement correction and fixation exist in veterinary surgery. It is important to have an understanding of the techniques, their indications, contraindications, prognoses, and potential complications. Surgery to correct other abomasal disorders such as abomasal obstruction and perforating abomasal ulcers in cattle and small ruminants do exist, but are far less common.

REFERENCES

1. Wittek T, Constable PD, Morin DE. Ultrasonographic assessment of change in abomasal position during the last three months of gestation and first three months of lactation in Holstein-Friesian cows. J Am Vet Med Assoc 2005;227(9):1469–75.

2. Trent AM. Surgery of the abomasum. In: Fubini SL, Ducharme NG, editors. Farm animal surgery. St Louis (MO): Saunders; 2004. p. 196–239.

3. Pentecost RL, Niehaus AJ, Anderson DE, et al. Outcome following surgical correction of abomasal displacement in lactating dairy cattle: a retrospective study of 127 cases (1999-2010). Journal of Veterinary Science & Animal Husbandry 2014;1(4):1.

4. Constable PD, St-Jean G, Koenig GR, et al. Abomasal luminal pressure in cattle with abomasal volvulus or left displaced abomasum. J Am Vet Med Assoc 1992; 201(10):1564–8.

5. Wittek T, Constable PD, Furll M. Comparison of abomasal luminal gas pressure and volume and perfusion of the abomasum in dairy cows with left displaced abomasum or abomasal volvulus. Am J Vet Res 2004;65(5):597–603.

6. Constable PD, St Jean G, Hull BL, et al. Prognostic value of surgical and postoperative findings in cattle with abomasal volvulus. J Am Vet Med Assoc 1991; 199(7):892–8.

7. Meylan M. Prognostic indicators in cattle with right-sided displacement of the abomasum and abomasal volvulus. Schweiz Arch Tierheilkd 1999;141(9):413–8 [in German].

8. Constable PD, St Jean G, Hull BL, et al. Preoperative prognostic indicators in cattle with abomasal volvulus. J Am Vet Med Assoc 1991;198(12):2077–85.

9. Garry FB, Hull BL, Rings DM, et al. Prognostic value of anion gap calculation in cattle with abomasal volvulus: 58 cases (1980-1985). J Am Vet Med Assoc 1988; 192(8):1107–12.

10. Boulay G, Francoz D, Dore E, et al. Preoperative cow-side lactatemia measurement predicts negative outcome in Holstein dairy cattle with right abomasal disorders. J Dairy Sci 2014;97(1):212–21.

11. Buczinski S, Boulay G, Francoz D. Preoperative and postoperative L-lactatemia assessment for the prognosis of right abomasal disorders in dairy cattle. J Vet Intern Med 2015;29(1):375–80.

12. Simpson DF, Erb HN, Smith DF. Base excess as a prognostic and diagnostic indicator in cows with abomasal volvulus or right displacement of the abomasum. Am J Vet Res 1985;46(4):796–7.

13. Kalaitzakis E, Roubies N, Panousis N, et al. Evaluation of ornithine carbamoyl transferase and other serum and liver-derived analytes in diagnosis of fatty liver and postsurgical outcome of left-displaced abomasum in dairy cows. J Am Vet Med Assoc 2006;229(9):1463–71.

14. Klein J, Darvin ME, Muller KE, et al. Serial non-invasive measurements of dermal carotenoid concentrations in dairy cows following recovery from abomasal displacement. PLoS One 2012;7(10):e47706.

15. Reynen JL, Kelton DF, LeBlanc SJ, et al. Factors associated with survival in the herd for dairy cows following surgery to correct left displaced abomasum. J Dairy Sci 2015;98(6):3806–13.

16. Ichijo T, Satoh H, Yoshida Y, et al. Prognostic judgment at post-surgery by biochemical parameters in beef cattle with left displaced abomasum. J Vet Med Sci 2014;76(10):1419–21.

17. Braun U, Feller B, Hassig M, et al. Ultrasonographic examination of the omasum, liver, and small and large intestines in cows with right displacement of the abomasum and abomasal volvulus. Am J Vet Res 2008;69(6):777–84.

18. Wittek T, Tischer K, Gieseler T, et al. Effect of preoperative administration of erythromycin or flunixin meglumine on postoperative abomasal emptying rate in dairy cows undergoing surgical correction of left displacement of the abomasum. J Am Vet Med Assoc 2008;232(3):418–23.

19. Wittek T, Tischer K, Korner I, et al. Effect of preoperative erythromycin or dexamethasone/vitamin C on postoperative abomasal emptying rate in dairy cows undergoing surgical correction of abomasal volvulus. Vet Surg 2008;37(6):537–44.

20. Sickinger M, Doll K, Roloff NC, et al. Small volume resuscitation with hypertonic sodium chloride solution in cattle undergoing surgical correction of abomasal volvulus. Vet J 2014;201(3):338–44.

21. St Jean GD, Hull BL, Hoffsis GF, et al. Comparison of the different surgical techniques for correction of abomasal problems. OMP CONT EDUC PRACT 1987; 9(11):F377–82.

22. Trent AM. Surgery of the abomasum. Agri Pract 1992;13(9):12–4.

23. Baird AN, Harrison S. Surgical treatment of left displaced abomasum. OMP CONT EDUC PRACT 2001;23(10):S102–8.

24. Jorritsma R, Westerlaan B, Bierma MP, et al. Milk yield and survival of Holstein-Friesian dairy cattle after laparoscopic correction of left-displaced abomasum. Vet Rec 2008;162(23):743–6.

25. Mulon PY, Babkine M, Desrochers A. Ventral laparoscopic abomasopexy in 18 cattle with displaced abomasum. Vet Surg 2006;35(4):347–55.

26. Seeger T, Kumper H, Failing K, et al. Comparison of laparoscopic-guided aboma-sopexy versus omentopexy via right flank laparotomy for the treatment of left abomasal displacement in dairy cows. Am J Vet Res 2006;67(3):472–8.
27. Sterner KE, Grymer J, Bartlett PC, et al. Factors influencing the survival of dairy cows after correction of left displaced abomasum. J Am Vet Med Assoc 2008; 232(10):1521–9.
28. Wren G. In-clinic displaced abomasum surgery. Bovine Veterinarian 1993;4–8.
29. Fubini SL, Ducharme NG, Erb HN. A comparison in 101 dairy cows of right paral-umbar fossa omentopexy and right paramedian abomasopexy for treatment of left displacement of the abomasum. Can Vet J 1992;33(5):318–24.
30. Wallace CE. Left abomasal displacement -a retrospective study of 315 cases. Bov Pract 1975;10:50–8.
31. Mather MF, Dedrick RS. Displacement of the abomasum. Cornell Vet 1966;56(3): 323–44.
32. Kelton DF, Garcia J, Guard CL, et al. Bar suture (toggle pin) vs open surgical abo-masopexy for treatment of left displaced abomasum in dairy cattle. J Am Vet Med Assoc 1988;193(5):557–9.
33. Robertson JM, Boucher WB. Treatment of left displacement of the bovine abomasum. J Am Vet Med Assoc 1966;149(11):1423–9.
34. Pearson H. The treatment of surgical disorders of the bovine abdomen. Vet Rec 1973;92(10):245–54.
35. Gabel AA, Heath RB. Correction and right-sided omentopexy in treatment of left-sided displacement of the abomasum in dairy cattle. J Am Vet Med Assoc 1969; 155(4):632–41.
36. Roy JP, Harvey D, Belanger AM, et al. Comparison of 2-step laparoscopy-guided abomasopexy versus omentopexy via right flank laparotomy for the treatment of dairy cows with left displacement of the abomasum in on-farm settings. J Am Vet Med Assoc 2008;232(11):1700–6.
37. Wittek T, Locher LF, Alkaassem A, et al. Effect of surgical correction of left dis-placed abomasum by means of omentopexy via right flank laparotomy or two-step laparoscopy-guided abomasopexy on postoperative abomasal emptying rate in lactating dairy cows. J Am Vet Med Assoc 2009;234(5):652–7.
38. Wittek T, Furll M, Grosche A. Peritoneal inflammatory response to surgical correc-tion of left displaced abomasum using different techniques. Vet Rec 2012; 171(23):594.
39. Hull BL. Closed suturing technique for correction of left abomasal displacement. Iowa State Univ Vet 1972;34(3):142–4.
40. Rutgers LJ, Van der Velden MA. Complications following the use of the closed su-turing technique for correction of left abomasal displacement in cows. Vet Rec 1983;113(12):255–7.
41. Grymer J, Sterner KE. Percutaneous fixation of left displaced abomasum, using a bar suture. J Am Vet Med Assoc 1982;180(12):1458–61.
42. Janowitz H. Laparoscopic reposition and fixation of the left displaced abomasum in cattle. Tierarztl Prax Ausg G Grosstiere Nutztiere 1998;26(6):308–13 [in German].
43. Newman KD, Anderson DE, Silveira F. One-step laparoscopic abomasopexy for correction of left-sided displacement of the abomasum in dairy cows. J Am Vet Med Assoc 2005;227(7):1142–7, 1090.
44. van Leeuwen E, Janowitz H, Willemen MA. Laparoscopic positioning and attach-ment of stomach displacement to the left in the cow. Tijdschr Diergeneeskd 2000; 125:391–2 [in Dutch].

45. Christiansen K. Laparosckopisch kontrollierte operation des nach links verlagerten Labmagens (Janowitz-operation) ohn Ablegen des Patienten. Tierärztl Praxis 2004;66.
46. Babkine M, Desochers A, Boure L, et al. Ventral laparoscopic abomasopexy on adult cows. Can Vet J 2006;47(4):343–8.
47. Vogel SR, Nichols S, Buczinski S, et al. Duodenal obstruction caused by duodenal sigmoid flexure volvulus in dairy cattle: 29 cases (2006-2010). J Am Vet Med Assoc 2012;241(5):621–5.
48. Mulon PY, Desrochers A. Surgical abdomen of the calf. Vet Clin North Am Food Anim Pract 2005;21(1):101–32.
49. Tulleners EP, Hamilton GF. Surgical resection of perforated abomasal ulcers in calves. Can Vet J 1980;21(9):262–4.
50. Braun U, Schnetzler C, Dettwiler M, et al. Ultrasonographic findings in a cow with abomasal lymphosarcoma: case report. BMC Vet Res 2011;7:20.
51. Buczinski S, Belanger AM, Francoz D. Ultrasonographic appearance of lymphomatous infiltration of the abomasum in cows with lymphoma. J Am Vet Med Assoc 2011;238(8):1044–7.
52. Wittek T, Constable PD, Morin DE. Abomasal impaction in Holstein-Friesian cows: 80 cases (1980-2003). J Am Vet Med Assoc 2005;227(2):287–91.
53. Tschuor AC, Muggli E, Braun U, et al. Right flank laparotomy and abomasotomy for removal of a phytobezoar in a standing cow. Can Vet J 2010;51(7):761–3.

Intestinal Surgery

André Desrochers, DMV, MS[a],*, David E. Anderson, DVM, MS[b]

KEYWORDS

- Cattle • Surgery • Intestine • Jejunum • Colon • Enterectomy

KEY POINTS

- The short mesentery in cattle makes intestinal exteriorization challenging.
- Duodenal sigmoid flexure volvulus is suspected if there is extreme hypochloremic alkalosis.
- Cattle with jejunal hemorrhage syndrome (JHS) have a poor prognosis.
- Intraoperative clot fragmentation should be favored with JHS rather than enterectomy.
- The prognosis is better for animals with ileal flange volvulus rather than mesentery root torsion.

Intestinal surgery in cattle is challenging because it is often done with the animal standing under sedation. Because of the abdominal pain and state of shock, affected animals will be prone to move constantly or even lay down. Moreover, it is technically demanding and can rarely be performed without assistance, unlike most common surgeries in cattle. Decision-making is crucial and appropriate technical technique is essential to improve success rate.

DECISION-MAKING

Doing an exploratory laparotomy in cattle is easy, fast, and inexpensive. There are less consequences if revealed to be unnecessary compared to other species. However, an unnecessary laparotomy could be harmful to a critical patient that could have been medically treated. Before making the decision to favor a surgical or medical approach, information must be gathered and the case approached in a logical manner: (1) review the possible causes of abdominal pain relevant to the particular case; (2) recognize the indications for immediate surgery; (3) determine if surgery is an option given the cost, facilities, and surgical abilities; (4) establish medical treatment before or during surgery; (5) if surgery is postponed, determine in advance a precise time and list criteria to be monitored to help decision-making; and (6) establish and present to

The authors have nothing to disclose.
[a] Department of Clinical Sciences, Faculty of Veterinary Medicine, Université de Montréal, 3200 Sicotte, St-Hyacinthe, Quebec J2S 7C6, Canada; [b] Large Animal Clinical Sciences, University of Tennessee, C247 Veterinary Teaching Hospital, 2407 River Drive, Knoxville, TN 37996, USA
* Corresponding author.
E-mail address: andre.desrochers@umontreal.ca

the client a most realistic prognosis and cost estimate. A systematic approach based on adequate signalment and history, complete physical examination, and judicious choice of ancillary tests are the tools available to clinicians.

Frequent clinical signs and physical findings include colic, distended abdomen, tachycardia, and shock. A very distended abdomen requires rapid assistance. A stomach tube should be passed to decompress the rumen. If no free gas is coming out of the tube, it might be a frothy bloat or intestinal volvulus. Abnormal findings at rectal palpation are presence of fresh blood, absence of feces, tension band, distended small bowel, distended cecum, or a mass among small bowels. Ileus and peracute enteritis can be easily confused with jejunal obstruction. Usually, the small bowel will be distended primarily with fluids and easily palpable per rectum. Tension bands may also be palpated. In volvulus, intestines are severely distended with gas occupying the pelvic cavity. Intussusception is difficult to identify precisely but usually is suspected if a hard mass is felt among distended small bowels. Jejunal hemorrhage syndrome (JHS) might have a similar rectal examination finding except that the rectum is filled with ripe raspberry-like feces in variable quantity. Animals with enteritis may have a fever and show other clinical signs or laboratory results compatible with it (ie, leukopenia). Finally, the heart rate is a good indicator of the severity of the condition but should be correlated with other findings. A cow with mildly distended small bowel and a heart rate of 80 beats per minute (bpm) does not need immediate assistance. However, a cow with a distended organ and heart rate of 100 bpm and dehydrated needs immediate assistance.

Ultrasound imaging is very helpful to evaluate the abdomen in cattle.[1,2] Presence of severely distended and empty intestines at the ultrasound examination indicates obstruction (**Fig. 1**). Surgery is indicated even if the cause if not clearly identified at this point.

PREOPERATIVE CONSIDERATIONS

The surgeon must decide if the procedure will be performed standing, or on lateral or sternal recumbency. If the animal is down, the decision is easy. If the animal is standing, the decision is often based on surgeon's training and experience. If the animal is

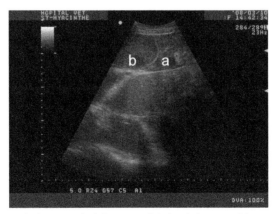

Fig. 1. Transabdominal ultrasound of the ventral right abdomen with a curvilinear probe on an adult Holstein cow. The jejunal loops are distended, occupying most of the ultrasound field (b). The presence of empty jejunal loops (a) adjacent to distended loops is compatible with intestinal obstruction.

weak, the surgery is performed with the animal in left lateral recumbency. Sternal re-cumbency is an option but the animal must be secured to prevent it from standing during the surgery (**Fig. 2**). Doing the surgery on a secured recumbent animal has the main advantage of doing the manipulation without worrying if the animal lies down, kicks, or moves constantly while suturing the intestines. However, securing an animal on lateral recumbency is difficult in a field setting. Moreover, exteriorization of bowels is more difficult on a laterally recumbent animal.

Preoperative analgesia is provided to the patient before invading the abdomen. Flunixin meglumin, ketoprofen, butorphanol, meloxicam, or ketamine stun[3] is frequently used for standing gastrointestinal (GI) surgery in cattle. If the surgery is per-formed standing, sedation must be used cautiously so the animal will not lie down. The authors rarely use sedation unless the behavior of the animal is aggressive or will pre-vent safe manipulation of the bowels. Broad spectrum antibiotics must be given before the surgery and repeated during the procedure if it lasts longer than 2 hours. Regional block or paravertebral block is preferred, allowing the surgeon to extend the incision at his or her convenience. If the animal is in shock and there is electrolytes imbalance, fluids are given before and during the procedure. Blood transfusion must be considered in some severe cases of JHS. Avoid any high-volume oral fluids if the abdomen is distended.

PRINCIPLES OF BOVINE INTESTINAL SURGERY

The cranial part of the descending duodenum courses cranially from the pylorus to the ansa sigmoidea duodenalis medial to the liver. The descending duodenum then courses caudally, wraps around the omental curtain, and turns cranially to the ascending duodenum. This portion of the duodenum courses cranially to the root of the mesentery medial to the omentum and joins the jejunum. The entire duodenum is contained by 2 mesenteries: mesoduodenum and omentum. The jejunum is restricted by a short mesentery except for the distal third of the jejunum and proximal segment of the ileum, which are suspended by a long mesenteric segment often referred to as the jejunoileal flange. This segment can be easily exteriorized from the abdomen but the remainder of the jejunum and ileum are poorly exteriorized because of the short mesentery. Although the demeanor of cattle allows for standing

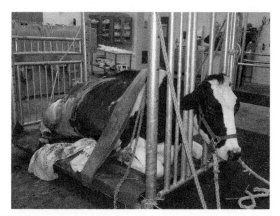

Fig. 2. This adult Holstein cow was unable to stand because of electrolytes imbalance. Intes-tinal obstruction was suspected. The animals is secured in sternal recumbency and surgically prepared for a right flank laparotomy.

paralumbar fossa laparotomy, excessive tension on the mesentery will likely stimulate the patient to lie down and interfere with surgical procedures.

Enterectomy

A cow has a short mesentery, therefore, traction on it is painful and the animal may go down at any moment. This short mesentery precludes adequate exteriorization of some segments of the small bowel. Only the portion to be resected should be exteriorized to avoid excessive traction and contamination during the resection-anastomosis (**Fig. 3**). Infiltration of 2% lidocaine into the mesentery where resection is planned may decrease the pain of traction. The mesenteric vessels (arteries and veins) are ligated using mass ligation with absorbable suture material (United States Pharmacopeia [USP] 3 chromic gut, USP 1 polyglactin 910), being sure not to compromise the blood supply to the intestine to be preserved. Mass ligation is required because cattle do not have a well-defined arcuate vascular anatomy (as do horses) and the fatty mesentery renders vessel identification impossible.[4] The sutures are placed in an overlapping pattern such that double ligation of the vessels is accomplished (**Fig. 4**A). This technique may be performed rapidly. However, it is impossible to effectively ligate all the vessels. It will be completed on complete resection of the intestinal segment. Stapling instrumentation is highly unreliable for occlusion of mesenteric vessels because of the large amount of fat normally found in the intestinal mesentery of cattle. Ligasure (Covidien, Medtronics, Minneapolis, MN, USA) is an electrocautery device that will seal vessels through a specially designed forceps. It

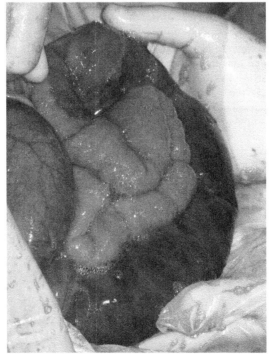

Fig. 3. Loops of jejunum are exteriorized through a right flank laparotomy. Pink empty loops are adjacent to an obstructed reddish segment of jejunum. The obstruction was caused by a large hematoma typically found in the JHS.

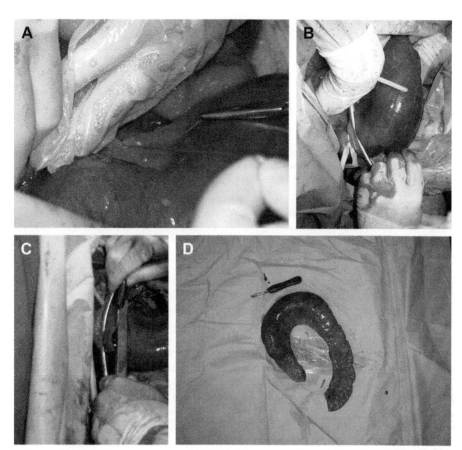

Fig. 4. (*A*) Ligatures are blindly placed in the fatty mesentery to decrease excessive bleeding during intestinal resection. (*B*) A Penrose drain and a Doyen forceps are placed on the sound portion of the jejunum. (*C*) A second Doyen forceps is placed on the resected portion. The resection is performed by incising between the 2 Doyen forceps. (*D*) The resected loop of jejunum and the hematoma within.

seals vessels up to 7 mm in diameter. It is efficient and safe but expensive to use. Moreover, the machine is not meant to be used in a field situation.

After completion of mesentery ligation and transection, Doyen intestinal forceps are used to occlude the lumen of the normal and abnormal bowel (**Fig. 4**B–D). When exteriorization allows it, thirty centimeters of healthy bowel adjacent to the affected portion are also resected. The proximal segment of bowel is carefully exteriorized to its maximum length and the Doyen forceps are removed. Distended orad intestine can be decompressed through the enterectomy site with special care to avoid contamination of the incision or abdomen with ingesta. This procedure will lessen the severity of postoperative ileus and shorten convalescence. The 2 segments of intestine are reunited by end-to-end or side-to-side anastomosis with an absorbable suture material (USP 2–0 for adult, USP 3–0 to 4–0 for calves with polyglactin 910 or polydioxanone) using a single or 2-layer suture pattern.[5] A simple full-thickness, continuous suture provides better apposition and less lumen diameter reduction (**Fig. 5**). The anastomosis is performed in 2 to 3 overlapping simple continuous suture lines, each

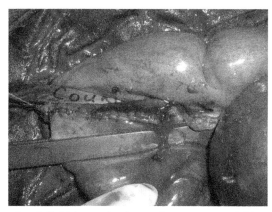

Fig. 5. Two overlapping full-thickness simple continuous sutures (180° each) were used for the anastomosis.

placed in one-half of one-third of the circumference, so that a purse-string effect is not created. A 2-layer technique consists of a simple continuous suture involving the mucosa and submucosa, followed by a Cushing or Lembert pattern. The initial suture line should be placed at the mesenteric attachment because this is the most likely site for leakage to occur. Some surgeons prefer using a full-thickness, simple interrupted suture when segments to anastomose are of significantly different diameter (**Fig. 6**). After the anastomosis, the mesentery is sutured in a continuous pattern with a USP 0 absorbable suture material (see **Fig. 6**). The affected intestine is thoroughly washed with sterile isotonic fluids, checked for the presence of leakage, and replaced into the abdomen. Carboxymethylcellulose gel can be applied over the anastomosis site to prevent adhesions.

Enterotomy

A simple enterotomy will allow removal of a foreign body into the lumen or to take a full-thickness biopsy at a specific area of the GI tract. Two suturing techniques for closure of a jejunal enterotomy were compared in cattle. Although the stapling

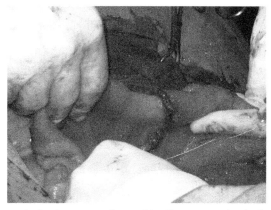

Fig. 6. Simple interrupted sutures were favored by the surgeon to do the anastomosis. The mesentery is sutured in a simple continuous manner.

technique was faster (TA 55 with 3.5 mm staples), enterotomy suture with 1-layer inter-rupted Gambee technique resulted in fewer adhesions and thickening of the intestinal wall. At 13-weeks postsurgery, the lumen diameter reduction was similar between both suture techniques.[6] As previously described, a simple continuous suture followed by a Lembert or Cushing will provide a watertight suture with minimal lumen reduction.

GENERAL GUIDELINE FOR POSTOPERATIVE MANAGEMENT

All intestinal surgery is classified as clean-contaminated surgery and some are clearly infected because of a peritonitis. The antibiotics regimen will vary according to this classification. The authors usually recommend 5 days of broad spectrum antibiotics after any intestinal resection. Antibiotics can be continued for 2 weeks if there is a peri-tonitis. Dehydration and electrolytes imbalances should be corrected rapidly with intravenous (IV) fluids. Any oral fluids administration must be avoided until the animal is passing feces.

Pain management is often neglected postoperatively in cattle. Ileus is caused by electrolytes imbalance and pain, and will delay normal recovery. A variety of nonste-roidal antiinflammatory drugs (NSAIDs) are available depending on the countries. They are frequently used to control pain after abdominal surgeries in cattle. To the authors' knowledge, there are no publications on the effect of NSAIDs on intestinal motility. However, preoperative flunixin (2.2 mg/kg) has improved postoperative recovery after an omentopexy.[7] In the authors' clinics, it is routine procedure to administer NSAIDs preoperatively and the day after. It should be repeated cautiously on anorexic animals because of potential abomasal ulceration. Butorphanol is opioid with less effect on the abomasum. Although expensive, it can be given at a dosage of 0.05 mg/kg 3 times a day. Lidocaine drip has been used in horses to treat postoperative ileus. The authors use a bolus of 1.3 mg/kg of lidocaine at a rate of 0.05 mg/kg per minute.[8]

Duodenum Outflow Problems

The first portion of the duodenum is the cranial part leaving the pylorus going toward the liver cranially and dorsally. It forms a cranial sigmoid flexure at the level of the gall bladder and continues caudally to the descending duodenum. At the caudal aspect of the greater omentum, it forms the caudal flexure while running cranially and medially to the ascending duodenum. Exteriorisation of the duodenum is limited to the cranial and descending duodenum. The duodenum can be affected in many ways, from simple ileus to perforation.[9,10]

Any intervention on the duodenum is difficult because only the oral part of the cranial duodenum and a portion of the descending duodenum can be exteriorized. Three types of obstruction are reported: functional, intraluminal or extraluminal, and strangu-lation. Phytobezoar or trichobezoar, and foreign bodies, were reported to cause intra-luminal obstruction, whereas adhesions and liver abscesses may cause extraluminal obstruction.[9-15] Strangulation of the caudal flexure of the duodenum was reported in 3 cows during late pregnancy because the uterus had passed through a rent in the mesoduodenum.[16,17] A duodenal obstruction caused by a malposition of the gall-bladder was also reported.[18]

Clinical Signs

The clinical signs are variable depending on the origin of obstruction. If there is no strangulation of the duodenum, the onset of clinical signs is slow with progressive distension of the ventral abdomen. This distension is caused by the enlargement of the abomasum and the rumen. Those animals are usually severely dehydrated, with an elevated heart rate, and transabdominal rectal palpation is unrewarding except from the lack of feces. A small ping behind the last right ribs has been identified in volvulus of the sigmoid flexure.[19] Ultrasound examination specifies which segment of the duodenum is obstructed and locates the origin of the obstruction. The cranial duodenum is often severely distended (8 cm of diameter) with an enlarged abomasum but the rest of the GI tract is empty.

Clinical Pathologic Findings

Duodenal obstruction should be suspected if there is a severe hypochloremic hypokalemic metabolic alkalosis: serum chloride of 70 mmol/L (normal around 100 mmol/L), total serum carbon dioxide of 44 mmol/L (normal 30 mmol/L), and serum potassium of 3 mmol/L (normal of 4–5 mmol/L).[5,9,19,20] Depending on the location of the obstruction, liver enzymes may also be increased.[18,19] Chloride ruminal contents are elevated (>30 mmol/L).[20]

Surgery

If the cause cannot be determined, a temporary diagnosis of ileus is given and a large volume of IV fluids is administered for 12 to 24 hours. Depending on the dehydration, up to 40 to 60 L of physiologic saline are administered intravenously. Hypokalemia is treated with 100 to 200 g or oral potassium chloride. The animal is observed by monitoring the heart rate, fecal output, and GI motility with ultrasound.

Duodenal problems are approached through a standard right laparotomy. The length of the incision may vary from 20 to 40 cm depending on the procedure. A simple enterotomy can be performed on the cranial and descending duodenum to remove a foreign body (**Fig. 7**) or trichobezoar. However, any obstruction involving the sigmoid flexure of the duodenum is difficult because it cannot be exteriorized. A laterolateral bypass between the cranial and descending duodenum is the only alternative (**Fig. 8**).[19,20]

Recently, a new condition was described as a volvulus of the sigmoid flexure of the duodenum.[19] The origin of the condition is unknown. A similar presentation was reported by van der Velden in the 1980s.[20] Asynchronous motility of the cranial duodenum was suspected. This is a surgical condition and diagnosis is confirmed during the laparotomy. Surgical findings are an enlarged abomasum and cranial duodenum. The sigmoid flexure is severely distended with gas and a volvulus can be palpated at

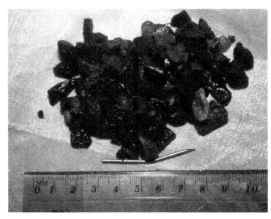

Fig. 7. Gravels and a 14-gauge hypodermic needle were recovered through an enterotomy of the duodenum on an adult Holstein cow.

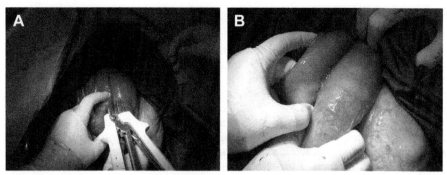

Fig. 8. (*A*) Surgical stapling (Gastrointestinal anastomosis, Medtronic, Minneapolis, MN) is being used to create a laterolateral bypass between the cranial and descending duodenum. (*B*) The duodenoduodenal bypass is finished and ready to be replaced in the abdomen.

its root, close to the neck of the gall bladder, on the visceral part of the liver (**Fig. 9**). The volvulus is reduced and cranial duodenal content is milked through the flexure to ensure that it is functional. If the viability of the sigmoid flexure is in doubt, a laterolateral duodenal bypass must be performed between the cranial duodenum and the descending duodenum.[19] The prognosis for any duodenal obstruction is generally good after cause and electrolytes imbalance are corrected.

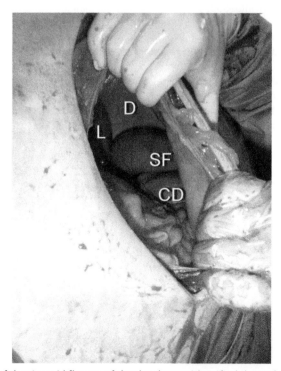

Fig. 9. Volvulus of the sigmoid flexure of the duodenum identified through a right flank incision on a standing adult cow. CD, cranial duodenum; D, diaphragm; L, liver; SF, sigmoid flexure.

INTUSSUSCEPTION

Intussusception refers to the invagination of 1 segment of intestine into an adjacent segment of intestine. The invaginated portion of intestine is termed the intussusceptum, and the outer, or receiving, segment of intestine is termed the intussuscipiens (**Fig. 10**). Intussusception occurs sporadically in cattle of all ages, breeds, and gender and may be seen at any time during the year.[21,22] However, in a case-control epidemiologic study of 336 cattle, intussusception occurred most commonly in calves less than 2 months old, Brown Swiss cattle seemed to be overrepresented and Hereford cattle seemed to be underrepresented compared with Holstein cattle.[21] Although the inciting cause is rarely identified, intussusception may occur secondary to enteritis, intestinal parasitism, sudden changes in diet, mural granuloma, or abscess (**Fig. 11**), intestinal neoplasia (especially adenocarcinoma), mural hematoma, heavy work load,[23] and administration of drugs that affect intestinal motility.[24–28] Any focal disturbance of intestinal motility may facilitate the invagination of an orad segment into an aborad segment of intestine. Intussusception involving the caecum was reported in 51 calves, of which 40 had diarrhea.[29] Intussusception occurs most commonly in the distal portion of the jejunum but intussusception has been found affecting the proximal jejunum, ileum, cecum, and spiral colon.[21,24,26–37] In a review of 336 intussusceptions in cattle, 281 affected the small intestine, 7 were ileocolic, 12 were cecocolic, and 36 were colocolic.[21]

Clinical Signs

Cattle affected with intussusception demonstrate clinical signs of abdominal pain (restlessness, kicking at the abdomen, lying down, getting up frequently, and assuming abnormal posture) for up to 24 hours after the onset of disease. Cattle are frequently anorectic, lethargic, and reluctant to walk. After the initial signs of abdominal pain subside, affected cattle become progressively lethargic, recumbent, and show apparent depression. Abdominal distention becomes apparent after 24 to 48 hours duration. This is caused by gas and fluid distention of the forestomach and intestines, and sequestration of ingesta within the gastrointestinal tract results in progressive dehydration and electrolyte depletion. Heart rate will increase

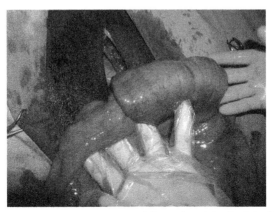

Fig. 10. A jejunal intussusception is exteriorized through a right flank incision on a standing adult cow.

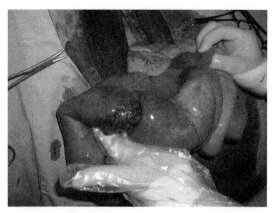

Fig. 11. Intussusception was reduced by gently pulling on the segments. However, a granuloma is present and the segment must be resected.

proportionally to abdominal pain, intestinal necrosis, and dehydration. Fecal production may be normal for up to 12 hours after the occurrence of the intussusception but minimal fecal production is noted after 24 hours duration. Passage of dark scant feces or only mucus is often observed with intussusception.

Clinical Pathologic Findings

Hemoconcentration is usually present (increased packed cell volume and total proteins), and an inflammatory leukogram may be seen if ischemic necrosis of the intussusceptum has occurred. Often, changes in the white blood cell count and differential are minimal, and changes in peritoneal fluid constituents are not seen because the intussusceptum is isolated by the intussuscipiens. Hypochloremic, metabolic alkalosis is found with serum biochemistry analysis. Hyponatremia, hypokalemia, hypocalcemia, azotemia, and hyperglycemia also may be found. The magnitude of these changes depends on the location and duration of the lesion. Increased blood urea nitrogen (BUN) can be observed the more orad the intussusception. Proximal jejunal intussusception causes rapid and severe dehydration, electrolyte sequestration, and metabolic alkalosis. Most lesions occur in the distal jejunum and may require more than 48 hours to develop these changes. Elevation of rumen chloride concentration (>30 mEq/l) may be found if fluid distention of the rumen is present.

Diagnosis

Diagnosis of intussusception is usually confirmed during exploratory laparotomy. The intussusception can be felt as a hard sausage-like structure during rectal palpation[34] but distention of multiple loops of small intestine is most commonly identified. These rectal palpation findings are similar to those found in JHS. In the authors' experiences, an intussusception may be present for 48 hours or more in adult cattle without intestinal distention being found during rectal palpation. It depends on its location and the severity of the obstruction. Some animals will still pass a certain amount of feces. In calves and small ruminants, percutaneous palpation and ultrasonographic examination of the abdomen may be used to identify intestinal distention and, possibly, the intussusception.[29,38] Transabdominal and rectal ultrasound can also be used in adult cattle with the appropriate equipment. The intussusception has a typical target-like image on ultrasound with distended orad bowels and adjacent free fluid.[33,39] It should be suspected in cattle with a history of abdominal pain and abdominal distention, scant feces consisting of blood and mucus, and palpable distention of the intestine. Differential diagnoses include JHS, functional ileus, trichobezoar, foreign bodies, intestinal incarceration or strangulation, vagal syndrome, intestinal neoplasia, fat necrosis, and jejunoileal flange volvulus. Abomasal ulcers might be included in the differential if dark feces are observed.

Treatment

Affected cattle must be stabilized before surgical intervention is performed. Fluid therapy should be aimed at replacing fluid and electrolyte deficits. Surgical correction may proceed after the patient has been assessed as a suitable candidate. Most of these animals will have some degree of peritonitis. Broad spectrum antibiotics against gram-negative or gram-positive, as well as anaerobic, bacteria must be administered preoperatively. The regimen can be adjusted postoperatively related to surgical findings. Intra-abdominal surgical manipulations are painful demand appropriate preoperative analgesia. NSAIDs are given preoperatively, along with butorphanol (0.05 mg/kg S.C.). Right paralumbar fossa exploratory laparotomy is the surgical approach of choice for treatment of intussusception. Most small intestines of cattle have a short mesentery, preventing adequate exteriorization of the intussusception through a ventral midline incision. Also, the attachments of the greater omentum limit exposure with this approach. Most often, diagnostic exploratory laparotomy is performed with the cow standing after regional anesthesia. Tension on the mesentery of the small intestine results in pain and cattle may attempt to lie down during the procedure. Of 35 cattle having standing, right paralumbar fossa laparotomy for resection of intussusception, 14% became recumbent and 26% attempted to become recumbent during the surgery.[21] Preoperative planning should include anticipation of this possibility. When intussusception is suspected and the animal is of high perceived economic value, right paralumbar fossa celiotomy may be performed with the patient under general anesthesia and in left lateral recumbency. The intussusception may be more difficult to elevate through the incision in recumbent cattle because the fluid-filled bowel gravitates away from the surgical site. However, isolation and resection of the intussusception can be done without risk of the animal lying down during the procedure and with minimal risk of contamination of the abdomen.

Surgical removal by resection and anastomosis is the treatment of choice for intussusception. The intussusception is exteriorized from the abdomen and isolated using a barrier drape and moistened towels. Manual reduction of the intussusception is not recommended because of the risk for rupture of the intestine during manipulation, probable ischemic necrosis of the intestine after surgery, possible reoccurrence of the intussusception, and prolonged ileus caused by motility disturbance and swelling in the affected segment of bowel. However, if the intussusception is in the spiral colon, resection and anastomosis in this area is difficult. Manual reduction only can be successful.[32] Successful resection of a segment of the proximal loop of the ascending colon is reported.[40] The affected segment was resected and a side-to-side anastomosis was performed between the base of the caecum and the spiral colon.

Postoperative management should be directed to prevent dehydration, maintain optimal blood electrolyte concentration, control for infection and inflammation, and stimulate appetite. IV fluids are beneficial during the first 24 hours after surgery. The authors routinely perform rumen transfaunation 12 to 24 hours after surgery to stimulate forestomach motility and appetite. Large volume of oral drenching must avoided until normal output of feces is observed. Food should not be withheld after surgery. Administration of butorphanol tartrate (0.02–0.04 mg/kg, IV) may help with pain-induced ileus by providing mild visceral analgesia without direct adverse effects on intestinal motility. Lidocaine drip for the first 24 to 48 hours must be considered to improve gut motility and control pain.[8]

Prognosis

The prognosis for return to productivity after surgical correction of intussusception is variable and depends somewhat on the duration of the lesion and its location. Cattle respond favorably to surgery if operated on within 48 hours of the onset of the disease. Cattle presenting with severe dehydration (>12%), tachycardia (heart rate>120 bpm), severe decrease in serum chloride concentration (Cl) less than 80 mEq/l, and severe abdominal distention are considered to have a poor prognosis for survival. If viscera rupture is present at the time of surgery, the prognosis is grave. In a case-control, multicenter study in which surgery was attempted, 85 of 143 cattle with small intestinal intussusception, 0 of 4 with ileocolic, 10 of 11 with cecocolic, and 10 of 20 with colocolic were discharged from the hospital.[21] Overall, 31% of the animals diagnosed with intussusception were discharged from the hospital. In a case series, only 4 out of 20 animals diagnosed with jejunal intussusception were discharged from the hospital.[28] However, many animals were presented in an unfavorable clinical state demanding immediate euthanasia. Eleven underwent surgery and 4 were discharged 8 days after the surgery.[28] The extent and long duration of the condition before presentation negatively influenced the outcome.[28] In another case series on 12 adult bullocks, all survived right flank resection and anastomosis of jejunum or ileal intussusception. They passed feces within 24 hours.[23] Early recurrence has been reported in a calf.[38]

HEMORRHAGIC JEJUNAL SYNDROME

This syndrome has been recognized in adult dairy cows involving intraluminal and intramural intestinal hemorrhage, necrosis with subsequent clot formation, and intestinal obstruction. It is referred to as JHS, hemorrhagic bowel syndrome, intraluminal-intramural hematoma, bloody gut, or hemorrhagic enteritis.[41–44]

In the search for the cause of this disease, much speculation has fallen on Clostridium perfringens type A.[41,42] C perfringens type A was suspected as a cause or contributing factor in this disease because this organism has been cultured from the intestinal contents or feces of a large number of cows affected with JHS.[42,45–47] However, evidence regarding pathogenicity of these isolates has not been produced that links C perfringens type A to development of JHS. Moreover, C perfringens type A is also found in the gastrointestinal tract of cattle without causing clinically apparent disease.[48,49]

At present, it is thought that JHS is a multifactorial disease.[41,42,46] Proposed risk factors include feeding of silage or total mixed ration (TMR), feeding finely ground corn in the ration, early stage of lactation, high level of production, and free-choice feeding. These factors may create an environment in which stress, excess gastrointestinal starch, and subclinical rumen acidosis allow overgrowth of C perfringens type A bacteria in the gastrointestinal tract. C perfringens type A produce α-toxin, and some may produce a beta2 toxin.[50,51] In a retrospective study on 37 cattle, C perfringens type A was isolated of all the 20 samples (feces, blood clot, intestine).[47] A subsample of 10 was further analyzed for toxins in which α-toxin was isolated in all and beta2 toxin in 1 sample.[47] Excess grain or starch in the small intestine is more likely to lead to sudden bacterial overgrowth.[41,42,48,49,52] This passage of grain particles into the small intestine may be a factor in the pathogenesis of JHS in dairy cows fed high grain TMR. Excess mixing of TMR causing finely powdered corn was suspected to be related to an outbreak of clinical cases of JHS on 1 farm.[42]

Aspergillus fumigatus has been incriminated as the primary agent of JHS. *A fumigatus* is a fungus that sporulates abundantly causing no harm in immunocompetent animals. It was isolated from affected animals but not from normal animals. Moreover, *A fumigatus* seems to cause a similar disease in humans.[53] A gliotoxin was detected in animals infected with *A fumigatus*. It is hypothesized that the gliotoxin can potentiate *A fumigatus*.[52]

Clinical Signs

The physical presentation is variable depending on the onset of clinical signs. The condition has been reported in beef and dairy breeds, with a predilection for Holstein and Brown Swiss.[46,47,54–56] Brown Swiss were significantly overrepresented in 1 study.[56] Clinical signs of this peracute disease include recumbency, dehydration, shock, abdominal distension, anorexia, abdominal pain, and lack of feces or the production of tarry feces with blood clots. In many cases, the cow is found dead. Affected cows are usually in early lactation, producing large quantities of milk, and are fed silage or TMR.

The most common clinical findings are: hemorrhagic diarrhea with clots of dark blood or absence of feces, colic, tachycardia, white mucosa, right ventral distension, rumen atony, lack of intestinal motility, and variable right-sided ping.[46,47,56,57] Abdominal examination per rectum may reveal distended jejunum, depending on the location of the blood clot. A mass can also be palpated in some animals.

Clinical Pathologic Findings

Results are variable depending on the stage and severity of the disease. On hematology, a left-shift leukogram is often observed. Hematocrit and total protein are usually within normal limit even though a significant amount of blood may have been lost.[46,47,54] The most significant changes are on the chemistry profile. Typically, the affected animals will have a hypochloremic, hypokalemic, metabolic alkalosis accompanied by an elevated BUN (mean = 12.6 mmol/L, n = 1.67–6.51 mmol/L) with a normal creatinine and an elevated glucose (mean = 11.7 mmol/L, n = 2.6–4.9).[46,47,52] Liver enzymes (Succinate dehydrogenase, Lactate dehydrogenase, Gamma-glutamyl transferase) can also be increased because of the absorption of toxins from intestinal damage.[46]

Diagnostics

The history, the clinical findings and laboratory results are usually enough to confirm the diagnosis. The differential should include winter dysenteriae (coronavirus), intussusception, and abomasal ulcers. Transabdominal ultrasound examination of the intestinal tract is helpful to confirm the diagnosis but even more helpful to find an obstruction. Braun and colleagues[55] performed ultrasound on 63 cows with hemorrhagic bowel syndrome (HBS). Their findings included fluid and fibrin between jejunal loops, increased jejunal diameter (mean: 6.76 cm, n = 2–4 cm)[1] with postobstruction empty loops, absence of motility, heterogeneous hyperechoic intraluminal material corresponding to blood clots, and abomasal distension.[55] Similar findings were reported by other investigators (**Fig. 12**).[46,47]

Treatment

Before any surgical intervention, the animal's hemodynamic status and electrolytes imbalance must be stabilized. Large-volume (20–40L) isotonic solution or blood transfusion (6–12L) can be administered before surgery. Hypokalemia is a common finding. Some of these animals are recumbent before or after the surgery with a S-shaped

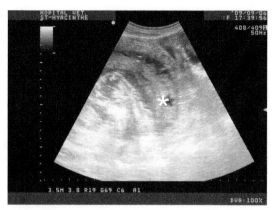

Fig. 12. Transabdominal ultrasound of the right ventral abdomen with a curvilinear abdominal probe on an adult Holstein cow. The animal was later diagnosed with JHS. The intraluminal hematoma in the jejunum (*asterisk*).

neck which is typical of the hypokalemic syndrome in cattle. It can certainly worsen the ileus. However, the surgery cannot be delayed because it may takes a few days to correct the hypokalemia.

Medical treatment is achieved if the animal is still passing feces and there are no signs of obstruction at the ultrasound. Specific treatment of the condition includes oral administration of mineral oil (4L Semel in die up to 3 days) and intramuscular or IV B-lactam. Nonsteroidal anti-inflammatory drugs are routinely given to control visceral pain. IV slow lidocaine infusion has been used in cattle to control visceral pain and improve GI motility. It is part of the authors' medical treatment protocol and postoperative treatment.[8] If the animal stops passing feces or an obstruction is suspected at the palpation per rectum or transabdominal ultrasound examination, surgery is elected.

Through a right paralumbar fossa approach, the affected segment of jejunum is easily identified. A firm, distended, intrajejunal mass of variable length will obstruct the lumen with orad jejunal distension (see **Fig. 3**). There are 3 surgical options: aboral fragmentation and massage of the clot, enterotomy, and resection anastomosis. The decision is based on the length of the clot and the integrity of the jejunal wall (**Fig. 13**).

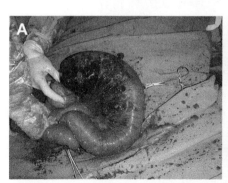
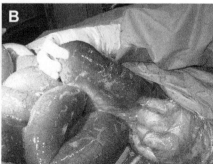

Fig. 13. JHS in an adult cow. (*A*) The exteriorized segment is compromised and must be resected. (*B*) The bluish color of the affected segment is from the intraluminal hematoma. The serosa and the mesentery are relatively sound. Therefore, manual breakage and progressive massage of the hematoma must be attempted to relieve the obstruction.

Prompt laparotomy and manual massage must be favored, especially in field conditions (**Fig. 14**).

Enterotomy is rarely done by itself because the clot is adhered to the submucosa over a significant length (20–30 cm). If manual massage failed or the affected segment is disrupted, then resection-anastomosis must be performed as described previously. The intestine diameter discrepancy between preobstruction and postobstruction can be considerable. The enterectomy site must be of equal diameter before achieving the anastomosis. To achieve this, the angle of the jejunal incision may vary between the preobstruction and postobstruction segment. Any restriction at the anastomosis site will prevent orad blood clot to pass through and increase recurrence (**Fig. 15**). A latero-lateral anastomosis should be considered if the surgeon is concerned about the expected anastomosis diameter.

Postoperative Care and Prognosis

Fluids or blood are usually continued until the animal is passing feces in large amount or to correct previous blood analysis abnormalities. Antibiotics (B-lactam) are given for at least 5 days. Depending on contamination during the procedure or the presence of peritonitis, it can be combined with an antibiotic effective against gram-negative bacteria. Mineral oil will be administered daily postoperatively until the animal is passing feces. NSAIDs are given at least 24 hours after the procedure and can be prolonged if needed. IV lidocaine drip will also be given for 24 to 48 hours to improve motility. In general, the animal will pass feces 24 to 36 hours after the procedure.

The prognosis for survival is fair and recurrence frequent. In a study on 11 beef and dairy cattle, exploratory laparotomy was performed on 7 animals but treatment was not

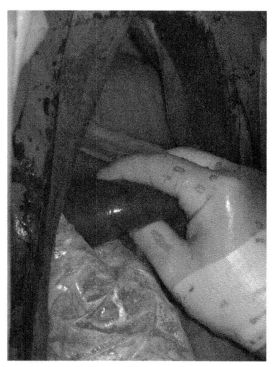

Fig. 14. Manual massage of the hematoma secondary to a JHS.

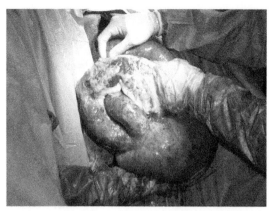

Fig. 15. Second laparotomy following a recurrence of obstruction of a JHS 72 hours after a jejunal resection anastomosis. Fibrin is covering distended loops of jejunum which are already adhered.

pursued because of economic restriction or severity of the condition. Ten were euthanized and 1 died.[54] Twenty-two dairy cows form the same herd were diagnosed and treated for HBS.[46] Seven out of 8 animals treated medically died. Of the 13 that underwent surgery, 4 were euthanized because of the extent of the disease. Manual clot fragmentation, enterotomy, and resection anastomosis was attempted on the remaining 9 but only 5 survived for an overall survival rate of 23%.[46] In another study, medical treatment was successful in 2 out 5 animals and 18 out of 30 animals survived after a surgical procedure; resection anastomosis (14 out of 20), clot fractionation (4 out of 18), and intraoperative euthanasia (2).[47] Peek and colleagues[56] described the surgical findings and outcomes of 31 dairy cattle. Eighteen of the 31 (58%) that were surgically treated were discharged. Recurrence of JHS was observed on the 5 animals that died within a year. According to the investigators, clot fractionation was associated with a better prognosis than enterotomy or resection anastomosis.[56] In another study on 65 cows with JHS that underwent right-flank laparotomy, 23 survived.[57] All these results clearly show that prognosis is fair to grave depending on the severity of the disease. Although resection anastomosis seems appealing to resolve the problem, it is clearly not a guarantee of success with a significant chance of recurrence.

INTESTINAL VOLVULUS

Volvulus refers to the rotation of viscera around its mesenteric attachment. Torsion refers to the rotation of viscera around its own (or long) axis. Although torsion of the abomasum and uterus are found in cattle, torsion of the small intestine is rare. Small intestinal volvulus may occur in different forms.[58–60] The most severe forms of intestinal volvulus originate from the root of the mesentery and involve the entirety of the small intestine and mesenteries (**Fig. 16**). Volvulus of the root of the mesentery causes obstruction of venous outflow and arterial blood supply to the intestines. Ischemic necrosis of the intestine occurs rapidly, which causes metabolic acidosis, shock, and death. Volvulus of the jejunoileal flange refers to volvulus of the mid-to-distal jejunum and proximal ileum in which the mesentery is long (**Fig. 17**). This long mesentery and associated bowel has been termed the flange and it may rotate about its mesentery without involving the remaining small intestine. Often, arterial occlusion is not found with volvulus of the jejunoileal flange, possibly because extensive fat

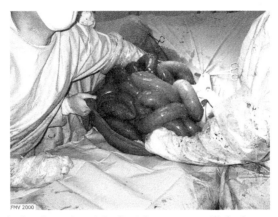

Fig. 16. Jejunal volvulus through a right flank laparotomy. All the loops of the jejunum are severely distended with gas because of the mesenteric root torsion. It is exteriorized to allow intraabdominal manipulation and reduction of the intestinal volvulus.

deposits within the mesentery may prevent compression of the muscular wall of the arteries until the volvulus becomes severe. However, obstruction of outflow of venous blood may be equally detrimental because of mural edema, shunting of blood away from the mucosa, and progressive ischemia.

Cattle of any breed, age, or sex may be affected by intestinal volvulus at any time during the year. In a review of 190 cattle having intestinal volvulus, dairy breeds were at a higher risk of developing volvulus compared with beef breeds.[58] This difference was thought to be associated with differences in management. Neither lactation nor gestation was identified as a risk factor, and calves were not found to be at an increased risk compared with adult cattle. In a separate study of 100 cattle having intestinal volvulus, 86 were calves between 1 week and 6 months old.[61]

Clinical Signs

Cattle having volvulus of the root of the mesentery may be found dead with severe abdominal distention. Early in the course of the disease, affected cattle demonstrate

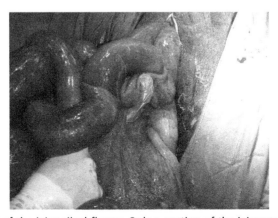

Fig. 17. Volvulus of the jejunoileal flange. Only a portion of the jejunum is distended and the its long mesentery predisposing to volvulus can be observed.

acute, severe abdominal pain (kicking at the abdomen, rolling, lying down and getting up frequently, grunting) and have marked elevation in heart rate (>120 bpm) and respiratory rate (>80 bpm). The rapid progression of the disease precludes development of significant dehydration but cardiovascular shock is usually present.

Cattle having volvulus of the jejunoileal flange may present similarly to cattle having volvulus at the root of the mesentery. However, these cattle often demonstrate clinical signs consistent with acute intestinal obstruction rather than cardiovascular shock. Cattle show signs of abdominal pain, are tachycardic (80–120 bpm), and pass minimal feces. Cattle may be dehydrated at the time of examination.

Clinical Pathologic Findings

Because of the rapid onset and progress, cattle having intestinal volvulus may not demonstrate change in serum biochemistry or hematology data. The changes expected with intestinal volvulus are consistent with intestinal obstruction, stress, and dehydration, including azotemia, hypocalcemia, hyperglycemia, and a leukocytosis with a mild left shift.[58] In the early stages of the disease, cattle develop alkalemia with normal serum potassium concentration. As cardiovascular compromise and intestinal ischemia proceed, cattle develop metabolic acidosis and hyperkalemia. Cattle having the shift to acidosis and hyperkalemia have a poor prognosis for survival.[58]

Diagnosis

Diagnosis of intestinal volvulus is by exploratory laparotomy. Rectal palpation reveals multiple loops of distended intestine filling the caudal abdomen and excessive tension on the intestinal mesentery. Simultaneous auscultation and percussion of the abdomen yields multifocal pings of variable pitch and location. Findings of scant feces, abdominal pain, sudden onset of abdominal distention, and multiple loops of distended intestine on rectal palpation in cattle are highly suggestive of intestinal volvulus. Differential diagnoses include intussusception, cecal volvulus, abomasal volvulus, intraluminal obstruction, and severe indigestion.

Treatment

Immediate surgical correction is the treatment of choice. IV fluids should be administered to treat cardiovascular shock but preparation for surgery should not be delayed. The volvulus must be corrected before irreversible ischemic injury or thrombosis of the mesenteric arteries has occurred. A right paralumbar fossa laparotomy with the cow standing is the approach of choice. Restoration of normal anatomic position of the intestines is more easily done with the patient standing. Cattle that are thought to be at great risk of becoming recumbent during surgery should be placed under general anesthesia, in left lateral recumbency, and the laparotomy performed through the right paralumbar fossa. The presence of the volvulus and the direction of the twist are assessed by palpating the root of the mesentery and, in the case of jejunoileal flange volvulus, following this ventrally to the location of the twist. The intestinal mass is gently derotated, being careful not to cause rupture of the viscera. This procedure may require exteriorization of various portions of the intestinal mass. After correction of the volvulus, the intestinal tract should be examined for evidence of nonviable bowel. If the intestine is compromised (arterial thrombosis, blackened serosa, friable wall of the affected segment, mural edema), then intestinal resection and anastomosis is indicated (see previous discussion of intussusception). Also, exploration of the abdomen should be done to rule out the presence of a second lesion (eg, abomasal displacement, fecalith, intussusception, anomalous fibrovascular bands, and peritonitis).

Postoperative management is directed toward maintaining optimal hydration, electrolyte, and acid-base status. Antibiotics and anti-inflammatory drugs are indicated. Ileus may be seen during the first 48 hours after surgery but the use of prokinetic drugs should be weighed against the risk of leakage at the site of the anastomosis if intestinal resection was performed. Passage of large volumes of diarrhea within 24 hours after surgery is considered to be a favorable prognostic indicator.

Prognosis

Prognosis varies with the severity and duration of the lesion. Prognosis for survival for cattle having volvulus of the root of the mesentery (44%) is less than for volvulus of the jejunoileal flange (86%).[58] Overall, dairy cattle have a better prognosis for survival (63%) than beef cattle (22%). This difference is presumed to be because dairy cattle are observed more frequently and, therefore, treatment sought earlier in the progression of the disease. Of 92 cattle in which surgical correction of intestinal volvulus was attempted, 13 were euthanatized during surgery, 25 died within 24 hours after surgery, 13 died between 2 and 7 days, and 41 (45%) survived.[61]

TRICHOBEZOARS

Intraluminal obstruction of the intestinal tract of cattle, sheep, and goats is most commonly caused by a trichobezoar, phytobezoar, or enterolith.[62,63] These foreign bodies form in the rumen or abomasum and may pass into the intestinal tract where they become lodged within the small intestine or spiral colon. Hairballs (trichobezoar) are caused by frequent ingestion of hair. This is seen most commonly in cattle infested with lice or mange, or during the spring when shedding of the winter hair coat occurs. Phytobezoars and enteroliths form around undigested materials (eg, nylon fibers, cotton fabric). In a necropsy survey of 166 dead calves less than 90-days-old in Western Canada, 56 calves died because of perforation of an abomasal ulcer.[64] Calves having an abomasal ulcer were 2.74 times more likely to have an abomasal hairball. Calves less than 31 days old and having an abomasal ulcer were 3.81 times more likely to have an abomasal hairball. However, the investigators were unable to establish a causative relationship between the presence of abomasal hairballs and a perforating ulcer. During a study of confined cattle being fed a roughage-limited diet, cows began biting hair from each other's hair coats and developed multiple ruminal hairballs (2–10 hairballs weighing 0.2–3.8 kg each).[65] The investigators speculated that the cows began grazing hair because of the lack of roughage in the diet, boredom, and high stocking density. One report describes clinical findings in 2 sheep having 107 individual hairballs.[66] The investigators speculated that pruritus or some unknown dietary deficiency was the cause of excessive ingestion of the wool.

Clinical Signs

Animals affected with ruminal or abomasal bezoars may be observed to have decreased appetite, weight loss, decreased fecal production, lethargy, and apparent depression. Multiple bezoars present in the rumen or abomasum of calves, sheep, and goats may be found during transabdominal palpation or on abdominal radiographs. When an obstruction of the small intestine or spiral colon occurs, affected animals initially show clinical signs of abdominal pain (restlessness, kicking at the abdomen, lying down and getting up frequently, arching the back, and stretching out of the legs while standing) and progress to recumbency and apparent depression. Progressive bloat or abdominal distention and lack of fecal production are noted.

Clinical Pathologic Findings

Serum biochemistry analysis reveals hypokalemic, hypochloremic, metabolic alkalosis, the severity of which depends on the duration and location of the lesion. These changes are most severe with proximal intestinal obstruction and become more severe with increasing duration. If ischemic necrosis of the intestinal wall has occurred, an inflammatory leukogram with increased numbers of immature neutrophils may be seen. As peritonitis develops and organic acids are released into the blood stream, the serum biochemistry changes to a metabolic acidosis with relative hyperkalemia. These changes are consistent with a poor prognosis. Perforation of an abomasal ulcer or rupture of the intestine and contamination of the abdomen with ingesta carries a poor to grave prognosis.

Diagnosis

In affected cattle, serum biochemistry changes are consistent with intestinal obstruction. Rumen chloride concentration may be elevated (rumen Cl > 30 mEq/l). The cause of intraluminal obstruction is rarely palpable per rectum but small intestinal distention may be palpable. Ultrasonographic examination of the abdomen may be useful in calves and small ruminants. Intraluminal intestinal obstruction should be suspected in cattle with recurrent rumen tympanites, which is transiently responsive to decompression and is associated with minimal fecal production. Differential diagnoses include intussusception, vagus indigestion syndrome, intestinal lymphosarcoma, fat necrosis, intestinal entrapment around anomalous fibrovascular bands, and volvulus of the jejunoileal flange.

Treatment

Trichobezoars, phytobezoars, or enteroliths located within the rumen are unlikely to cause clinical signs unless the number and magnitude of the foreign bodies is severe (eg, 2 sheep in which hairballs accounted for >10% of the animals' body weight).[66] A cow suffered esophageal obstruction after suspected attempted regurgitation of a rumen trichobezoar.[67] Ruminal foreign bodies are removed via a left paralumbar fossa celiotomy and rumenotomy. Abomasal hairballs may cause pyloric obstruction, which leads to rapid onset of abdominal distention. The authors prefer to perform a right paramedian or ventral paracostal laparotomy to exteriorize the abomasum. An abomasotomy is performed along the greater curvature of the abomasum, the foreign bodies removed, and the abomasum is closed with absorbable synthetic suture material (eg, 0 polydioxanone, polyglycolic 910) using 2 layers of an inverting suture pattern. When obstruction of the duodenum, jejunum, or spiral colon is suspected, a right paralumbar fossa celiotomy and exploration of the abdomen should be performed. The foreign body is found by exteriorizing a segment of normal or distended intestine and tracing this segment oral or aboral, respectively, until the obstruction is found. This segment of intestine is exteriorized from the abdomen, isolated using moistened surgical towels, and an enterotomy performed (**Fig. 18**). After removal of the foreign body, the enterotomy is closed with absorbable suture material (eg, 2–0 polydioxanone, polyglactin 910) using 2 lines of an inverting suture pattern. The enterotomy may be closed transversely to maximize the lumen of the affected segment of intestine and minimize the tension endured by the suture line during contraction of the intestinal wall. When the perceived economic value of the affected cow is high, surgery may be performed

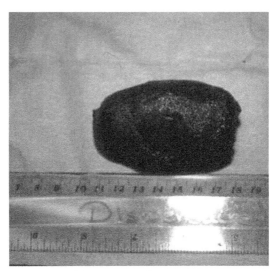

Fig. 18. A trichobezoar removed from proximal jejunum on an Angus heifer.

with the patient under general anesthesia. This will minimize the risk of ingesta contamination of the abdomen during surgery.

IV fluid therapy is based on the clinical estimate of dehydration, severity of intestinal lesions identified at surgery, and severity of serum biochemistry changes. In general, cattle should receive 20 to 60 L of isotonic saline, intravenously, over 12 hours. The authors routinely add calcium (1 mL of 23% calcium gluconate/kg body weight) and dextrose (to create a 1.25% solution) to the IV fluids. NSAIDs (banamine, 1 mg/kg body weight, IV, every 12 hours for 3 days) and antibiotics (for 3–5 days) also are administered.

Prognosis

The prognosis for return to productive use is based on the animal's body condition, presence of visceral perforation or peritonitis, and ability to perform surgical removal of the foreign body without contaminating the abdomen.

INCARCERATION, ENTRAPMENT, INTERNAL HERNIATION

A loop of jejunum or any organs can be trapped in a rent through the mesentery, mesocolon, around the umbilical vein, or simply caught between adhesions. The outcome is variable depending on the severity of the obstruction. It can be a simple ileus to a strangulated segment of intestines. There are many case reports in the literature showing the infinite possibilities of internal herniation, including incarceration of the jejunum in the epiploic foramen,[68] prolapse of the jejunum through a rectal tear,[69] jejunal incarceration in a partially everted urinary bladder,[70] strangulation of the jejunum by a persistent urachus,[71] or around a persistent round ligament of the liver.[72] Strangulation of the caudal sigmoid flexure of the duodenum was described in 2 late-pregnant cows. The uterus was trapped through the mesoduodenum caudally causing an oral obstruction without significant vascular strangulation.[16] It was hypothesized that the mesoduodenal defect was developmental. Manual reduction was impossible. Transection and end-to-end anastomosis were successfully performed on both animals.[16]

Gut tie is a jejunal incarceration around the ductus deferens in castrated steers.[73–75] It could be related to excessive manual traction on the testicle during castration creating a rent in the mesoductus and allowing jejunum to wrap around the ductus deferens causing strangulation. The clinical signs are similar to any intestinal obstruction. Abdominal palpation per rectum will show mucus or a small amount of feces, distended jejunum, and a small-diameter tight band crossing the caudal abdominal cavity toward the inguinal rings. Although manual rupture of this band per rectum has been reported,[75] surgery is often indicated to precisely cut the ductus and evaluate intestinal viability. Prognosis is generally good, depending on the viability of the affected portion of the jejunum.

The ileum is rarely affected or rarely needs surgical attention. Jejunoileal or ileocecal intussusception,[29,33] volvulus[76] and persistent vitellointestinal duct in a calf[77] have been reported. Biopsy of the ileum for the diagnosis of paratuberculosis[78] or its cannulation to study digestion of different nutrient has been reported.[79,80] Ileal impaction has been described in 22 cows.[81] The cause is unknown, however, because animals were mainly affected during fall and winter, it is hypothesized that winter type of feeding is a significant contributing factor. The affected animals had signs of mild colics, absent or scant feces, and dilated jejunum at rectal palpation and ultrasound. Exploratory laparotomy was necessary to confirm the diagnosis. In 19 animals, the ingesta was broken down and massaged aborally into the caecum. In a few animals, typhlotomy or enterotomy was necessary to decompress and remove the impaction. A side-to-side ileocecal anastomosis had to be performed in 6 animals to prevent recurrence. The short-term and long-term prognosis was considered good.

REFERENCES

1. Braun U. Ultrasound as a decision-making tool in abdominal surgery in cows. Vet Clin North Am Food Anim Pract 2005;21:33–53.

2. Braun U, Nuss K, Knubben-Schweizer G, et al. [The use of ultrasonography for diagnosing the cause of colic in cows. A review]. Tierarztl Prax Ausg G Grosstiere Nutztiere 2011;39:289–98 [in German].

3. Coetzee JF, Gehring R, Tarus-Sang J, et al. Effect of sub-anesthetic xylazine and ketamine ('ketamine stun') administered to calves immediately prior to castration. Vet Anaesth Analg 2010;37:566–78.

4. Levine SA, Smith DF, Wilsman NJ, et al. Arterial and venous supply to the bovine jejunum and proximal part of the ileum. Am J Vet Res 1987;48:1295–9.

5. Fubini SL, Trent AM. Small intestine surgery in cattle. In: Fubini SL, Ducharme NG, editors. Farm animal surgery. St Louis (MO): Elsevier; 2004. p. 240–8.

6. Steiner A, Waldvogel A, Wicki P, et al. Comparison of staple and Gambee techniques for enterotomy closure in the normal bovine jejunum. Zentralbl Veterinarmed A 1992;39:193–203.

7. Gieseler T, Wittek T, Furll M. Effects of preoperative flunixin meglumine in cows with left abomasal displacement (LDA). Tierarztl Prax Ausg G Grosstiere Nutztiere 2008;36:15–9 [in German].

8. Nichols S. Postoperative assessment: ileus and pain management. 2011 ACVS Veterinary Symposium. Illinois, November 3–5, 2011.

9. Braun U, Steiner A, Gotz M. Clinical signs, diagnosis and treatment of duodenal ileus in cattle. Schweiz Arch Tierheilkd 1993;135:345–55.

10. Weaver AD. Duodenal perforation and abdominal abscess in a cow. J Am Vet Med Assoc 1989;195:1603–5.

11. Steiner A, Muller L, Pabst B. An unusual complication after the partial resection of the ascending duodenum of a cow. Tierarztl Prax 1989;17:17–20 [in German].
12. Cebra CK, Cebra ML, Garry FB. Gravel obstruction in the abomasum or duodenum of two cows. J Am Vet Med Assoc 1996;209:1294–6.
13. Anderson DE. Surgical diseases of the small intestine. Vet Clin North Am Food Anim Pract 2008;24:383–401, viii.
14. Mullowney PC, Whitlock RH. Traumatic duodenitis in a dairy cow. Vet Rec 1978; 103:557–8.
15. Braun U, Schnetzler C, Previtali M, et al. Duodenal ileus caused by a calf feeding nipple in a cow. BMC Vet Res 2011;7:2.
16. Koller U, Lischer C, Geyer H, et al. Strangulation of the duodenum by the uterus during late pregnancy in two cows. Vet J 2001;162:33–7.
17. Muggli E, Lesser M, Braun U, et al. Herniation of the gravid uterus through a mesoduodenal defect and concurrent omental hernia in a cow. Vet Surg 2014;43:91–4.
18. Boerboom D, Mulon PY, Desrochers A. Duodenal obstruction caused by malposition of the gallbladder in a heifer. J Am Vet Med Assoc 2003;223:1475–7, 1435.
19. Vogel SR, Nichols S, Buczinski S, et al. Duodenal obstruction caused by duodenal sigmoid flexure volvulus in dairy cattle: 29 cases (2006-2010). J Am Vet Med Assoc 2012;241:621–5.
20. van der Velden MA. Functional stenosis of the sigmoid curve of the duodenum in cattle. Vet Rec 1983;112:452–3.
21. Constable PD, St Jean G, Hull BL, et al. Intussusception in cattle: 336 cases (1964-1993). J Am Vet Med Assoc 1997;210:531–6.
22. Pearson H. Intussusception in cattle. Vet Rec 1971;89:426–37.
23. Yadav GU, Bhikane AU, Aher VD, et al. Standardization of diagnostic procedures and operative methodology in clinical cases of intussusception in bovines. Intas Polivet 2009;10:4–7.
24. Archer RM, Cooley AJ, Hinchcliff KW, et al. Jejunojejunal intussusception associated with a transmural adenocarcinoma in an aged cow. J Am Vet Med Assoc 1988;192:209–11.
25. Milnes EL, McLachlan A. Surgical management of small intestinal intussusception associated with jejunal adenocarcinoma in a dairy cow. N Z Vet J 2015;63: 288–90.
26. Okamoto M, Itoh H, Koiwa M, et al. Intussusception of the spiral colon associated with fibroserous granulation in a heifer. Vet Rec 2007;160:376–8.
27. Payton J. Perforating duodenal sarcoma and intussusception in a cow. J Am Vet Med Assoc 1954;124:351–2.
28. Silva Filho AP, Afonso JAB, Souza JCDA, et al. Clinical and pathological analysis in 20 cases of intussusception in cattle. Veterinaria e Zootecnia 2010;17:422–31 [in Portuguese].
29. Doll K, Klee W, Dirksen G. Cecal intussusception in calves. Tierarztl Prax Ausg G Grosstiere Nutztiere 1998;26:247–53 [in German].
30. Dabas VS, Mistry JN, Suthar DN, et al. Intussusception in cross-bred cows: a review of 10 cases. Indian J Vet Surg 2014;35:50–2.
31. Dharmaceelan S, Senthilkumar S, Jayakumar K, et al. Jejuno-jejunal intussusception in kangeyam bullocks: a report of two cases. Intas Polivet 2008;9:149–50.
32. Hamilton GF, Tulleners EP. Intussusception involving the spiral colon in a calf. Can Vet J 1980;21:32.
33. Karapinar T, Kom M. Transrectal ultrasonographic diagnosis of jejunoileal intussusception in a cow. Irish Vet J 2007;60:422–4.

34. Kushwaha RB, Gupta AK, Bhadwal MS, et al. Intestinal obstruction due to intussus-ception in cattle: a clinical study of twenty cases. Indian J Vet Surg 2012;33:63–5.
35. Lee DB, Shin SM, Lee KC, et al. Surgical management of an ileocecocolic intussus-ception in a Korean native calf: a case report. Veterinarni Medicina 2013;58:645–9.
36. Shinde MM. Intussusception in cross-bred cattle: a study of nine cases. Indian J Vet Surg 1996;17:52.
37. Strand E, Welker B, Modransky P. Spiral colon intussusception in a three-year-old bull. J Am Vet Med Assoc 1993;202:971–2.
38. Pravettoni D, Morandi N, Rondena M, et al. Repeated occurrence of jejuno-jejunal intussusception in a calf. Can Vet J 2009;50:287–90.
39. Sheikh I, Tyagi SP, Adarsh K, et al. Usefulness and limitation of ultrasonography in the diagnosis of intestinal intussusception in cows. Vet Med Int 2011;2011: 584387.
40. Horne MM. Colonic intussusception in a Holstein calf. Can Vet J 1991;32:493–5.
41. Godden S, Frank R, Ames T. Survey of Minnesota dairy veterinarians on the occurrence of and potential risk factors for jejunal hemorrhage syndrome in adult dairy cows. Bov Pract 2001;35:97–103.
42. Kirkpatrick MA, Timms LL, Kersting KW, et al. Case report - jejunal hemorrhage syndrome of dairy cattle. Bov Pract 2001;35:104–16.
43. st-Jean G, Anderson DE. Intraluminal-intramural hemorrhage of the small intes-tine in cattle. In: Howard JE, Smith RA, editors. Current veterinary therapy; food animal practice. 4th edition. Philadelphia: WB Saunders Co; 1999. p. 539.
44. Anderson BC. 'Point source' haemorrhages in cows. Vet Rec 1991;128:619–20.
45. Ceci L, Paradies P, Sasanelli M, et al. Haemorrhagic bowel syndrome in dairy cat-tle: possible role of *Clostridium perfringens* type A in the disease complex. J Vet Med Ser A 2006;53:518–23.
46. Dennison AC, VanMetre DC, Callan RJ, et al. Hemorrhagic bowel syndrome in dairy cattle: 22 cases (1997-2000). J Am Vet Med Assoc 2002;221:686–9.
47. Francoz D, Babkine M, Couture Y, et al. Haemorrhagic intestinal syndrome in cattle: retrospective study of 37 cases. (Gastro-enterologie) [French]. Medecin Veterinaire du Quebec 2005;35:65–72.
48. Songer JG. Clostridial enteric diseases of domestic animals. Clin Microbiol Rev 1996;9:216–34.
49. Songer JG. Clostridium perfringens type A infection in cattle. Proceedings of the Thirty Second Annual Conference American Association of Bovine Practitioners. Nashville (TN): 1999.
50. Bunting M, Lorant DE, Bryant AE, et al. Alpha toxin from *Clostridium perfringens* induces proinflammatory changes in endothelial cells. J Clin Invest 1997;100: 565–74.
51. Gustafson C, Tagesson C. Phospholipase C from *Clostridium perfringens* stimu-lates phospholipase A2-mediated arachidonic acid release in cultured intestinal epithelial cells (INT 407). Scand J Gastroenterol 1990;25:363–71.
52. Elhanafy MM, French DD, Braun U. Understanding jejunal hemorrhage syn-drome. J Am Vet Med Assoc 2013;243:352–8.
53. Sockett DC. Hemorrhagic bowel syndrome. Mid Atlantic Nutrition Conference. Maryland, March 24–25, 2004. p. 139–145.
54. Abutarbush SM, Radostits OM. Jejunal hemorrhage syndrome in dairy and beef cattle: 11 cases (2001 to 2003). Can Vet J 2005;46:711–5.
55. Braun U, Forster E, Steininger K, et al. Ultrasonographic findings in 63 cows with haemorrhagic bowel syndrome. Vet Rec 2010;166:79–81.

56. Peek SF, Santschi EM, Livesey MA, et al. Surgical findings and outcome for dairy cattle with jejunal hemorrhage syndrome: 31 cases (2000-2007). J Am Vet Med Assoc 2009;234:1308–12.

57. Braun U, Schmid T, Muggli E, et al. Clinical findings and treatment in 63 cows with haemorrhagic bowel syndrome. Schweiz Arch Tierheilkd 2010;152:515–22.

58. Anderson DE, Constable PD, St Jean G, et al. Small-intestinal volvulus in cattle: 35 cases (1967-1992). J Am Vet Med Assoc 1993;203:1178–83.

59. Fubini SL, Smith DF, Tithof PK, et al. Volvulus of the distal part of the jejunoileum in four cows. Vet Surg 1986;15:150–2.

60. Tulleners EP. Surgical correction of volvulus of the root of the mesentery in calves. J Am Vet Med Assoc 1981;179:998–9.

61. Rademacher G, Dirksen G, Klee W. Diagnosis, treatment and prognosis of intestinal torsion in cattle. Tierarztl Umsch 1995;50:271–6 [in German].

62. Pearson H. The treatment of surgical disorders of the bovine abdomen. Vet Rec 1973;92:245–54.

63. Pearson H, Pinsent PJN. Intestinal obstruction in cattle. Vet Rec 1977;101:162–6.

64. Jelinski MD, Ribble CS, Campbell JR, et al. Investigating the relationship between abomasal hairballs and perforating abomasal ulcers in unweaned beef calves. Can Vet J 1996;37:23–6.

65. Cockrill JM, Beasley JN, Selph RA. Trichobezoars in four Angus cows. Vet Med Small Anim Clin 1978;73:1441–2.

66. Ramadan RO. Massive formation of trichobezoars in sheep. Agri Pract 1995;16:26–8.

67. Patel JH, Brace DM. Esophageal obstruction due to a trichobezoar in a cow. Can Vet J 1995;36:774–5.

68. Deprez P, Hoogewijs M, Vlaminck L, et al. Incarceration of the small intestine in the epiploic foramen of three calves. Vet Rec 2006;158:869–70.

69. Charmillot B. Prolapse of the jejunum through perforated rectum in a cow. Enterectomy. Schweizer Archiv fur Tierheilkunde 1976;118:553–6 [in French].

70. Frazer GS. Uterine torsion followed by jejunal incarceration in a partially everted urinary bladder of a cow. Aust Vet J 1988;65:24–5.

71. Mesaric M, Modic T. Strangulation of the small intestine in a cow by a persistent urachal remnant. Vet Rec 2003;153:688–9.

72. Ducharme NG, Smith DF, Koch DB. Small intestinal obstruction caused by a persistent round ligament of the liver in a cow. J Am Vet Med Assoc 1982;180:1234–6.

73. Lores M, Haruna JA, Ortenburger A. Bilateral 'gut-tie' in a recently castrated steer. Can Vet J 2006;47:155–7.

74. Norman T. 'Gut-tie' in steers. Vet Rec 1997;140:687–8.

75. Wolfe DF, Mysinger PW, Carson RL, et al. Incarceration of a section of small intestine by remnants of the ductus deferens in steers. J Am Vet Med Assoc 1987;191:1597–8.

76. Cecen C, Celimli N, Kabakaya GU, et al. Volvulus of the distal jejunum and ileum and mesenteric torsion in a calf. Cattle Pract 2007;15:97–9.

77. Strachan WD, Tremaine WH, Holdsworth DM, et al. Persistent vitellointestinal duct in a calf. Vet Rec 1997;140:629–30.

78. Gilardoni LR, Paolicchi FA, Mundo SL. Bovine paratuberculosis: a review of the advantages and disadvantages of different diagnostic tests. Rev Argent Microbiol 2012;44:201–15.

79. Allen AJ, Park KT, Barrington GM, et al. Development of a bovine ileal cannulation model to study the immune response and mechanisms of pathogenesis of paratuberculosis. Clin Vaccin Immunol 2009;16:453–63.
80. Harmon DL, Richards CJ. Considerations for gastrointestinal cannulations in ruminants. J Anim Sci 1997;75(8):2248–55.
81. Nuss K, Lejeune B, Lischer C, et al. Ileal impaction in 22 cows. Vet J 2006;171: 456–61.

Surgery of the Umbilicus and Related Structures

Aubrey N. Baird, DVM, MS

KEYWORDS

- Umbilical hernia • Umbilical remnants • Umbilical mass • Umbilical abscess
- Ruminant umbilical surgery

KEY POINTS

- Umbilical hernias (or masses) are not uncommon conditions seen in all ruminants, that can range from simple hernias to umbilical remnant abscesses.
- Umbilical surgery can be performed in ruminants with the aid of sedation and local anesthesia or general anesthesia depending on the condition, size of the animal, and facilities available.
- Ruminants do not often have umbilical masses associated with a patent urachus or incarcerated intestine.
- Ruminants will occasionally be born with or develop an open hernia, which requires emergency treatment to provide the best chance for survival.

The calf is the ruminant most commonly treated for umbilical hernia (or mass) in most practices in the United States, but all ruminants share the same umbilical anatomy and can be affected by umbilical conditions. Techniques described in this article concern calves, but can apply to any ruminant species. A retrospective review of ruminants with congenital defects presented to a teaching hospital determined umbilical hernias to be the most common congenital defect in cattle and the second most common in goats.[1] A survey of nearly 1000 farms reported that, over a 10-year period, almost 16% of the farms had sheep with umbilical hernias, making it the third most reported congenital condition on those farms (behind entropion and brachygnathia inferior).[2] Another review of approximately 3000 lambs found umbilical hernia to be the second most common congenital defect, yet still affecting less than 0.5% of all the lambs born.[3] Sheep and goats are affected by umbilical hernias, but they more often present with abdominal wall hernias from blunt trauma, which respond to closure similar to umbilical hernias.[4] That study reported more sheep affected by hernias than goats, but no comparison was made to the clinic population so it is difficult to determine differences in prevalence.[4]

The author has nothing to disclose.
Large Animal, Department of Veterinary Clinical Sciences, Purdue University College of Veterinary Medicine, Lynn Hall, 625 Harrison Street, West Lafayette, IN 47907-2026, USA
E-mail address: abaird@purdue.edu

UMBILICAL REMNANTS

Any discussion of umbilical surgery or umbilical masses would be remiss if it did not describe the normal umbilical area and related anatomy (**Fig. 1**). The umbilicus provides circulation and waste disposal in the fetal calf through placental attachment. The paired umbilical arteries are found on either side of the bladder. They carry oxygen-poor blood from the fetus. After birth, these arteries become the lateral ligaments of the bladder. Infection of 1 or both of the umbilical arteries is called omphaloarteritis. They are normally thick-walled, with clotted blood inside. Any abscess will be appreciated to be an enlargement of the artery that is otherwise a consistent diameter for the entire length of the structure. The urachus is a fetal continuation of the bladder taking waste to the allantoic sac. It should atrophy shortly after birth and disappear in the normal calf. The umbilical vein courses from the umbilicus cranially into the liver. It delivers oxygen-rich blood and nutrients to the fetus through the liver and ductus venosus. It normally becomes the round ligament of the liver (falciform ligament). Any of these structures can become infected and be associated with umbilical masses.[5] Infected umbilical remnants can be associated with an enlarged umbilicus that can be partially reducible or nonreducible; it can drain purulent exudate frequently or intermittently. Occasionally, an abnormal umbilical remnant can be discovered when repairing what is thought to be a simple reducible hernia.

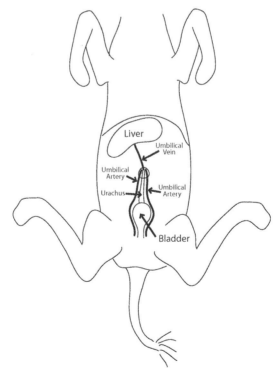

Fig. 1. The normal umbilical remnants in the calf that may become infected and be associated with umbilical masses. (*From* Baird AN. Umbilical surgery in calves. Vet Clin North Am Food Anim Pract 2008;24(3):469; with permission.)

The tissue making up the normal umbilical cord seen at birth is the urachus and umbilical vein. The umbilical arteries retract into the abdomen as the cord is stretched at birth. Good hygiene, although sometimes difficult to accomplish, is critical at calving to prevent ascending infections of the umbilical cord. Dipping the umbilicus with strong iodine or other antiseptic solution is important, although not easily done in some management situations. Although a calving area that can be watched closely is helpful in some situations, such a confinement area can become a source of infection toward the end of the calving season if strict attention is not paid to cleaning and disinfection. Therefore, calving on clean fresh pasture may be superior to having a calving lot or barn.

EXAMINATION AND CLASSIFICATION

The most important part of examination of umbilical masses by the practitioner is manual palpation. First, a size-appropriate restraint should be provided. Young calves can frequently simply be held with 1 arm around the neck and a hand on the tail. Bigger calves may require 2 people to accomplish the same restraint. Calves may be placed in lateral recumbency by use of physical restraint alone or combined with a casting rope. The author prefers to use a rope tightened round the calf's flank rather than more elaborate patterns required to cast adult cattle. Even larger and more fractious calves may require squeeze chute restraint. The presence of infected umbilical remnants is often easier to determine in the recumbent calf. The author routinely palpates calves while in dorsal recumbency as they are being prepared for surgery. The abdominal relaxation in recumbency allows deeper palpation, which may help to identify enlargement of the urachus or umbilical vein within the abdominal cavity. The author has found that the abscessed remnant must still be large to determine its presence reliably on palpation. When the practitioner suspects the presence of a large abscess, he or she can then make the initial body wall opening into the abdominal cavity cranial or caudal to the umbilical mass opposite the enlarged abdominal structure palpated.

The umbilical mass should be palpated to determine if the calf shows any signs of pain when the mass is being manipulated. One should thoroughly examine for the presence of any discharge or scab that would indicate previous drainage and then try to reduce the mass while paying particular attention to structures within the mass that may be movable, and reduce into the abdominal cavity. It is helpful if one can identify if the movable contents of the mass are omentum or sections of intestine. Also, one can occasionally palpate adhesions of the hernia contents to the hernia sac. Umbilical masses can be classified as nonreducible, reducible, or partially reducible. If reducible (or partially reducible), the hernia ring should be evaluated for thickness and completeness and the size of the body wall defect should be assessed. A nonreducible mass may indicate an abscess that is either a large cavity full of thick, purulent exudate or multiple foci of infection surrounded by fibrous tissue. One is frequently tempted to simply lance and drain an umbilical abscess. However, that method should be undertaken with caution because the result could be formation of an abomasal fistula in the case of a Richter's hernia, or alternatively, evisceration or enterotomy in the case of an incorrect diagnosis. One may wish to aspirate the suspected abscess or perform an ultrasound examination.

ULTRASONOGRAPHIC EXAMINATION

Ultrasound examination of the umbilicus has been described elswhere.[6] Ultrasonography of an umbilical mass may provide good information before surgical resection or an attempt to lance and drain an abscess. Interpretation of ultrasonography of the umbilical remnants can be challenging to the inexperienced clinician. Appropriately interpreted ultrasonography may help the practitioner to select which umbilical mass cases they wish to treat surgically in the field.

As ultrasound capabilities become more commonplace and practitioners become more experienced with its use, it has become more useful in examination of umbilical masses and related umbilical remnants. This diagnosis aids in planning for abdominal surgery related to umbilical masses. One study found a strong correlation between ultrasonographic and physical examination of umbilical abnormalities at surgery or post mortem. However, adhesions were present yet undetected in nearly one-half of those cases.[7]

A generous area of ventral abdomen and flank should be clipped for best imaging. Some scans may be done successfully using alcohol to provide contact for the probe. Many young calves can be examined with minimal physical restraint in a standing position. Some believe the standing position makes the umbilical remnants easier to examine.[7] The practitioner should develop a systematic method of examination. One suggestion is to image the caudal umbilicus and remnants caudal to the umbilicus, then the cranial umbilicus and remnants cranial to the umbilicus. Last, the liver should be imaged to determine whether umbilical vein abnormalities extend into the liver or whether there are liver abscesses present.[8]

The type probe used varies with the size of the animal and operator comfort. One can use the knowledge of the anatomy of the umbilical remnants described in this article to evaluate those structures ultrasonographically. Keep in mind that the umbilical remnants may not be present in a normal calf, and abscesses or enlargement of the remnants as imaged by ultrasound are significant findings. The practitioner will quickly develop expertise in the technique when it is followed by surgical exploration and direct observation.

This author does not perform ultrasound examinations in most of these cases. At this time, the ultrasound examinations are reserved for sick calves or the ones whose physical examination findings indicate potential complications. He and his colleagues choose to keep the ultrasound machine out of harm's way when performing preoperative examination of the fractious calf and to not spend valuable anesthesia or sedation time when preparing the calf for surgery. When we choose not to perform an ultrasound examination, we take the approach that we are prepared to explore the abdomen and appropriately treat whatever lesion is present.

RESTRAINT

Umbilical surgery may be performed successfully in ruminants with either sedation and local anesthesia or general anesthesia. The method chosen depends mainly on the practitioner's preference with consideration to size and temperament of the animal, expected difficulty of the procedure, and facilities. Many umbilical procedures can be done as field procedures, whereas others are better performed in a clinic setting. Sedation and general anesthesia techniques are not covered in this article.

General anesthesia prevents patient movement when performing a difficult, complicated surgery. General anesthesia can also be useful in cases of less complicated surgeries where the surgeon is inexperienced, thereby reducing postoperative infections resulting from contamination by subcutaneous or umbilical remnant abscesses. The author currently uses general anesthesia predominantly for several reasons. First, in his teaching hospital environment, they want the veterinary student to get as much hands-on experience as possible with umbilical surgery, and for their initial experience to be positive. Second, their cases may take longer to perform either because of student involvement or because they operate more complicated cases referred from the general practitioner. Keep in mind that calves operated with sedation and local anesthesia tend to become restless during prolonged procedures. Finally, cases seen at referral institutions tend to be older, larger calves, which are more difficult to handle safely without general anesthesia. However, in a practice situation where time and expense are critical, the author would not hesitate to surgically treat young calves with the umbilical conditions described in this article with sedation, local anesthesia, and physical restraint.

INCISION AND CLOSURE

One report claims a good outcome in calf hernias 2 to 5 cm with a snugly applied abdominal support bandage as an alternative to surgery. This technique may be useful in young calves with small hernias, but it is not detailed in this article on umbilical surgery.[9]

Before surgical preparation and incision, any draining umbilical mass should be sutured closed to prevent contamination of the surgical site (**Fig. 2**). In heifers, a simple elliptical skin incision is made around the umbilical mass. Caution should be taken with location of the skin incision to ensure adequate skin remains to allow skin closure without tension. The subcutaneous tissue is dissected around the umbilical mass until the glistening white external sheath of the rectus abdominis muscle is exposed. A small body wall incision (just large enough for the surgeon to insert a finger into the abdominal cavity to palpate for any structures associated with the mass) is made on the midline either cranial or caudal to the mass. The location of the initial incision is based on surgeon preference. When one suspects an abscess of an umbilical remnant caudal or cranial to the mass, it is reasonable to make the initial body wall incision opposite the suspected abscess. Some investigators prefer to make the initial incision lateral to the mass; however, this author is more comfortable with the incision on the midline.[10] The surgeon dissects around the hernia sac or mass with another elliptical incision through the body wall musculature while using fingers or instruments to retract associated structures out of harm's way. The body wall incision is continued cranially or caudally, avoiding abscesses or infected fetal remnants. Most commonly, caudal extension is needed to treat lesions involving the urachus. The midline body wall closure is by the method of surgeon's choice. Suture choice depends largely on the size of the calf. The author routinely uses #1 Vicryl with a simple continuous pattern after placing 1 to 2 near-far-far-near tension sutures. The subcutaneous tissue is closed with absorbable suture in a simple continuous pattern. The skin closure may be done in a simple

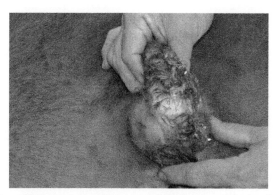

Fig. 2. Preoperative photograph showing an umbilical mass with purulent discharge that should be sutured to close the draining tract and limit contamination of the surgical site.

continuous pattern using nonabsorbable suture to be removed in 10 to 14 days or with absorbable suture if the practitioner or owner so desires. However, most calves that owners wish to have corrected surgically warrant a recheck and suture removal.

The male calf presents more of a challenge because of the preputial orifice being close to the umbilicus. The elliptical skin incision is only useful when the umbilical mass is less than 3 cm in diameter. For most umbilical masses in males, a half-moon or semilunar skin incision is more appropriate (**Fig. 3**). The skin incision is centered over the umbilicus with the concave side directed caudally (**Fig. 4**). Caudal reflection of the sheath is usually adequate to allow an elliptical body wall incision. The semilunar skin incision also allows caudal extension of the skin incision on either side of the sheath and prepuce as a paramedian incision. The caudal paramedian skin incision allows reflection of the sheath and prepuce to the contralateral side. The elliptical body wall incision can then be extended as needed. This approach allows access caudally to any urachal abscess or umbilical artery infections without damaging the elastic tissues of the prepuce or the penis itself. The body wall closure is the same as the female. If the skin incision has been extended as a paramedian, the subcutaneous closure is done longitudinally on the line of the paramedian skin incision. Occasional tacking sutures will be helpful to obliterate dead space where the prepuce has been reflected. The subcutaneous closure of the semilunar incision is done transversely. The underline will have a dimple and not be very cosmetically pleasing immediately after the surgery. However, the long-term result is very acceptable. The skin closure is again surgeon's preference. It is wise to place the first suture at the cranial most aspect of the semilunar incision and work caudally from that point on each side. This makes it much easier to accomplish an even closure.

Some surgeons suggest performing closed herniorrhaphy rather than opening the peritoneal cavity. This option is only viable if there are no infected umbilical structures within the abdomen requiring removal. Closed herniorrhaphy is an option to correct small simple umbilical hernias that are easily reduced. After elliptical incision through and removal of the skin, the hernia sac is inverted into the abdominal cavity and the edges of the hernia are closed with appositional or overlapping suture. A reason for closed herniorrhaphy is to avoid potential peritoneal contamination.[11] Thirty-four simple reducible hernias treated at a teaching hospital were repaired surgically with either an open or closed technique. The surgery time was shorter with the closed technique and the complication rate was lower (5% vs 21%).[12] The complication rate seems to be high for simple hernias in that report, and the author is not aware of other literature

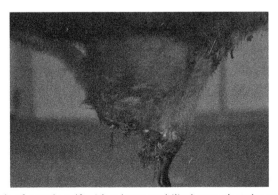

Fig. 3. Photograph of a male calf with a large umbilical mass that the author would treat surgically using the semilunar skin incision.

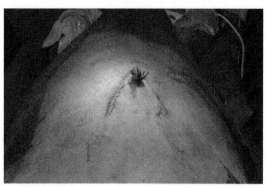

Fig. 4. Intraoperative photograph of the skin closure of the semilunar incision used to treat an umbilical mass in a male calf.

with similar findings. Although it is worth consideration in a field setting for a simple hernia, it may be more critical to select a good environment and be mindful of aseptic technique for a field repair. The author has not appreciated such a complication rate, even with repair of infected umbilical masses, much less simple reducible hernias.

One may consider doing a mesh herniorrhaphy in cases of hernias exceeding 15 cm diameter or for a second surgery when previous closure failed.[11] There have been a number of different materials and techniques used in small ruminant hernia repair.[13–15] The mesh may be placed inside the muscular body wall in a retroperitoneal fashion and secured by mattress sutures. In some cases, the mesh is placed between the incised edges of the hernia ring.[11] Yet another technique is to place the mesh as a patch over the closure of the hernia ring subcutaneously. Use of mesh increases the cost of the procedure and the chance of postoperative infection.

The author frequently has mesh implants available for very large hernias, but they are rarely necessary in ruminants. Other technique to decrease tension on the abdominal wall when closing large defects including fasting the calf for 24 hours or more before repairing the hernia and the use of tension-relieving sutures. Larger hernias are closed with more tension sutures and less with continuous suture patterns.

SIMPLE HERNIAS

The case most frequently treated umbilical disorder in the field is the simple hernia. This hernia can easily be reduced completely and has no associated infected remnants. Classically, simple hernias either contain small intestine (enterocele) or omentum (epiplocele) that is easily replaced in the abdominal cavity by depressing the hernia sac. The contents slide with little to no resistance from the hernia sac into the abdomen, and when the sac is released, the contents return readily. It is important to note the size of the body wall rent when the hernia is reduced. Most simple hernias successfully treated in the field will be no more than 3 fingers in size and have a hernia ring that seems to be thick and is easily palpated. Although the practitioner in the field setting may shy away from performing surgery on calves that have larger hernias, they can certainly be treated successfully.

This author suggests that only first-time repairs of umbilical disorders be attempted in a field setting. When incisional hernias occur or abscesses form after hernia repair, referral is recommended. Often repeat surgeries benefit from an experienced surgeon as well as the superior immobilization with general anesthesia, adequate assistance, and the availability of surgical equipment found in a hospital setting.

OMPHALOPHLEBITIS

Infection of the umbilical vein is easily identified on entering the abdominal cavity. A deep abdominal ligature is usually sufficient to completely resect the abnormal portion of the umbilical vein completely. In cases where the abnormal vein extends into the liver parenchyma, marsupialization of the vein is indicated.[10,16] This possibility justifies a bigger area of surgical preparation than one might think necessary. Marsupialization of the vein can be done at the cranial end of the skin incision or through a separate body wall incision cranial to the skin incision. This author prefers marsupialization through a separate stab incision because it leads to fewer incisional complications. The risk of abdominal contamination is minimal when properly covering the end of the vein during relocation. The separate stab also compliments the semilunar incision described earlier in male calves. The abnormal vein is dissected free at the umbilicus and covered with a surgical sponge and glove to prevent contamination of the abdomen with contents of the abscess. A circular skin incision is made cranial to the umbilical incision and just to the right of the midline. This positioning allows the vein to exit the abdominal cavity directly ventral to the liver. The size of the circular skin incision is determined by the size of the umbilical vein that will exit the body wall. The external rectus sheath is then either incised in a circular fashion or simply in a linear manner and bluntly enlarged to accommodate the cut end of the affected vein. The vein is usually sutured with minimal tension to the external rectus sheath using 10 to 12 simple interrupted absorbable sutures. A second layer of sutures secures the vein to the skin, again with simple interrupted sutures using nonabsorbable or delayed absorbable material. The vein can be flushed to stimulate drainage and healing, although this technique is not without potential complications. The practitioner should never flush under pressure because the ductus venosus could become patent and allow flush solution and contaminated exudate to enter the systemic circulation.[16] The calf should receive systemic antibiotics postoperatively. Frequently, establishing ventral drainage is all that is needed to allow the infection of the vein to resolve. Owners should be informed that a second surgery may be required after the infection has resolved, to resect the vein and close the defect in the body wall. This is most commonly required after marsupialization at the cranial extent of the ventral midline incision. However, the author has found that few of the calves that have a marsupialization have required a second surgery. The healed vein usually atrophies, and the defect in the body wall seals over nicely. One is justified in being concerned about the band of umbilical vein leading to entrapment of intestine, such as has been reported with other umbilical remnants.[17,18] However, the author has never seen this complication or any such report in the literature.

URACHUS

The most commonly infected umbilical remnant is the urachus. The calf is less likely to have a patent urachus draining urine like some other large animal species. Any abnormal urachus in the calf is nearly always an abscess, although urachal cysts have been reported in calves, which present with a nonreducible, fluctuant umbilical mass.[19] The calf may have an umbilical mass that periodically drains purulent exudate with minimal abscess within the abdominal cavity. Alternatively, the mass outside the body wall may be small and the abscess inside the abdominal cavity may be much larger than the calf's urinary bladder. Some calves may present with pollakiuria. The frequent urination of small volumes is related to the urachal remnant not allowing the bladder to decompress fully and therefore the animal has the frequent urge to urinate. One can occasionally determine the presence of an urachal abscess in young calves by deep transabdominal palpation. This palpation becomes more difficult as the calf grows larger. It is easier to palpate bigger calves in dorsal recumbency while sedated or under general anesthesia. This is the type case where ultrasound examination, which is discussed elsewhere in this article, is very helpful. The author does not routinely use ultrasonography for the calf umbilicus, although he acknowledges the value of the technique. He and his colleagues take the approach that the animal needs surgery and they will correct the problems they find at surgery. However, it could be argued that ultrasonography could be helpful in determining which cases might be too involved for the practitioner to operate with sedation and local anesthesia only in a field setting. As for the surgical excision of the urachal abscess, the skin and body wall incision is made as described. One must continue the body wall incision caudally to allow the apex of the bladder to be exteriorized. The author packs off the apex of the bladder and attached urachus with moist towels. The urachus and tip of the bladder should be resected. Leaving a portion of the urachus may lead to a urachal diverticulum that does not empty completely at urination and therefore could contribute to cystitis. The author places stay sutures using 0 monofilament suture on either side of the bladder near the apex. The tip of the bladder and urachus are sharply resected near the apex. Suction is used to remove the urine from the bladder. In the absence of suction, one could aspirate the urine using a large syringe. Some surgeons prefer placing doyen forceps across the bladder rather than stay sutures. The author uses 0 or 2-0 Vicryl to close the mucosa in a simple continuous pattern making every effort not to penetrate the mucosa. He then closes the seromuscular layer with an inverting pattern, such as a Cushing or Lembert, with the same suture material. This closure should achieve a fluid-tight seal that does not leak urine.

Older cattle (frequently yearlings) can experience perforation of a persistent urachus. These animals have uroperitoneum and may present with abdominal distension. The owner may not have noticed any abnormal clinical signs though pollakiuria may have been present. The animal that has uroperitoneum will develop azotemia and uremia. Rectal palpation of these animals usually reveals an elongated, cylindrical bladder; the palpater will not be able to reach around the apex. Extremely sick animals may be treated by draining the abdominal fluid while administering intravenous fluids. One should be careful not to remove abdominal fluid too rapidly without giving intravenous fluids because the rapid fluid shift may lead to hypovolemic shock. The author treats these animals by way of a standing left flank laparotomy. After incision into the abdominal cavity, urine dorsal to the ventral aspect of the incision will pour from the abdomen. The author and his colleagues purposefully do not drain additional urine from the abdomen. The urachal remnant will be attached to the ventral abdomen at the umbilicus. It can be grasped by wrapping it around the surgeon's hand to better apply traction. In this manner, it can be detached bluntly from the body wall. Frequently, the amount of fibrin associated with the urachus and abdominal floor is considerable. Exteriorizing the urachus and bladder apex through the flank incision will reveal rents in the urachus. The tip of the bladder is exteriorized at the incision site with relative ease. The urachus can then be resected and the bladder closed as described in the calf with an urachal abscess. Before closing the flank incision, a stab incision is made in the flank through which an equine nasogastric tube is placed into the abdominal cavity extending to the ventral abdomen. The tube is sutured in place and a 1-way valve is placed on the end of the tube. One-way valves can be created by attaching the cut fingertip end of a surgical or examination glove to the end of the tube. The tube allows the urine to slowly exit the abdominal cavity over a period of 3 to 5 days. Therefore, the animal may not need intravenous fluids to prevent shock owing to a fluid shift associated with rapid drainage of the abdominal fluid.

OMPHALOARTERITIS

Umbilical arteries are the least frequently infected umbilical remnant. Omphaloarteritis is difficult to differentiate from a urachal abscess by palpation. Pathogenesis of omphaloarteritis includes incomplete retraction of the arteries into the abdomen at birth and subsequent contamination of clotted blood within the arteries. When umbilical arteries are abscessed, they can be resected. The infected artery is dissected carefully from the bladder and any adhered omentum. After isolation of the artery, it can be ligated and resected. The author has treated a calf that presented for pollakiuria that had a large abscess of one umbilical artery, and no urachal abnormality.

UMBILICAL ABSCESS

Older calves frequently present with a nonreducible umbilical mass that can either be in the form of a thickened umbilical cord or a bigger ovoid mass. It is usually not painful when palpated. It may be draining purulent exudate or have signs of previous drainage, such as a scar or scab. Alternatively, no signs may exist of any break in the skin. This abnormality is not associated with a body wall defect or intraabdominal infections of the umbilical remnants; the abscess is confined external to the body wall. Calves tend to wall these off nicely and seldom show any clinical signs, but occasionally a calf with a large abscess will be unthrifty. Those described as a thickened cord usually contain several small areas of abcessation surrounded by fibrous tissue. Often, these abscesses become less noticeable as the calf grows. The true umbilical abscesses may be treated by opening the abscess and allowing it to drain. However, one should be very careful to be sure the calf actually has an abscess without involvement of other structures. Ultrasonography or aspiration with a needle and syringe should be performed before opening the abscess. The purulent exudate present in the umbilical abscess will usually be thick. Therefore, one must use a 16- or 14-gauge needle to aspirate because smaller needles seldom yield positive results. Long-term results may be better when these abscesses are treated with surgical resection rather than drainage because lancing the abscess still requires repeated lavaging to achieve proper healing and to prevent the abscess from resealing when it still contains infected exudate.

OTHER CONDITIONS

A Richter's (or parietal) hernia may be mistaken for an abscess by the most experienced of practitioners. The Richter's hernia contains 1 wall of a luminal organ in the hernia. These hernias are often associated with an intense inflammatory reaction and frequently edema. The calf will not show signs of intestinal obstruction; the normal flow of ingesta continues because only 1 wall of the intestine is entrapped in the hernia. In calves, the most frequent section of intestine entrapped in the Richter's hernia is the abomasum. As such, if one mistakes the Richter's hernia for an umbilical abscess and treats by establishing drainage, one will create an abomasal fistula. Occasionally, a fistula will form without intervention.[20] The calf that has an abomasal fistula draining ingesta will develop electrolyte abnormalities that may complicate anesthesia necessary to repair the fistula. If such a fistula occurs, the surgical treatment of choice is to make an elliptical incision and perform an en bloc resection of the fistula.[21] The practitioner should close the abomasum as any luminal organ and then close the body wall routinely. Fistula repair in adult cattle after an abomasopexy technique has been described using wire tension sutures through the entire body wall, with stents. This technique is used because of tension on the closure and contamination of the surgical site. That specific repair is beyond the scope of this discussion on umbilical surgery.

The calf that develops an abomasal fistula secondary to a complicated umbilical hernia is nearly always a candidate for primary closure as described for standard umbilical surgery.

Another umbilical abnormality rarely seen at birth is an omphalocele. An omphalocele occurs when 1 of the 4 body folds fails to migrate normally in embryologic development. This condition is described as having the appearance of a hernia covered by a paper-thin membrane (amnion) rather than hair. One can usually appreciate the presence of small intestine in the hernia, and sometimes a portion of the liver. If the cow is allowed to clean the calf without human intervention, she may actually rupture the amnion and cause an open hernia exposing abdominal viscera. This condition has been reported in kittens, humans, goats,[22] and calves.[23] Although in humans it is frequently associated with other congenital anomalies (especially cardiac abnormalities), concurrent congenital anomalies have not been described in veterinary reports. These cases usually present as newborn calves because of owner concern about the "hairless hernia" or because the amnion has ruptured, causing evisceration. However, the author has treated 1 calf that had grown to be 400 pounds before the open hernia developed and the owner sought veterinary care. The treatment for this condition is herniorrhaphy, as is the treatment for calves with open hernias unrelated to omphalocele. More important than the ultimate treatment is the initial first aid delivered by the attendant who first sees the affected calf. If the tissue covering the hernia is still intact, the hernia should be reduced and an abdominal bandage placed before transport to a veterinarian or calling a practitioner to the farm is necessary to prevent evisceration and contamination. This procedure can certainly be a field procedure because the newborn calf is small enough to restrain safely in dorsal recumbency and a line block is adequate anesthesia. Another calf with an omphalocele treated by the author arrived at his clinic at less than 6 hours of age. Although the closed omphalocele was noted immediately at birth, before placing an abdominal bandage, the hernia became open as the cow aggressively cleaned the calf. When the calf arrived at the clinic, she was held in dorsal recumbency on the floor, and the herniated small intestine was found to be nonreducible through the defect in the body wall, congested, desiccated, and grossly contaminated. Under local anesthetic, the body wall defect was elongated cranially after minimal clipping and preparation. The intestine was cleaned quickly and placed in a sterile palpation sleeve (**Fig. 5**). The sleeve containing

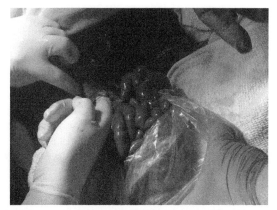

Fig. 5. Photograph of the congested small intestine in an open hernia of a newborn calf. The intestine is being cleaned and placed into a sterile palpation sleeve before being returned to the abdominal cavity as an emergency procedure.

the intestine was placed into the abdominal cavity and the skin and body wall were closed as 1 layer with continuous sutures. The ventral abdomen was then clipped and prepped appropriately for surgery. The sutures used to close the abdomen were then removed, and the incision was slightly elongated to allow easy retrieval of the palpation sleeve containing the previously herniated intestine. The condition of the intestine improved while in the abdominal cavity and was determined to be viable. The intestine was cleaned thoroughly and returned to the abdomen. Carboxymethyl-cellulose was placed in the abdominal cavity to decrease adhesion formation before the incision was closed routinely. The calf was treated with antibiotics and antiinflam-matories. She had a low-grade fever but was doing well enough clinically to be dis-charged from the hospital 4 days after surgery. She developed an incisional hernia that was repaired at 2 months of age. A limited exploration of the abdominal cavity at that time revealed no adhesions or other abnormalities. The heifer went on to show well at the regional level and be a successful brood cow.

SUMMARY

Ruminants of all types requiring umbilical surgery can be affected by a number of different conditions. However, the practitioner should be able to correct any of these conditions surgically, especially in young animals, as a field procedure if appropriate restraint and environment are available. Like other aspects of veterinary practice, the individual must decide what services he or she wishes to offer clients in their practice and which ones will be referred. The objective of this article is to equip veterinarians who wish to treat umbilical masses surgically with the information they need.

REFERENCES

1. Gangwar AK, Devi KS, Singh AK, et al. Congenital anomalies and their surgical correction in ruminants. Adv Anim Vet Sci 2014;2(7):369–76.
2. Greber D, Doherr M, Drogemuller C, et al. Occurrence of congenital disorders in Swiss sheep. Acta Vet Scand 2013;55(27):1–7.
3. Bonca GH, Cristescu A, Mircu C, et al. Clinical observations regarding the inci-dence of some heredopathies in two sheep populations from pure-breed Turcana and Turcana cross breed. Lucrari Stiintifice - Universitatea de Stiinte Agricole a Banatului Timisoara, Medicina Veterinara 2012;45(4):97–102.
4. Al-Sobayil FA, Ahmed AF. Surgical treatment for different forms of hernias in sheep and goats. J Vet Sci 2007;8(2):185–91.
5. Baxter GM. Umbilical masses in calves: diagnosis, treatment, and complications. Compendium on Continuing Education for the Practicing Veterinarian 1989;11(4):505–13.
6. Watson E, Mahaffey MB, Crowell W, et al. Ultrasonography of the umbilical struc-tures in clinically normal calves. Am J Vet Res 1994;55(6):773–80.
7. Staller GS, Tulleners EP, Reef VB, et al. Concordance of ultrasonographic and physical findings in cattle with an umbilical mass or suspected to have infection of the umbilical cord remnants:32 cases (1987-1989). J Am Vet Med Assoc 1995;206:77–82.
8. Steiner A, Lejeune B. Ultrasonographic assessment of umbilical disorders. Vet Clin North Am Food Anim Pract 2009;25:781–94.
9. Fazili MR, Buchoo BA, Bhattacharyya HK, et al. Uncomplicated (simple) umbilical hernia in crossbred dairy calves: management with or without surgery. Indian Vet J Surg 2013;34(2):111–4.

10. Trent AM, Smith DF. Surgical management of umbilical masses with associated umbilical remnant infections in calves. J Am Vet Med Assoc 1984;185(12): 1531–4.
11. Potter T. Umbilical masses in calves. UK Vet 2007;12(3):1–5.
12. Sutradhar BC, Hossain MF, Das BC, et al. Comparison between open and closed methods of herniorrhaphy in calves affected with umbilical hernia. J Vet Sci 2009; 10(4):343–7.
13. Abass BT. Bovine tunica vaginalis: a new material for umbilical hernioplasty in sheep. Iraqi J Vet Sci 2008;22(2):69–76.
14. Vilar JM, Corbera JA, Spinella G. Double-layer mesh hernioplasty for repairing umbilical hernias in 10 goats. Turk J Vet Anim Sci 2011;35(2):131–5.
15. Remya V, Kumar N, Mohan D. Polyproylene mesh aided hernioplasty for repair of umbilical hernia in a goat. Intas Polivet 2015;16(1):39–41.
16. Steiner A, Christoph JL, Oertle C. Marsupialization of umbilical abscesses with involvement of the liver in 13 calves. Vet Surg 1993;22(3):184–9.
17. Hylton WE, Rousseaux CG. Intestinal strangulation associated with omphaloarteritis in a calf. J Am Vet Med Assoc 1985;186(10):1099.
18. Baxter GM, Darien BJ, Wallace CE. Persistent urachal remnant causing intestinal strangulation in a cow. J AM Vet Med Assoc 1987;191(5):555–8.
19. Lischer CJ, Iselin U, Steiner A. Ultrasonographic diagnosis of urachal cyst in three calves. J Am Vet Med Assoc 1994;204(11):1801–4.
20. Fubini SL, Smith DF. Umbilical hernia with abomasal-umbilical fistula in a calf. J AM Vet Med Assoc 1984;184(12):1510–1.
21. Field JR. Umbilical hernia with abomasal incarceration in a calf. J Am Vet Med Assoc 1988;192(5):665–6.
22. Gahlod BM, Raut BM, Raghuwanshi DS, et al. Congenital umbilical defect in kid with intestinal evisceration. Vet World 2008;1(5):147.
23. Baird AN. Omphalocele in two calves. J Am Vet Med Assoc 1993;202(9):1481–2.

Urolithiasis

Ricardo Videla, DVM, MS, Sarel van Amstel, BVSc, MMedVet*

KEYWORDS

- Ruminant urolithiasis • Veterinary urinary blockage • Urinary obstruction ruminants
- Urinary obstruction goat/sheep • Urolithiasis goat/sheep

KEY POINTS

- Urolithiasis is one of the most common emergencies in goats and, unless treated, is fatal.
- Amputation of the urethral process, with or without urine acidification, is usually unsuccessful.
- In the case of struvite stones, tube cystostomy gives the best results.
- In the case of calcium stones, survey radiographs are valuable to select an appropriate treatment plan.

RISK FACTORS AND UROLITH COMPOSITION

Several factors play a role in the development of urolithiasis, including anatomy of the urethra, age, sex, breed, water restriction, geographic location, and season. The urethra of the male ruminant is tortuous and narrow, thus facilitating lodging of uroliths at the sigmoid flexure, and more commonly in the urethral process of small ruminants.[1] Females are rarely affected, most likely because they have a shorter and wider urethra that facilitates passage of uroliths. Early neutering was suggested as a predisposing factor because it may result in underdevelopment of the urethra and decreased urethral lumen.[2] The first step for the development of urinary calculi is the presence of a nidus, usually formed by urinary tract debris, casts, mucoprotein, cells, or bacteria, followed by precipitation of minerals, which is favored by concentrated urine.[3] In a study of uroliths from 832 goats, 44% contained more than 70% calcium carbonate, making this the most common type.[4] Goats older than 1 year of age and breeds of African descent are at a greater risk of developing calcium carbonate uroliths than Anglo-Nubian, Nubian, and Toggenburg breeds.[4] Nevertheless, other urolith types can affect very young small ruminants, putting every age category at risk. Geographic location and diet also have an effect on urolith composition. A study that evaluated 354 urinary calcium carbonate stones from goats revealed that 27% had been collected in the Midwest, 15% in the southeast, 11% in the Northeast, and only 4% from the

The authors have nothing to disclose.
Large Animal Clinical Sciences, College of Veterinary Medicine, The University of Tennessee, 2407 River Drive, Knoxville, TN 37996, USA
* Corresponding author.
E-mail address: svanamst@utk.edu

Southwest.[4] Calcium carbonate stones occur more commonly in animals fed forage or grass,[4] calcium oxalate stones are associated with ingestion of oxalate-containing plants, struvite stones (magnesium ammonium phosphate) are associated with consumption of grain, and silica stones are more common in the Western United States and Canada where grasses have higher silica concentrations. Urine pH also plays an important role, since alkaline pH favors the development of calcium carbonate, struvite, and apatite stones.[3]

CLINICAL SIGNS

Clinical signs vary depending on species, degree of obstruction, and duration of blockage. Small ruminants suffering from a complete blockage of the urethra often show severe signs of discomfort such as abnormal stance, straining to urinate, kicking at the abdomen, teeth grinding, vocalizing, and anorexia. Other signs may include pulsation of the urethra (visible in the perineum), tail swishing, tachycardia, and tachypnea. A distended bladder can often be palpated in the caudal abdomen. Cattle, on the other hand, tend to show more subtle signs, such as anorexia and elevation of the base of the tail. Urolithiasis is common enough that it should be considered as a top differential in any male ruminant with colic. It is not unusual for goat and sheep owners to suspect constipation and gastrointestinal disease based on the clinical signs.

Animals suffering from a partial obstruction may experience more subtle signs, which are often accompanied by stranguria, polakiuria, and/or hematuria. The presence of edema around the prepuce or scrotum and in the caudal ventral abdomen are indicative of urethral rupture. Bladder rupture should be suspected if the animal seems to be depressed and the signs of pain dissipate, and when bilateral abdominal distention is observed. If unattended, obstructive urolithiasis causes severe uremia and death eventually.

The physical examination should include exteriorization of the penis, when possible. The following technique can be used to exteriorize the penis in small ruminants. The animal is restrained, with or without sedation, in a sitting position and 3 mL of a 2% lidocaine solution infused into the preputial opening. This maneuver desensitizes the prepuce and glans penis. The sigmoid flexure is pushed cranially, while the preputial skin is moved caudally. This maneuver exposes the preputial mucosa with the tip of the penis, which is firmly grabbed with a gauze sponge and pulled outward. Sedation may be required to exteriorize the penis and perform initial diagnostic tests. These authors prefer to use diazepam (0.1–0.3 mg/kg intravenously) as an anxiolytic and for urethral relaxation. Other commonly used sedatives are acepromazine (0.05–0.1 mg/kg, intravenously) or xylazine (0.05–0.1 mg/kg intravenously). However, both of these drugs may enhance hypotension and xylazine promotes diuresis; thus, their use is not recommended until the obstruction is relieved.

ANCILLARY DIAGNOSTIC TESTS

Time is important when dealing with cases of urolithiasis, because delaying treatment can lead to complications that can worsen the prognosis. Transabdominal ultrasonography, using a 3.5- or 5-MHz transducer, is a valuable tool to assess bladder size and the presence of free fluid in the abdomen, which indicates bladder rupture. This modality is also useful to evaluate the kidneys and to identify stones within the urinary system. The diameter of the bladder of affected goats usually ranges from 4 to 15 cm, depending on the animal's breed and size.[5] Regardless of size, a bladder that appears round with a thin wall should increase suspicion of urinary blockage. Bloodwork abnormalities are commonly associated with urolithiasis.

Assessment of blood urea nitrogen, creatinine, and electrolytes are valuable to support the diagnosis, determine chronicity, establish prognosis, and aid in implementation of supportive care to stabilize metabolic derangements. Abnormalities include hemoconcentration, azotemia, hyponatremia, and hyperkalemia. These changes are most likely associated with reduced glomerular filtration rate and compromised renal tubular reabsorption and tubular secretion. Other abnormalities may include hypochloremia, hypocalcemia, and hyperphosphatemia. Nevertheless, these changes are not always present early on, because ruminants seem to benefit from salivary secretions to better manage uremia, hyperphosphatemia, and hyperkalemia.[6]

Plain radiographs are sometimes performed in an attempt to determine the location of the blockage, the number of stones, and the radiolucency of the stones, which can be useful in determining the prognosis, and establishing the treatment and postoperative management. The disadvantage of obtaining radiographs on admission include time, cost, and the fact that only radiopaque calculi (calcium carbonate, calcium oxalate, silicate, etc) can be visualized. Therefore, radiographs are usually recommended in cases where radiopaque stones are suspected based on geographic region[7] or diet. It is recommended to obtain 2 lateromedial projections, one with both pelvic limbs pulled cranially (toward the elbows) and one with both pelvic limbs pulled caudally to allow visualization of the urethra and bladder without superposition of the bones of the pelvic limbs.[7]

INITIAL CARE

The ultimate goal is to allow urine excretion, which in most cases can only be achieved with surgical treatment. In some instances, amputation of the urethral process (vermiform appendage) at the connection with the glans may resolve the obstruction, followed by treatment with orally administered ammonium chloride to acidify the urine in an attempt to dissolve struvite stones. Ammonium chloride, 450 mg/kg every 24 hours, was successful at lowering the urine pH to less than 6.5.[8] The authors prefer to check urine pH daily and use ammonium chloride to effect because it is unpalatable, often having a negative effect on appetite, and it can cause metabolic acidosis if used extensively. Unfortunately, the rate of reoccurrence is high in cases treated medically because ruminants typically develop several small stones rather than a single urolith, making it likely that another stone will get lodged in the urethra before urolith dissolution can be achieved with urine acidification.

A soft urinary catheter can be inserted in the urethra in an attempt to localize the blockage; however, the presence of the urethral diverticulum at the level of the ischial arch hinders passage of a catheter into the bladder.[9] Retrograde hydropulsion is not recommended because it is often unsuccessful and could exacerbate damage to the urethra.

Hyperkalemia should be addressed, especially if greater than 6 mmol/L, to decrease the risk of fatal cardiac arrhythmias. Therapy with insulin and dextrose can be implemented to favor shifting of potassium intracellularly. Calcium gluconate decreases the risk of arrhythmias by increasing the threshold potential, but its effect is temporary. Fluid therapy is indicated after resolution of the obstruction to address dehydration, restore kidney function, and flush the urinary system. Normal saline (0.9%) is usually recommended because hypochloremia and hyponatremia are common in these patients; however, treatment should be based on electrolyte status. Nonsteroidal antiinflammatory drugs can be useful to decrease inflammation of the urethra and prevent formation of strictures, but should be used with caution until renal perfusion is reestablished. Their use is discouraged in cases with severe azotemia to prevent further damage to the kidneys. Antimicrobials may be used off label to prevent infections associated with a compromised urinary system and/or surgical treatment.

TREATMENT

Urolithiasis is often a difficult and challenging problem. Cost and other factors that may influence a successful outcome are important to consider. Chronic obstruction may cause bladder rupture or atony, which often result in azotemia and electrolyte changes and backing up of urine, thus predisposing to hydronephrosis. It is also important to look for signs of urethral rupture, such as perineal and/or ventral swelling because that may dictate the best treatment option, which would include urine diversion techniques as the primary treatment approach or perhaps culling in case of breeding animals.

The primary food and water source could also be used as basis for developing a treatment plan. Struvite (magnesium ammonium phosphate) is often reversible in an acidic solution, whereas calcium stones, such as calcium carbonate or phosphate (apatite), are more stable and less likely to dissolve. If struvite is likely to be the cause of the obstruction, treatment options include cystocentesis and bladder irrigation with an acidic solution,[10] or tube cystostomy placed percutaneously, laparoscopically, or via laparotomy, and normograde hydropulsion followed by irrigation with an acidic solution.[11,12] **Fig. 1** presents a flow chart of possible treatment alternatives after tube cystostomy. If calcium stones (calcium carbonate or phosphate–apatite) are suspected as the primary cause of the obstruction, survey radiographs are useful to determine a treatment plan, because the urethra may be obstructed with a large number of stones (pearl string effect)[13] (**Fig. 2**). In such cases, better results may be obtained if another primary surgical approach such, as perineal urethrostomy,[14] bladder marsupialization,[9] urethroscopy, and laser lithotripsy[5] and vesicopreputial anastomosis (UTVCM, unpublished data) is used. In the case of calcium stones, survey radiographs may aid in selection of the best treatment plan based on number and anatomic location of stones (**Fig. 3**).

Amputation of the urethral process in small ruminants, with or without urine acidification, usually precedes these treatment options, but is typically only effective in

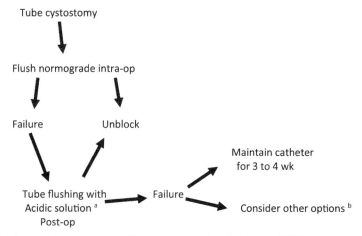

Fig. 1. Treatment plan for obstruction caused by struvite stones. [a] 76% success rate; urination, 11 days; hospitalization, 14 days; <20% reobstruction.[14] [b] Perineal urethrostomy, marsupialization, long term foley, vesico-preputial anastomosis.

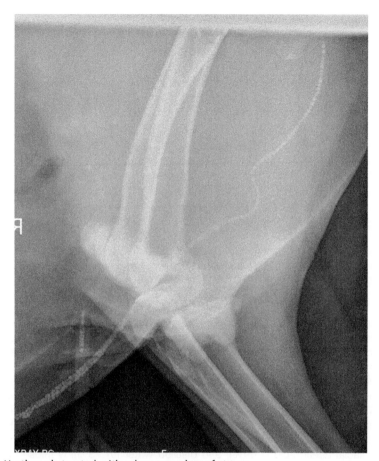

Fig. 2. Urethra obstructed with a large number of stones.

about 50% of cases, and the recurrence rate is 80% to 90% within hours or days.[15] Nevertheless, amputation of the urethral process should always be part of any treatment strategy because stones are often lodged there (**Fig. 4**). In some instances, the glans penis may show signs of necrosis, which may lead to stricture. The penis

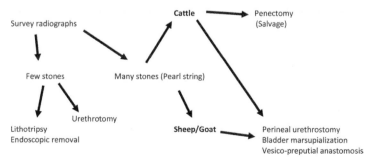

Fig. 3. Treatment plan for obstruction caused by calcium stones.

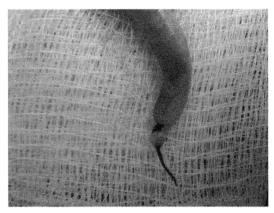

Fig. 4. Stone lodge in the urethral process.

should be exteriorized as previously explained, and the urethral process can then be removed obliquely with a pair of scissors. In animals with an intact frenulum, the urethral process is peeled away from the tip of the penis before amputation.[11]

Cystocentesis and Bladder Irrigation with an Acidic Solution

If obstruction is suspected to be caused by struvite stones, cystocentesis and bladder irrigation with an acidic solution, such as Walpole's solution, is an option.[10] This procedure was carried out in 25 concentrate-fed goats with a median age of 9 months. The goats were placed in left or right lateral recumbency, and an ultrasound-guided cystocentesis was performed using a 1.5- to 3.5-inch, 18-gauge needle to which a 30-inch extension set was attached, and urine was aspirated using a 60-mL syringe. To ensure that the needle remains within the bladder, the tip should be visible on ultrasound at all times. A volume of 120 to 500 mL of urine is removed and the pH determined. Fifty milliliters of Walpole's solution (pH 4.5 and composed of sodium acetate [1.16%], glacial acetic acid [1.09%], and distilled water [97.75%]) is infused into the bladder and, after waiting about 2 minutes, a second urine sample is obtained and the pH measured. Decompression of the bladder and administration of Walpole's solution is repeated until a urine pH of 4 to 5 is achieved. The cystocentesis needle is left in place during the procedure.[10] The urethral obstruction initially resolved in 20 of the 25 goats with this treatment; however, obstruction recurred in 6 of the 20, and only 9 of 13 goats in which long-term follow-up information was available returned to their intended use.[10]

TUBE CYSTOSTOMY
Percutaneous

Percutaneous tube cystostomy is primarily used as a cost-saving procedure, because it usually eliminates the need for general anesthesia, or it can be performed in situations where general anesthesia is not available, or as a time-saving procedure compared with other surgical interventions.[11,16–19] However, the incidence of complications is high.[15] The procedure was carried out, as follows, in 12, 4 to 8-month-old male goats in which overdistention of the bladder was confirmed on abdominal palpation. With the animal in right lateral recumbency, a 1-cm incision was made through the skin 3 to 4 cm left lateral to the penis and 3 to 4 cm cranial to the scrotum. The abdominal cavity was penetrated using blunt dissection. A subcutaneous tunnel was created using a straight hemostat, and a Foley catheter was pulled through the tunnel. A 5-mm Kirschner wire was inserted into the Foley until it penetrated through the end. The Foley with the wire was then pushed through the abdominal opening until it was felt to be up against the bladder wall. The wire with the Foley was then pushed through the bladder wall using a sudden thrust, and the cuff inflated using 5 mL of saline. The Foley catheter was anchored to the skin. Follow-up treatment included ammonium chloride given orally. All the animals started urinating after 5 to 9 days, and the catheters were removed after 12 to 15 days.[17] In another approach, the animal remains standing and after an anesthetic line block in the caudal left flank, a 2-cm vertical incision is made into the abdomen. Using an index finger, a catheter attached to a cannula, such as a teat cannula of which the tip had been sharpened, is guided into the abdomen. The cannula is moved ventrally to the dorsal surface of the bladder, at which point it is thrust into the bladder. Urine flow should start immediately, after which the cannula is moved deeper into the bladder. The catheter is fixed to the skin on the outside.[16] This technique was used on 7 goat kids and 3 lambs. Surgical time ranged from 9.7 to 18 minutes.[16] Urine flow stopped in 2 goat kids after 3 to 4 days and this was due to kinking and collapse of the tubing. The mean time to normal urine flow was 7 days for the remaining 8 animals.[16]

Another study found that percutaneous tube cystostomy resulted in a reduced time to, and an increased requirement for, a second surgical intervention.[15] Failure resulted from tube displacement from the bladder, persistent obstructive urolithiasis, recurrence of obstructive urolithiasis, and urethral rupture.[15] In that study, 8 goats in which the percutaneous tube cystostomy failed subsequently underwent a second procedure, and had adhesions between loops of the small intestine, and between the small intestine and bladder. This may have been due to leakage around the tube or the type of catheter used.[15]

Laparoscopic

Laparoscopic-assisted cystotomy has been described in 5 normal male sheep.[20] With the sheep in dorsal recumbency, a right paramedian 1.5-cm stab incision was made into the abdomen caudal to the umbilicus which allowed the insertion of a 10-mm trocar–cannula system. The abdomen was insufflated with CO_2 to an intraabdominal pressure of 13 mm Hg. The surgical table was tilted to a 20° head-down position to displace the abdominal viscera cranially until the bladder could be visualized. A second paramedian portal was made on the left side close to the teats. Using a 5-mm trocar–cannula system, a forceps was inserted through the portal and the bladder grasped at its apex and elevated to the inside of the body wall. A 3-cm incision was made in the inguinal area overlying the elevated bladder, which was pulled to the outside during desufflation of the abdomen. After placement of stay sutures, a cystotomy was performed and the bladder lavaged. After suturing the cystotomy site, the bladder was replaced in the abdomen. The sheep were repositioned in a head-down position and the abdomen reinflated. The bladder is again grasped with the forceps and a pigtail-tip balloon is inserted through a cannula. The balloon is inflated and the catheter fixed to the skin on the outside. There were no postoperative complications.[20]

Laparotomy

The most successful surgical method for treating obstructive urolithiasis in cattle and small ruminants is surgical tube cystostomy.[1,12,15] Cystotomy allows removal of stones from the bladder and urethral flushing.[12,15] Tube cystostomy establishes urinary diversion and facilitates reestablishment of urethral patency.[12,15,20] This procedure has been carried out in sheep, goats, cattle, camelids, and buffalo.[3,12,13,18,21] With the animal in dorsal recumbency, a paramedian incision is made immediately proximal to the pubis. The bladder is usually covered by omentum, except in camelids, and may contain a lot of fat, making it more difficult to visualize. Two stay sutures, which are used to exteriorize the bladder, are placed near the apex. A cystotomy is performed on the ventral surface, and suction of the urine removes the majority of the stones. The bladder trigone is palpated for additional stones. Normograde flushing is performed using a suitably size polypropelene catheter. With a finger deep in the trigone to prevent back flushing, saline is flushed through the catheter with gentle pressure in an effort to dislodge and remove any additional stones from the urethra. Normograde flushing is more likely to be successful in the case of struvite stones. Calcium stones are generally larger and tend to cause multiple blockages along the distal urethra, which makes normograde flushing ineffective. The cystotomy site is closed using a double inverting pattern. A purse string suture is placed away from the cystotomy site near the apex of the bladder. An 8-inch, 22-gauge Foley (female) catheter is pulled through a stab incision in the abdominal wall lateral and opposite to the caudal part of the abdominal incision. The Foley catheter is then inserted into the bladder through a stab incision in the center of the previously placed purse string suture, which is then tied. After inflation of the balloon, the bladder is pulled up against the abdominal wall and secured on the outside. The abdominal incision is closed. The bladder is flushed with saline to verify that there is no obstruction of flow through the Foley catheter. Overinflation of the catheter may result in discomfort and straining. By creating a diversion for urine flow through the catheter, inflammation in the urethra should subside over a few days postoperatively and facilitate passage of more stones; in some cases, the animal will start normal urination. If no urine has been observed to pass through the penis by 5 days postoperatively, the catheter can be clamped for up to 5 hours.[13,19] However, if the animal shows discomfort and straining without passing urine, the Foley catheter should be unclamped. Instillation of an acidic solution such as Walpole's or hemiacidrin (Renacidin) may aid in dissolving residual stones.[22] The authors would typically start infusing 30 mL of the solution, after which the Foley catheter is clamped for 30 minutes unless the animal is showing undue discomfort. More of the solution can be infused for longer periods of time during the following days. Once a good stream of urine is present, the clamp can be left in place for 24 hours and the animal observed for normal urination, at which time the Foley catheter can be removed.[13,19]

In 2 separate reports, urine flow was reestablished in a mean of 11 and 11.5 days.[1,3] If the animal is not able to urinate after 3 weeks, surgery to establish permanent urinary diversion has to be considered.[13] The success rate for tube cystotomies is more than 80% for sheep, but lower for goats because of the high incidence of calcium carbonate stones.[13] Other reports indicated success rates of 76% to 90% in the short term and 86% in the long term.[1,13] Rarely, the tube becomes dislodged and lost, and if this happens shortly after the initial placement, insertion of another tube may be difficult because of the absence of a walled off track between the bladder and abdominal wall. One of the major problems with surgical tube cystostomy is the cost associated with prolonged hospitalization.[12] For this reason, the authors recommend radiographs on presentation if calcium stones are suspected, because in these cases multiple stones are commonly present in the urethra (pearl string obstruction), and a tube cystostomy often does not resolve the obstruction.

Tube cystostomies have been used in other species including, old and new world camelids,[12] potbellied pigs (van Amstel, unpublished data, 2014), cattle, and buffalo.[18] Complications after tube cystostomy in camelids (n = 18) included an inability to restore a patent urethra (n = 5), development of uroperitoneum upon removal of the cystostomy catheter (n = 1), removal of the tube by the animal (n = 1), and development of testicular swelling (n = 1).[18] In 35 buffalo calves and 23 goats with obstructive urolithiasis treated with tube cystostomies, 80% of the calves and 86% of the goats made an uneventful recovery. Normal urination through the urethra returned

12 to 18 days postoperatively. Complications included urethral rupture in 5 calves and obstruction of the tube in 2 calves and 2 goats.[18] In 125 cases of urolithiasis (33% goats and 66% buffalo calves), follow-up on 88% of these cases reported catheter obstruction in 12% of animals and urethral rupture in 6%. Catheters were removed between 13 to 17 days, except in 12% of cases (all buffalo calves) in which catheters were remove after 1 month.[19]

Long-term tube cystostomy can be used when other techniques, such as stricture after perineal urethrostomy, have failed. The advantage of this technique is that the incidence of urine scald is less than with bladder marsupialization. The main problems associated with this approach is catheter loss or blockage with cellular debris or new stone formation. To prevent this, an 8-inch 22 F-gauge (female) catheter is used, and this should be replaced every 4 to 6 weeks. The catheter should be replaced as soon as possible after loss because of rapid narrowing of the tract into the bladder.

Bladder Marsupialization

Urinary bladder marsupialization may be an option where other surgical interventions have failed or when owners are not willing to accept the risk of reobstruction associated with other procedures.[23] Advantages include simplicity of the technique, and decreased hospitalization time and duration of treatment.[23] Although the success rate is relatively high (80%), all animals are affected by urine scald.[12] Other complications include bladder mucosa prolapse through the stoma and ascending infections.[12] Marsupialization is performed with the animal in dorsal recumbency. A 10-cm incision is made in the caudoventral abdomen approximately 3 cm lateral and parallel to the prepuce. The apex of the bladder is identified and exteriorized using gentle traction. A stay suture is placed at each end of the intended cystostomy, which is about 4 cm in length. A second 4-cm paramedian incision is made on the contralateral side from the prepuce. This incision is placed as far cranial as possible to limit urine scalding without creating excessive tension on the bladder. With the aid of the stay sutures, the apex of the bladder is positioned through the second abdominal incision, taking care not to trap any small bowel.[23] The most cranial, caudal, medial, and lateral aspects of the incision in the bladder is anchored to the abdominal wall. The serosa and muscular layers of the bladder is sutured circumferentially to the peritoneum and muscle of the abdominal incision. The mucosa of the bladder is then sutured to the skin in a simple interrupted pattern to ensure good mucosa-to-skin apposition.[12] In a study that included 19 goats, short-term postoperative complications included bladder mucosal prolapse and death in 2 goats. Long-term complications included cystitis and fibrotic stomal closure occurred in another 2 goats. Urine scald was reported in all surviving animals.[23]

Seven normal 3- to 6-month-old goats were used in a study to evaluate the outcome of bladder marsupialization.[23] Four goats survived to day 180. One goat was found dead at day 150 and had suppurative fibrinonecrotic cystitis with occlusion of the stoma. Another goat developed complete stomal stricture by day 120. The severity of the urine scald seemed to be directly related to the size of the stoma. Animals with larger stoma had a larger area of scald,[23] and vice versa. The mean stomal diameter was 2.25 cm immediately after surgery, and this decreased at a rate of 0.24 cm per month thereafter, and the mean stomal size was 0.53 cm by day 180. Clinical signs related to ascending infections were not observed in the 5 remaining goats.[23] Necropsy showed a tubular-shaped bladder, but all urinary tract organs were grossly normal. Histologic examination of the skin showed a superficial, proliferative perivascular dermatitis with chronic lymphoplasmacytic infiltration.[23]

PREPUBIC URETHROSTOMY

Prepubic urethrostomy is a surgical option to correct urine outflow obstruction after stricture formation associated with perineal urethrostomy in small ruminants. The surgical procedure was carried out in a sheep as follows. The previous urethrostomy site was freed by means of a circumferential incision, and the penis amputated distal to the strictured area. After a caudoventral midline incision, muscles from the medial aspect of the upper leg were cut and reflected from the pubis and ischium, and the prepubic tendon was transected. Bilateral pubic and ischiatic osteotomies were carried out and the pubis removed to expose the pelvic canal.[24] The perineal incision was closed and the pubis replaced and secured with stainless steel wire through predrilled holes. The prepubic tendon was sutured to the pubis through predrilled holes. The intrapelvic portion of the urethra was freed by means of blunt dissection and moved down to the caudal part of the abdominal incision. To prevent mechanical obstruction to urine flow, an angle of greater than 50° between the urethra and bladder should be maintained.[24] The urethralis muscle is used to secure the urethra to the abdominal wall. The abdominal wall is closed, taking care not to make it tight around the urethra. The urethral mucosa is spatulated for about 1 cm and then sutured to the skin, making sure that good apposition is achieved,[24] because this limits granulation and scar tissue formation. Other complications included incisional hernia presumably caused by sectioning of the prepubic tendon during the initial surgical procedure.[24] In that case, the sheep died 3 years after surgery, and pyelonephritis was suspected as the cause of death. In another case, prepubic urethrostomy was carried out in a 2-year-old Pygmy goat,[24] but osteotomies were not performed. The goat developed stricture at the urethral orifice 2 months after the surgery and was euthanized.[24] It was concluded that pubic osteotomy may not be needed in small ruminants because the intrapelvic urethra is long enough to be transposed without causing too much tension. In another case, prepubic urethrostomy was carried out after stricture of a previous perineal urethrostomy. It was described as a very invasive procedure that leaves a lot of dead space, and an intrapelvic abscess developed. The same case also developed severe urine scald (Van Amstel et al, unpublished data).

PERINEAL URETHROSTOMY

Perineal urethrostomy is a well-documented technique for the treatment of urolithiasis in cattle and small ruminants. A permanent opening is made in the urethra, and the anatomic location of the opening varies from "high" perineal urethrostomy located near the ischium to "low" located above the scrotum. These are regarded as salvage procedures because the incidence of stricture formation may be 45% to 78% within 8 months.[14,25] Low urethrostomies were reported in 7 Belgian Blue bulls. Three cases were regarded as successful, and were slaughtered 5 months after surgery. Two animals showed insufficient weight gain and were slaughtered 1 to 2 months after surgery. One animal died after 3 months of unknown causes, and another obstructed again.[26]

A modified proximal perineal urethrostomy uses the intrapelvic urethra because of its greater diameter as compared with the extrapelvic part. For this procedure, a 6- to 8-cm vertical incision is made from just above the ischium. The penile body is located through blunt and sharp dissection and freed from surrounding soft tissue to the level of the ischium.[14] Dissection between the penile body and dorsal penile vessels is carried out before transecting the penis 1 to 1.5 cm below the ischium. For identification and orientation during the procedure, a catheter is placed in the urethra.[14] Blunt dissection is continued to identify the retractor penis muscle, if present, and the ischiocavernosus muscle attachment to the penis. These are carefully transected, making sure not to cut into the penile body or urethra. Continue to separate any further attachments from the urethra until it is possible to slide a finger around the intrapelvic urethra. For this purpose, the tunica albuginea can be grasped. The area is vascular and a fair amount of hemorrhage can be expected. Next the urethra is opened, making sure that the incision remains centered and continued to just dorsal to the ischium. Using 3-0 monofilament absorbable suture and starting at the top of the incision, the urethral mucosa is sutured to the skin on either side to create a funnel. Sutures should be placed so as to create good skin to mucosa apposition. Any remaining skin wounds are closed.[14] In the study reported here, hemorrhage was the most common complication intraoperatively and postoperatively. Other complications included misdirected urine stream, obstructive urolithiasis, bladder atony, dysuria, dehiscence, delayed healing, renal failure and persistent cystitis.[14] Urethrostomy sites were patent and functional in 9 goats available for follow-up beyond 12 months.[14]

Mucosal grafts for reversal of stricture after perineal urethrostomy are not commonly performed but one report describes a successful outcome after buccal mucosal graft urethroplasty in a goat wether.[27]

PRESCROTAL URETHROTOMY

Prescrotal urethrotomy was reported in 25 calves suffering from obstructive urolithiasis affecting the sigmoid flexure.[28] The surgical procedure was carried out by making a 5-cm prescrotal incision lateral to the penis. The sigmoid flexure was freed using blunt dissection. The penis was ligated proximal and distal to the obstruction followed by a urethrotomy over the area of obstruction. The proximal ligating suture was removed and a flexible Rayle's catheter was passed from the urethrotomy site into the bladder to make sure no other stones were present in the proximal urethra. The catheter was removed and the urethrotomy site closed. The Rayles catheter armed with a flexible wire was then passed retrograde up the urethra into the bladder and sutured to the glans penis after removal of the wire guide. The tube was removed after 8 to 10 days. Complications developed in 4 animals including infection at the surgical site in 2 calves; another developed adhesions at the sigmoid curve with phimosis as a consequence, and another calf developed a ruptured urethra.[28] The rest of the calves retained their normal erection and breeding capability.[28]

Urethroscopy and Laser Lithotripsy

Urethroscopy and laser lithotripsy can be used successfully where urethral obstruction is caused by a small number of hard stones such as calcium carbonate or phosphate[5] (Bartges, unpublished data, 2013).

Vesicopreputial Anastomosis

This is a novel unreported technique (Department of Large Animal Clinical Sciences, College of Veterinary Medicine, University of Tennessee) to redirect urine flow after failure to reestablish urination after techniques such as tube cystostomy or perineal urothrostomy. This technique is carried out as follows. With the animal in dorsal recumbency, a rigid probe is inserted through the preputial opening to the end of the preputial sac. With this landmark as a guide, a 6- to 8-cm incision is made 1 cm lateral and parallel to the preputial skin so that the middle of the incision is in line with the end of the preputial sac. The abdominal cavity is opened and the urinary bladder located and 2 stay sutures placed through the apex without entering the lumen. The bladder is pulled through the abdominal incision for about 3 cm. The bladder wall is then sutured to the abdominal wall in such a manner so as to form a tight seal. Next, the caudal end of the preputial sac and penis are

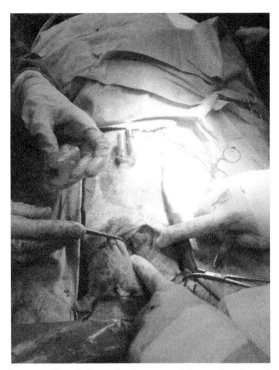

Fig. 5. A Foley catheter is placed through the preputial opening into the bladder and the balloon inflated.

freed from the skin and abdominal wall. A circumferential incision is made into the prepuce where the penis enters the preputial cavity. A prescrotal penile amputation (penectomy) is performed and the cranial transected portion of the penis removed. The opening in the prepuce is enlarged to where it can easily accommodate a 22-F gauge Foley catheter. Next, a similar size opening is made in the apex of the bladder. A 2-layer anastomosis between the preputial sac and the bladder is then performed making sure that good apposition between bladder and preputial mucosa is attained. An 8-inch 22-gauge Foley catheter is placed through the preputial opening into the bladder and the balloon inflated (**Fig. 5**). The Foley catheter is left in place for 3 to 4 weeks until healing has occurred. This technique can be used as a replacement for bladder marsupialization because urine scalding does not occur. Of the 4 cases performed using this technique, 1 goat died of hydronephrosis after stricture, 2 goats are doing well on follow-up 6 months after surgery, and the remaining goat had a second anastomosis performed after the first strictured.

Penile Amputation

Penile amputation is similar as described for perineal urethrostomy. In this technique the penis is transected in the perineal area (high or low) rather than creating a stoma. The distal part of the penis is left in place and not removed unless necrotic. This is a salvage procedure and is commonly done in cattle feedlots.

REFERENCES

1. Rakestraw PC, Fubini SL, Gilbert RO, et al. Tube cystostomy for treatment of obstructive urolithiasis in small ruminants. Vet Surg 1995;24(6):498–505.

2. Bani Ismail ZA. Effects of castration on penile and urethral development in Awassi lambs. Bulgarian J Vet Med 2007;10(No 1):29–34.
3. Ewoldt JM, Anderson DE, Miesner MD, et al. Short- and long-term outcome and factors predicting survival after surgical tube cystostomy for treatment of obstructive urolithiasis in small ruminants. Vet Surg 2006;35(5):417–22.
4. Nwaokorie EE, Osborne CA, Lulich JP, et al. Risk factors for calcium carbonate urolithiasis in goats. J Am Vet Med Assoc 2015;247(3):293–9.
5. Halland SK, House JK, George LW. Urethroscopy and laser lithotripsy for the diagnosis and treatment of obstructive urolithiasis in goats and pot-bellied pigs. J Am Vet Med Assoc 2002;220(12):1831–4.
6. Sockett DC, Knight AP, Fettman MJ, et al. Metabolic changes due to experimentally induced rupture of the bovine urinary bladder. Cornell Vet 1986;76(2):198–212.
7. Kinsley MA, Semevolos S, Parker JE, et al. Use of plain radiography in the diagnosis, surgical management, and postoperative treatment of obstructive urolithiasis in 25 goats and 2 sheep. Vet Surg 2013;42(6):663–8.
8. Mavangira V, Cornish JM, Angelos JA. Effect of ammonium chloride supplementation on urine pH and urinary fractional excretion of electrolytes in goats. J Am Vet Med Assoc 2010;237(11):1299–304.
9. May KA, Moll HD, Wallace LM, et al. Urinary bladder marsupialization for treatment of obstructive urolithiasis in male goats. Vet Surg 1998;27(6):583–8.
10. Janke JJ, Washburn KE, Bissett WT, et al. Use of Walpole's solution for treatment of goats with urolithiasis: 25 cases (2001-2006). J Am Vet Med Assoc 2009; 234(2):249–52.
11. Streeter RN, Washburn KE, McCauley CT. Percutaneous tube cystostomy and vesicular irrigation for treatment of obstructive urolithiasis in a goat. J Am Vet Med Assoc 2002;221(4):546–9, 501.
12. Ewoldt JM, Jones ML, Miesner MD. Surgery of obstructive urolithiasis in ruminants. Vet Clin North Am Food Anim Pract 2008;24(3):455–65, v.
13. Rings DM. Sheep and goat practice for the small animal practitioner. The North American Veterinary Conference, Small Animal and Exotics Orlando. Florida, 18–22 January, 2003: 539–542.
14. Tobias KM, van Amstel SR. Modified proximal perineal urethrostomy technique for treatment of urethral stricture in goats. Vet Surg 2013;42(4):455–62.
15. Fortier LA, Gregg AJ, Erb HN, et al. Caprine obstructive urolithiasis: requirement for 2nd surgical intervention and mortality after percutaneous tube cystostomy, surgical tube cystostomy, or urinary bladder marsupialization. Vet Surg 2004; 33(6):661–7.
16. Fazili MR, Malik HU, Bhattacharyya HK, et al. Minimally invasive surgical tube cystotomy for treating obstructive urolithiasis in small ruminants with an intact urinary bladder. Vet Rec 2010;166(17):528–31.
17. Kinjavdeker AP, Aithal HP, Pawde AM. Tube cystostomy for management of obstructive urolithiasis in goats. Indian Vet J 2010;87:137–8.
18. Tamilmahan P, Moshina A, Karthik K. Tube cystostomy for management of obstructive urolithiasis in ruminants. Vet World 2014;7.
19. Singh AK, Gangwar AK, Devil KS. Incidence and management of obstructive urolithiasis in buffalo calves and goats. Adv Anim Vet Sci 2014;2:503–7.
20. Franz S, Dadak AM, Schoffmann G. Laparoscopic-assisted cystotomy: an experimental study in male sheep. Vet Med 2009;8:367–73.
21. Duesterdieck-Zellmer KF, Van Metre DC, Cardenas A, et al. Acquired urethral obstruction in New World camelids: 34 cases (1995-2008). Aust Vet J 2014; 92(8):313–9.

22. Wolf C. Managing tube cystotomies in goats. In: Proceedings of the North American Veterinary Conference. 2006. p. 299–300.

23. May KA, Moll HD, Duncan RB, et al. Experimental evaluation of urinary bladder marsupialization in male goats. Vet Surg 2002;31(3):251–8.

24. Stone WC, Bjorling DE, Trostle SS, et al. Prepubic urethrostomy for relief of urethral obstruction in a sheep and a goat. J Am Vet Med Assoc 1997;210(7):939–41.

25. Haven ML, Bowman KF, Engelbert TA, et al. Surgical management of urolithiasis in small ruminants. Cornell Vet 1993;83(1):47–55.

26. Gasthuys F, Martens A, De Moor A. Surgical treatment of urethral dilatation in seven male cattle. Vet Rec 1996;138(1):17–9.

27. Gill MS, Sod GA. Buccal mucosal graft urethroplasty for reversal of a perineal urethrostomy in a goat wether. Vet Surg 2004;33(4):382–5.

28. Seddek AM, Bakr HA. New surgical technique for treatment of obstructive Penile urethrolithiasis without interference with breeding capability: clinical study on 25 calves. Pakistan Vet J 2013;33(3):385–7.

Surgical Procedures of the Genital Organs of Bulls

Tulio M. Prado, DVM, MS[a],*, Lionel J. Dawson, BVSc, MS[b], Jim Schumacher, DVM, MS[a]

KEYWORDS

- Bovine • Bull • Surgery • Genitalia • Fertility

KEY POINTS

- Injuries affecting the reproductive tract of bulls can cause pathologic changes that result in substantial economic and genetic losses to beef or dairy producers.
- Findings during a thorough physical examination are helpful indicators for the need to perform surgery and correct any abnormalities of the reproductive tract causing infertility.
- Injuries, diseases, or conditions of the reproductive tract of bulls can be managed surgically or treated to preserve the genetic potential of the bull.

PRESURGICAL CONSIDERATIONS

The majority of the reproductive tract abnormalities involving infertility in a bull are diagnosed via a thorough history and physical examination; seldom, a more in-depth diagnostic evaluation is required. The history should describe the bull's reproductive status and may include information such as conformation, gait, copulatory performance, drug therapy, behavioral changes, previous injuries, illnesses, or prior urogenital surgery.

Examination of the Genital Organs of the Bull

The penis and prepuce, from the sigmoid flexure to the glans penis, are examined easily with the bull adequately restrained. These structures, along with the scrotum and testes, should be evaluated visually and by palpation. Enlargements or restriction of movement inside the sheath should be considered abnormal (**Fig. 1**).[1,2]

The authors have nothing to disclose.
[a] Department of Large Animal Clinical Sciences, College of Veterinary Medicine, University of Tennessee, 2407 River Drive, Knoxville, TN 37996, USA; [b] Veterinary Clinical Sciences, Center for Veterinary Health Sciences, Oklahoma State University, 2065 West Farm Road, Stillwater, OK 74078, USA
* Corresponding author.
E-mail address: tprado@utk.edu

Vet Clin Food Anim 32 (2016) 701–725
http://dx.doi.org/10.1016/j.cvfa.2016.05.009
0749-0720/16/$ – see front matter © 2016 Elsevier Inc. All rights reserved.

vetfood.theclinics.com

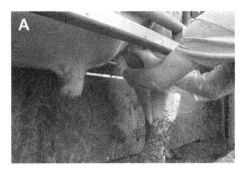
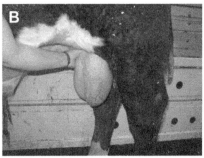

Fig. 1. Restraint of the bull (*A*) and evaluation of the external genitalia (*B*). General conformation of the scrotum and testicles, penis, sheath, and prepuce should be palpated and evaluated visually from the sigmoid flexure to the glans penis.

The penis and prepuce are examined after extending the penis manually by transrectal rectal massage or by electroejaculation. The bull's penis is most easily extended while the bull is mildly sedated. Massage of accessory sex glands, as well as manually straightening the sigmoid flexure after the bull is sedated, exposes the penis (**Fig. 2**). The penis can also be desensitized and extruded by anesthetizing the internal pudendal and middle hemorrhoidal nerve at the lesser sciatic foramen. An internal pudendal nerve block is indicated when anesthesia of the penis, prepuce, or retractor penis muscle is desired for any standing surgery.[3]

Palpation and ultrasonographic examination are important means of evaluating the accessory sex glands (**Fig. 3**). Ultrasonography can also be used to assess the physical status of cavernous tissue and to identify urethral abnormalities. Ultrasonographic examination of a penile hematoma may identify a rupture of the tunica albuginea.[4,5]

Other evaluations less commonly used include endoscopy, contrast radiographs of the cavernous spaces (cavernosography) for identifying a rupture or laceration of the tunica albuginea of the corpus cavernosum penis and also determining the cause of persistent impotence, and vascular shunts.[6,7] Urethral catheterization for obtaining fluid from the seminal vesicles for cytologic examination and culture.[8,9]

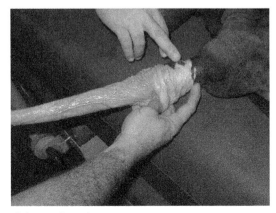

Fig. 2. Evaluation of the penis and prepuce.

A B

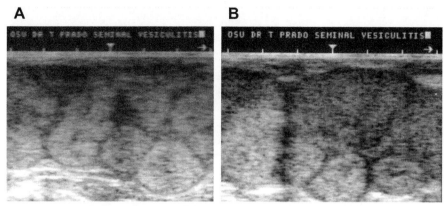

Fig. 3. (*A, B*) Ultrasound of seminal vesicles.

SURGERY OF THE PREPUCE AND PENIS

Any injury to the prepuce should first be allowed to heal, to control the inflammation and infection, for 6 to 8 weeks with sexual rest.[10] Reevaluation at 8 weeks allows an assessment of the need for surgery and the genetic and economic factors that influence whether the bull receives treatment.[10–12] Persistent frenulum, penile hematoma, and penile tumors, such as a fibropapilloma, are the 3 most common abnormalities for which surgery of the penis is indicated. Penile deviation and vascular shunts are less commonly encountered abnormalities.

Management of Preputial Injuries

A significant relationship seems to exist between a pendulous sheath and the tendency of habitual eversion of the prepuce (**Fig. 4**). Types of injuries to the prepuce can be categorized as lacerations, avulsions, contusions, frostbite, and abrasions (**Fig. 5**). Injury and infection lead to fibrosis and later to phimosis or stenosis of the prepuce (**Fig. 6**). Infection of the prepuce may sometimes lead to formation of an abscess, and the location of the abscess is usually midway between the preputial opening and the scrotum (**Fig. 7**). Bulls with a preputial abscess seldom recover to be used for breeding.[10–14]

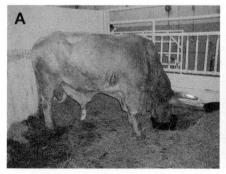
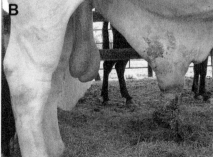

Fig. 4. (*A, B*) Pendulous sheath.

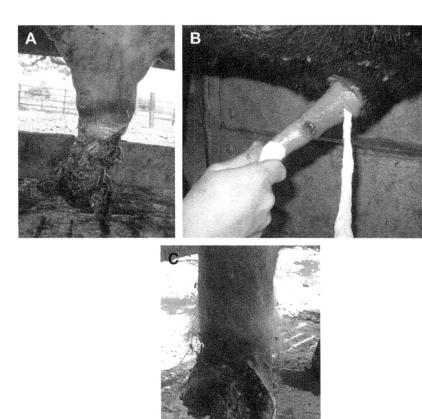

Fig. 5. Lacerations (*A*), avulsions (*B*), and contusions (*C*) of prepuce.

Preputial avulsions are the simplest of the preputial injuries. They usually happen when bulls are collected with an artificial vagina. The tear is 2 to 3 cm circumferentially located at the fornix, where the prepuce attaches to the penis. These tears are sutured with a simple interrupted suture pattern, using an absorbable suture (**Fig. 8**). Bulls need 2 weeks of sexual rest before their next collection.[10]

Acute preputial prolapse should be managed conservatively. Chronic preputial prolapse with severe edema and necrosis makes an accurate prognosis difficult at the time of initial examination, and a guarded prognosis must be given. Seven to 10 days of therapy may be required before an accurate prognosis can be determined. Reduction may not be possible if the prolapsed prepuce contains extensive areas of fibrosis causing stenosis.

Reducing edema promotes replacement of the prolapsed tissue into the sheath, which is the key to protecting the tissue from exposure and additional trauma. The authors massage the prolapsed preputial tissue with a formulation containing lanolin, scarlet oil, and oxytetracycline. This formulation protects the exposed tissue from dehydration, promotes epithelialization, and provides broad-spectrum antimicrobial treatment. The reduced prolapse is retained within the preputial cavity with a

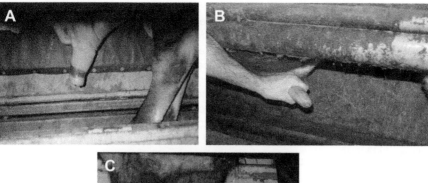

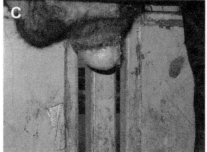

Fig. 6. (*A*) Phimosis caused by a stricture. (*B, C*) Phimosis caused by stenosis of the prepuce.

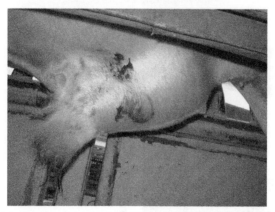

Fig. 7. A preputial abscess located midway between the preputial orifice and the base of the scrotum.

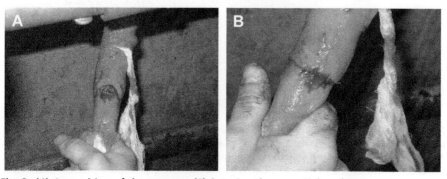

Fig. 8. (*A*) An avulsion of the prepuce. (*B*) Suturing the preputial avulsion.

purse-string suture or with a tape-and-tube retention device for 2 weeks, allowing the damaged prepuce to heal (**Fig. 9**).[10,13,14] Surgery is indicated if the bull is unable to retain the prepuce within the preputial cavity after the prepuce has healed. If prolapse becomes chronic, soak the prolapsed prepuce with a saturated solution of Epsom salt and then the lanolin–scarlet oil–oxytetracycline formulation. A rubber tube is placed into the lumen of the prolapsed prepuce, and a 2-inch stockinette tubular bandage (Lohmann and Rauscher, Jamesburg, NJ) is rolled over the prolapsed prepuce. Rolled elastic gauze is applied over the stockinette to reduce swelling. After the prepuce has healed, it should be amputated or reefed to permanently prevent habitual preputial prolapse.[10,13,15–18]

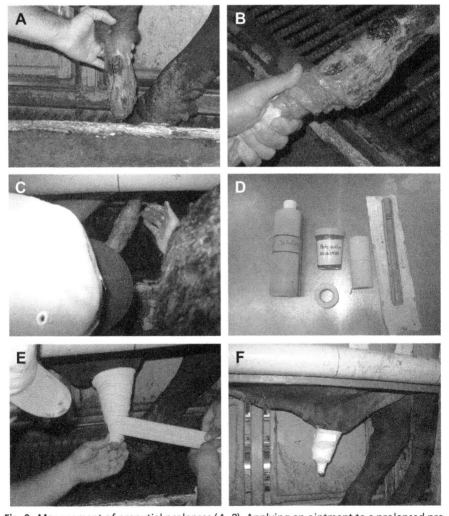

Fig. 9. Management of preputial prolapses (*A, B*). Applying an ointment to a prolapsed prepuce (*C*). Materials needed to maintain a prolapsed prepuce within the preputial cavity (*D*). Applying a bandage to the sheath to maintain a prolapsed prepuce within the preputial cavity (*E*). A bandaged sheath. The bandage maintains the prolapsed prepuce within the preputial cavity (*F*).

Preputial amputation

The prepuce is amputated by first inserting a plastic syringe case or tube into the preputial cavity; the prolapsed prepuce is then stabilized by inserting 2 thin Kirschner pins or long hypodermic needles at right angles to each other through the proximal healthy aspect of the prolapsed tissue and through the syringe case or tubing. A circumferential incision is directed diagonally to increase the circumference of the preputial lumen at the site of amputation, thereby decreasing the likelihood of preputial stenosis by formation of stricture. Another method used to decrease the likelihood of stenosis at the site of amputation is to remove a V-shaped segment of tissue at the area of amputation (**Fig. 10**). The edges of the healthy portion of the prepuce are sutured together with overlapping, interrupted horizontal mattress sutures. The stabilizing pins or needles and the plastic syringe case or tube are then removed. A preputial tape-and-tube retention device, as described, on management of preputial injuries, is applied to the surgical site and left for 1 to 2 weeks. Antimicrobial and antiinflammatory therapies are administered to the bull.[10]

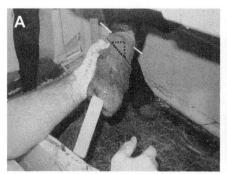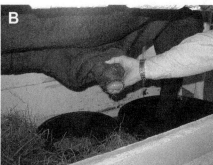

Fig. 10. Amputation of prepuce (*A*) and postoperative healing (*B*).

Reefing

For reefing, also known as segmental posthetomy or circumcision, surgery is performed under general anesthesia. After extending and preparing the penis and prepuce for septic surgery, a Penrose drain is placed around the penis and prepuce to serve as a tourniquet. The prepuce is incised circumferentially proximal and distal to the tissue to be removed, and connected by a longitudinal incision (**Fig. 11**). The integument prepuce between the 2 circumferential incisions is dissected from the underlying elastic tissue (**Fig. 12**). After removing the segment of integument, the remaining prepuce should be at least 1.5 times the segment of the free portion of the penis to allow the bull to be able fully extend its penis. The tourniquet is then removed and hemorrhaging vessels ligated. Subcutaneous tissue at the circumferential incisions is apposed with 4 simple interrupted sutures of 2-0 absorbable suture. Placing a "marker suture" on the proximal and distal circumferential incisions before beginning dissection ensures that the circumferential incisions are aligned when suturing commences. The preputial integument is sutured with the same suture in an interrupted horizontal mattress pattern (**Fig. 13**). The penis and prepuce are replaced into the preputial cavity and retained as described on management of preputial injuries. The bandage is removed after 3 to 4 days, and the bull is administered antimicrobial therapy for 1 week. Bulls undergoes sexual rest for 8 weeks and examined before allowing to resume natural breeding.[10]

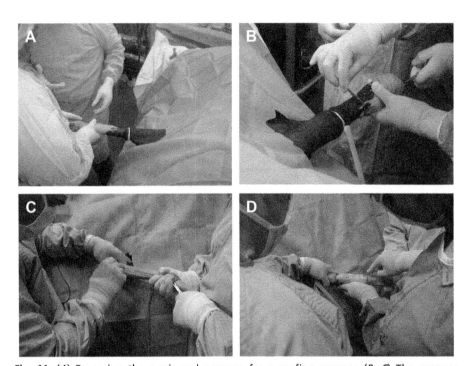

Fig. 11. (*A*) Preparing the penis and prepuce for a reefing surgery. (*B, C*) The prepuce is incised circumferentially proximal and distal to the tissue to be removed by reefing. (*D*) The proximal and distal circumferential incisions are connected by a longitudinal incision.

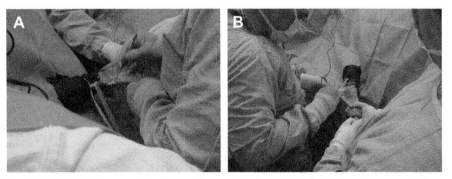

Fig. 12. (*A*) The integument between the proximal and distal incisions is removed from the underlying elastic tissue. (*B*) The integument between the proximal and distal incisions is removed from the underlying elastic tissue. This tissue is being removed using electrocautery.

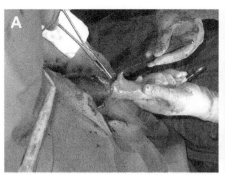
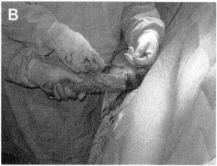

Fig. 13. (*A, B*) The proximal and distal sections of prepuce are approximated with interrupted horizontal-mattress sutures.

Preputial stoma

Preputial stoma is a novel surgical approach for semen collection in bulls with phimosis owing to preputial stenosis. After clipping and preparing the sheath for septic surgery, a longitudinal elliptical incision is made on the ventral aspect of the sheath proximal to the stenotic scar in the preputial cavity. The diameter of the stroma should sufficiently allow the free portion of the penis to extend, but not too much allowing the prepuce to prolapse. The skin within the elliptical incision is excised, and the peripenile elastic layers dissected through to the internal lamina of the prepuce. The prepuce is incised near the distal end of the elliptical incision. The free portion of the penis is exteriorized through the incision by grasping the glands penis with sponge forceps (**Fig. 14**). The preputial epithelium is apposed to the skin around the periphery of the stoma and sutured using a #0 absorbable suture in a simple interrupted pattern. A Penrose drain is sutured to the free portion of the penis to allow urine to drain away from the incision. Remove the Penrose 10 days after surgery (**Fig. 15**). Bulls should have no sexual activity nor attempts of semen collection for 8 weeks.[18]

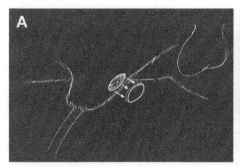
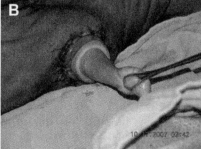

Fig. 14. (*A*) A stoma created caudal to a preputial stenosis. (*B*) Exteriorization of the penis through the stoma.

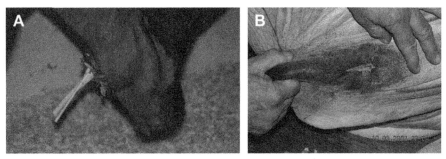

Fig. 15. Penrose drain protruding through a preputial stoma (*A*) and a healed preputial stoma (*B*).

Penile Fibropapilloma

Fibropapillomas can be removed with the bull restrained and standing, or ideally with the bull recumbent, sedated, and restrained on a rotating chute or tilt table.[11,19] The penis is extended, and the mass removed using a #15 or #10 scalpel blade, electrocautery, or a laser. The mass can also be removed using cryosurgery.[10,20] The surgeon must dissect carefully when the mass is adjacent the urethra, which can best be identified during dissection by passing a #8 Tomcat catheter into the urethra (**Fig. 16**).[10]

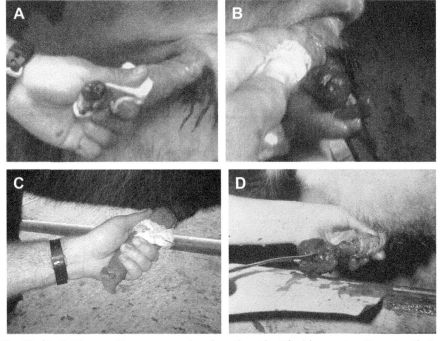

Fig. 16. (*A, B*) Fibropapilloma removed and urethra identified by passing Tomcat catheter into it. (*C*) A healing wound on the penis after removing a fibropapilloma. (*D*) The urethra is identified before excising a penile fibropapilloma by inserting a tomcat catheter into the lumen of the urethra. The urethra should be identified before removing a fibropapilloma to avoid damaging the urethra.

Persistent Frenulum

A persistent frenulum can be excised surgically, with the bull standing or recumbent, in a manner similar to that used to excise a fibropapilloma.[11] The penis is extended by grasping the frenulum, and the frenulum is resected using Mayo scissors. Bleeding is usually minimal, but may be controlled using electrocautery or ligation. The bull is sexually rested for 2 weeks (**Fig. 17**).[19]

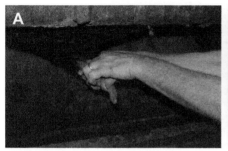
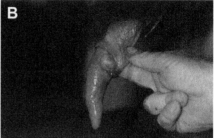

Fig. 17. (*A, B*) A persistent frenulum.

Penile Hematoma

Surgical intervention of large penile hematomas, caused by the impact of the penis against the cow's perineum during breeding, has been successful for bulls returning to service.[10,20–24] The rupture arises from the dorsal or crural canal of the tunica albuginea of the corpus cavernosum penis. Rarely, a penile hematoma occurs ventrally or at the midbody of the penis, and rarely disrupts the urethra.[22] Musser and colleagues[25] reported the incidence of surgical success in restoring copulatory function to be 80% in bulls with a hematoma of less than 20 cm in diameter. The success if the hematoma was greater than 20 cm in diameter was 75% with surgery but only 33% with conservative treatment (**Fig. 18**). Surgery to remove the blood clot, and possibly to suture the tunica albuginea, should be done within 10 days of the occurrence, before the blood clot gets organized.[10,21,23,24]

Surgery is performed under general anesthesia. The bull is placed in lateral recumbency and the sheath clipped and prepared for aseptic surgery (**Fig. 19**). An incision is made on the lateral aspect of the sheath, dorsal and lateral to the penis. The cavity of

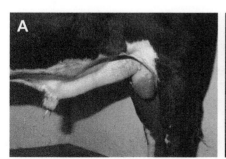
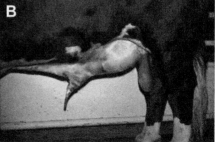

Fig. 18. Penile hematoma located at the base of the scrotum. (*A*) Less than 20 cm in diameter. (*B*) Greater than 20 cm in diameter.

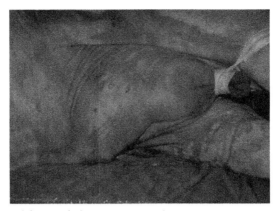

Fig. 19. Bull prepared for penile hematoma aseptic surgery.

the hematoma is opened, drained, and irrigated with sterile isotonic saline solution. The penis is exposed, debrided of fibrinous tissue and blood clots, and replaced within the sheath (**Fig. 20**). No benefit has been found in suturing the tear in the tunica albuginea. The subcutaneous tissues and skin are closed in 2 layers. No attempt is made to close the dead space to decrease the risk of developing restrictive adhesions. The bull should have sexual rest for 60 days and be examined again before allowing natural breeding.[10,25] The incidence of success of surgery decreases when bulls are allowed to breed less than 60 days after surgery, resulting in a recurrence of penile hematoma.[25]

The 4 possible sequelae to penile hematoma surgery are:

- Formation of an abscess at the surgical site, which may result in peripenile adhesions that restrict protrusion of the penis.
- Desensitization of the glans penis owing to damage to the dorsal penile nerves at the time of injury, during surgery, or from breakdown of adhesions involving the nerve during erection when the bull has returned to service. In this instance, the bull is unable to achieve intromission because the glans has no sensation, making the bull unable to locate the vulva (**Fig. 21**).
- Formation of peripenile adhesions that anchor the penis, even in the absence of postsurgical infections.
- The development of vascular shunts between the corpus cavernosum penis and the penile vasculature.[10]

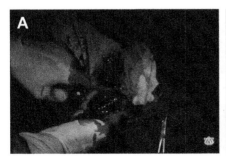
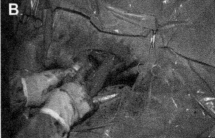

Fig. 20. (*A*) The capsule of the hematoma has been opened to exposed the clotted blood contained within. (*B*) Blood clots and fibrinous tissue within the capsule are being evacuated.

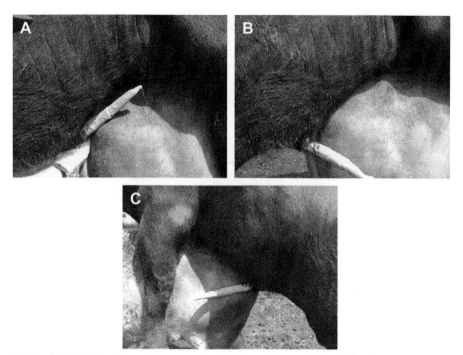

Fig. 21. (*A–C*) This bull is unable to penetrate the vagina owing to lack of sensation to the glans penis as a sequela of surgery to remove a penile hematoma.

Penile Deviation

The apical ligament of the penis is an extension of the tunica albuginea that provides dorsal strength and support to the erect penis. The 3 forms of penile deviation described in the bull occur because the apical ligament:

- Is too short, creating the rare S-shaped deviation,
- Is too long, creating a ventral deviation, or
- Slips to the left when the penis is erect, creating a corkscrew or spiral deviation.

The penis normally forms a spiral deviation after intromission when pressure maximizes within the corpus cavernosum penis at the moment of ejaculation. Bulls that develop a spiral deviation of the penis before intromission may have premature maximization of pressure within the corpus cavernosum penis (**Fig. 22**).[26]

Two surgical techniques have been described to reinforce the strength of the apical ligament:

- Splitting and interweaving the apical ligament (not be explained in this article because of the complication of formation of a vascular shunt),[11] and
- Autografting.

Autografting consists of using fascia from the tensor fascia lata muscle. For this technique, it is necessary to harvest an autogenous or homologous 2-cm wide, 20-cm long segment of fascia lata from the cranial borders of the biceps femoris muscle. The homologous strips of the fascia lata is harvested from fresh carcass and stored in 70% ethyl alcohol. All muscle, fat, and connective tissue are trimmed before

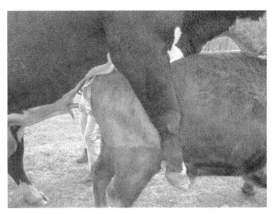

Fig. 22. Bull with corkscrew or spiral deviation.

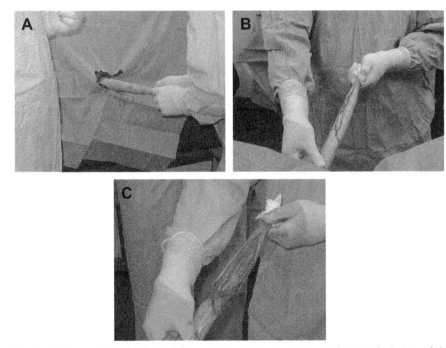

Fig. 23. (A) Preparation of the bull for aseptic surgery to correct corkscrew deviation of the penis. (B) Cutaneous incision on the dorsum of the penis to expose the apical ligament for correction of corkscrew deviation. (C) Exposure of the apical ligament and tunica albuginea for correction of corkscrew deviation.

preservation. Before use, the strip is soaked in normal saline for 30 minutes.[10,27] Carbon fiber material can also be used.[28]

For the surgery, after the penis and prepuce are prepared for aseptic surgery, an incision is made on the dorsal surface of the penis. The incision begins just caudal to where the apical ligament encircles the glans penis and extends to the level just before the point of attachment of the prepuce to the penis. In the proximal portion of the incision, the elastic tissue is incised to expose the apical ligament, which is then divided on midline to expose the tunica albuginea (**Fig. 23**). The autograft is trimmed to fit the dimensions of the exposed tunica albuginea and sutured to it using 2-0 absorbable suture (**Fig. 24**). The apical ligament is sutured with the same suture material and anchored to the autograft (**Fig. 25**). The external surface of the penis is closed with size 0 absorbable suture in a close spaced interrupted suture (**Fig. 26**). The bull is treated similarly to the other surgery and is withheld from service for 60 days.[10,27]

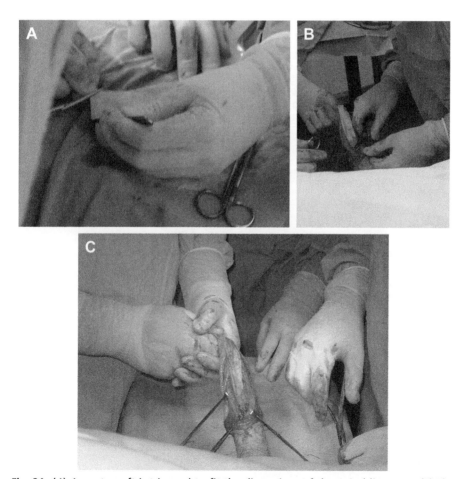

Fig. 24. (*A*) An autograft is trimmed to fit the dimensions of the apical ligament. (*B*) The autograft is sutured to the apical ligament and adjacent tunica albuginea. (*C*) The autograft is anchored to the apical ligament and tunica albuginea with sutures.

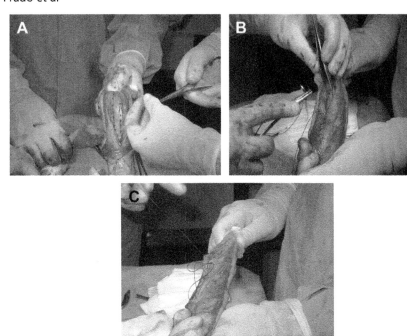

Fig. 25. (*A*) The autograft is anchored to the apical ligament and the tunica albuginea. (*B*) The longitudinal incision exposing the apical ligament is closed with sutures. (*C*) The longitudinal incision in the integument has been closed with sutures.

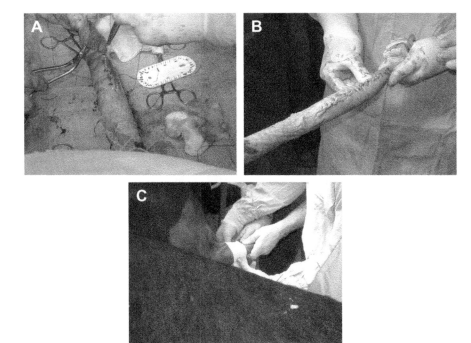

Fig. 26. (*A*) The longitudinal incision in the integument has been closed with sutures. (*B*) The longitudinal incision exposing the apical ligament has been closed completely. (*C*) A bandage is being applied to the sheath to retain the penis and prepuce within the preputial cavity.

Vascular Shunts

Vascular shunts are diagnosed by positive-contrast corpus cavernosography,[6,20,29–31] which is performed by taking serial radiographs of the penis as contrast medium is injected into the corpus cavernosum penis.[6,7,21]

Surgery to resolve a shunt is done by identifying and ligating the shunting vessel with #2-0 absorbable suture at its point of emergence from the corpus cavernosum penis. The ligature should include the superficial layer of the tunica albuginea. If identifying the communicating vessel is difficult, sterile dye, such as methylene blue, can be injected into the corpus cavernosum penis. The communicating vessel is identified as the dye escape from the corpus cavernosum penis. The bull is withheld from service for 30 to 45 days.[20]

Penile–Prepuce Translocation

Teaser bull describes an intact bull whose reproductive tract has been altered surgically to render it sterile and incapable of intromission. Although surgery to create a teaser bull cannot be classified as an elective surgery to restore fertility, a teaser bull is an excellent aid to enhancing fertility of a herd by improving heat detection so that artificial insemination can be better timed.[30]

Surgical procedures used to sterilize a bull are vasectomy or caudal epididymectomy, but neither of these procedures provides protection against transmission of venereal disease.[32–34] Surgical procedures that prevent intromission either allow protrusion, such as with penile–prepuce translocation, or only prevent protrusion, such aspenopexy.[35,36]

Bulls should be selected well before the breeding season to allow time for healing. Also, it is recommended that bull weight less than 272 kg (600 pounds). Large bulls are more difficult to handle and tend to experience more postoperative complications.[35]

Penile–prepuce translocation is the authors' preferred technique. In this procedure, the penis and prepuce are moved from the midline to an area in the left flank. Therefore, the procedure prevents intromission but does not prevent protrusion of the penis. For this reason, in the authors' opinion, bulls seem to maintain libido and function for

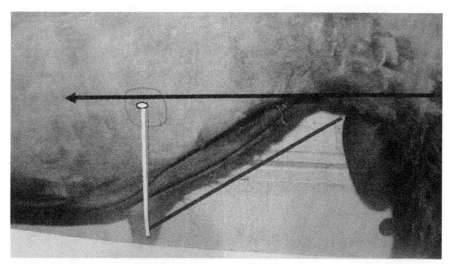

Fig. 27. A mark is made on the left flank, with the bull standing, at the proposed site of the circular incision.

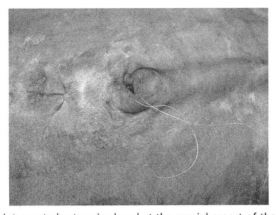

Fig. 28. A simple interrupted suture is placed at the cranial aspect of the preputial orifice.

a longer time than do bulls undergoing procedures that prevent protrusion of the penis.

Penile–prepuce translocation is performed with the bull anesthetized and in dorsal recumbency, but the site to which the preputial orifice is to be moved should be marked while the bull is standing because this site may shift when the bull is in dorsal recumbency. Failure to move the preputial orifice to the intended site may result in the bull being able to gain intromission.[10,35]

The authors mark the site for the circular incision, with the bull standing, by placing a piece of string between the base of the scrotum and the preputial orifice. Then, with the caudal end of the string held stationary at the base of the scrotum, the cranial end of the string is rotated to the left flank to the level of an imaginary horizontal line extending cranially from the left stifle. This site is dorsal to the fold of the left flank (**Fig. 27**).

The ventral aspect of the abdomen and the left flank are prepared for aseptic surgery. A simple interrupted suture is placed at the cranial aspect of the preputial orifice to serve as a reference when transferring the orifice to the left flank (**Fig. 28**). A circular skin incision, 4 cm in diameter, is made around the preputial opening. Then the skin is incised, on the midline from the caudal aspect of the circular incision just cranial to the scrotum. The prepuce is dissected from the abdominal wall, preserving the large blood vessels (**Fig. 29**).

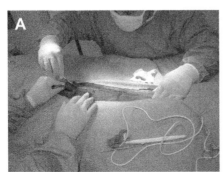
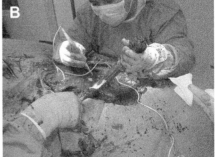

Fig. 29. (*A, B*) The penis and prepuce are dissected from the abdominal wall.

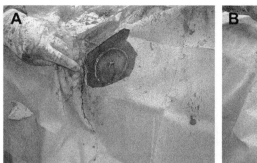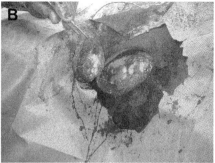

Fig. 30. (*A, B*) A circular incision made at the previously identified location, dorsal to the fold of the left flank.

A circular flank incision, the radius of which is similar to that of the incision encircling the preputial orifice, is made at the previously identified location, dorsal to the fold of the left flank (**Fig. 30**). The skin within the circular incision is excised, and a subcutaneous tunnel is created between the caudal end of the incision on the midline and the circular incision above the fold of the flank using a long sponge forceps or Knowles cervical forceps. The tunnel is enlarged to a size sufficient to accommodate the prepuce and penis without restriction by opening the jaws of the forceps. A sterile plastic sleeve is placed over the penis and prepuce and pulled through the tunnel (**Fig. 31**).

The subcutaneous tissue on the ventral midline is apposed with absorbable suture placed in a simple continuous pattern. The skin incision is closed using nonabsorbable suture inserted in a continuous Ford interlocking pattern. The circular portion of the wound on the midline is left unsutured. Using the previously placed skin suture as a guide, the cranial edge of the preputial orifice is aligned with the cranial edge of the circular flank incision, and the circular section of skin surrounding the preputial orifice is sutured to circular flank incision in 2 layers. The subcutaneous tissues are apposed with simple interrupted absorbable sutures, and the skin is apposed with a simple interrupted nonabsorbable sutures (**Fig. 32**). Bilateral caudal epididymectomy is performed before the bull is allowed to recover from anesthesia. The bull is treated after surgery as for other surgery of the penis and prepuce, and is withheld from service for 45 days.[10,35–38]

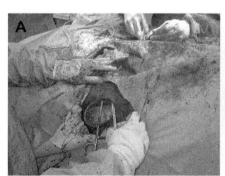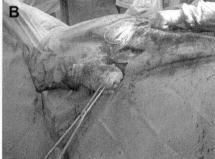

Fig. 31. (*A*) A tunnel is created between the caudal end of the midline incision and the circular incision. (*B*) The penis and prepuce are pulled through the tunnel.

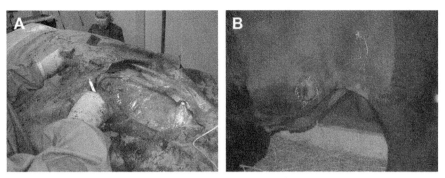

Fig. 32. (*A*) The ventral midline and circular incisions are closed in 2 layers with sutures. (*B*) The position of the preputial orifice after penile translocation.

SURGERY OF THE EPIDIDYMIS AND TESTES
Caudal Epididymectomy

For surgery, hair is clipped from the ventral aspect of the scrotum, the scrotum is scrubbed for aseptic surgery, and the site of incision is infiltrated with local anesthetic solution. The surgeon grasps the neck of the scrotum over 1 testis, forcing the testis ventrally. A 2-cm skin incision is made directly over the tail of the epididymis parallel to the scrotal raphe. The incision is extended through the common vaginal tunic to expose the tail of the epididymis. With dissection, the tail of the epididymis is freed from the testis and grasped with an Allis tissue forceps to exteriorize it. The deferent duct and the body of

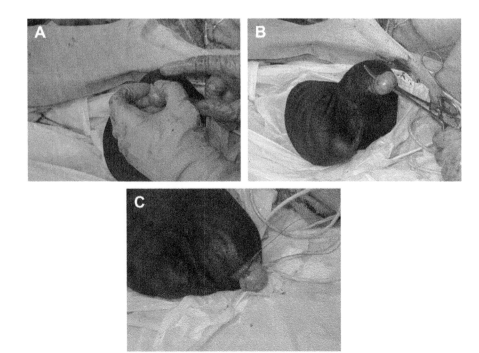

Fig. 33. (*A–C*) Caudal epididymectomy.

the epididymis are clamped with a hemostat to place a nonabsorbable suture around the epididymis proximal to each clamp; then the tail of the epididymis, which is the section between the clamps, is excised using scissors (**Fig. 33**). This procedure is repeated on the contralateral epididymis. The common vaginal tunic and the skin incision on the scrotum can be sutured or left unsutured to heal by second intention.[10,34–38]

Cryptorchidism

Bulls affected with cryptorchidism should not be used for breeding because cryptorchidism may be heritable. The undescended testis can be found within the abdomen, inguinal canal, or most commonly, subcutaneously in the inguinal region, which is termed an ectopic testis. The ectopic testis can be found on either side of the penis 15 to 30 cm cranial to the base of the scrotum and oriented with the long axis parallel to the penis.[39] Most affected bulls are affected unilaterally.

To remove an ectopic testis, an incision is made directly over the testis, the testis is exteriorized, and the spermatic cord is transected with scissors, after applying a transfixation ligature to the cord, or with an emasculator.[39] The descended testis is removed through a scrotal incision, and both surgical wounds are left unsutured to heal by second intention.

A retained abdominal testis can be removed through an inguinal, parainguinal, suprapubic paramedian, or flank approach. For each of these approaches, except the flank approach, the bull must be anesthetized. The authors prefer the parainguinal approach.[40]

Because cryptorchidism occurs much less commonly in bulls than in other domesticated mammals, in this article we refer to the equine reference because the procedure in the bull is identical to the stallion procedure.[40]

Unilateral orchidectomy

Trauma, inguinal herniation, torsion of the spermatic cord, unilateral hydrocele, hematocele, testicular neoplasia, and epididymitis or orchitis are all reasons for unilateral orchidectomy (**Fig. 34**). The swelling associated with inflammation and thrombosis of blood vessels of the testis accelerates the degeneration.[19,41] Medical treatments are often unsuccessful in returning the testis to normal function, and disease of one testis can cause temperature-induced dysfunction of spermatogenesis of the other testis that can result in permanent dysfunction of the nondiseased testis.

Unilateral orchiectomy is performed with the bull anesthetized and in lateral recumbency. The testis to be removed should be uppermost. The uppermost hind limb is abducted and secured, and the scrotum is prepared for aseptic surgery. An

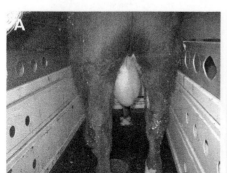 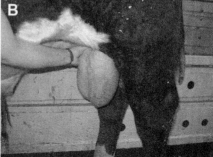

Fig. 34. (*A, B*) A bull with a hematocele of the left testis.

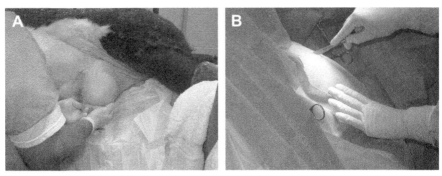

Fig. 35. (A) A bull in right lateral recumbency being prepared for aseptic excision of the testis as treatment for hematocele of the left testis. (B) A longitudinal incision in made in the scrotum over the left testis.

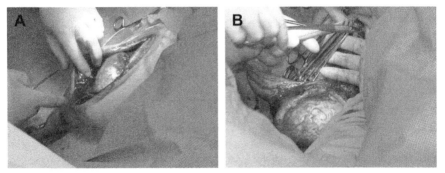

Fig. 36. (A) The diseased testis is dissected from surrounding fascia. (B) The vasculature and ductus deferens of the spermatic cord are double ligated and transected distal to the distal ligature.

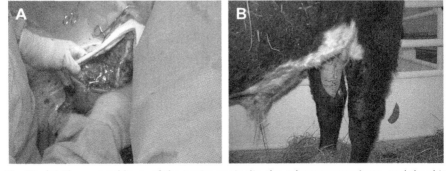

Fig. 37. (A) The parietal layer of the tunica vaginalis, the subcutaneous tissue, and the skin are closed separately with sutures. (B) The skin incision has been sutured.

elliptical incision is made over the entire length of the lateral aspect of that part of the scrotum overlying the diseased testis (**Fig. 35**). Removing a large portion of the scrotum with the elliptical incision decreases dead space when the incision is closed, thus decreasing the likelihood of formation of seroma. The testis, enclosed within the vaginal tunic, is dissected bluntly from surrounding fascia. The spermatic cord is double-ligated and transected using an emasculator (**Fig. 36**). The vaginal tunic, scrotal fascia, and subcutaneous tissues are closed separately using absorbable suture in a simple continuous suture pattern, and the scrotal skin is closed with an intradermal suture pattern using absorbable suture (**Fig. 37**).[41,42]

SURGERY OF THE ACCESSORY SEX GLANDS
Seminal Vesiculitis

Medical treatment for vesiculitis entails long-term antibiotic therapy, under the assumption that the cause is bacterial. Treated bulls often improve during treatment only to relapse after the course of therapy has been completed. Culling of affected bulls is usually the most cost-effective approach.[8,43]

Surgical removal of diseased glands is difficult, and for this reason the authors do not describe it in this article. The method for surgical correction has been described elsewhere.[43]

REFERENCES

1. Mosaheb MF, Ladds AH, Ladds PW. The pathology of the external genitalia of bulls in Northern Australia. Aust Vet J 1973;49:512–6.
2. Spitzer JC, Hopkins FM, Webster HW, et al. Breeding soundness examination of yearling beef bulls. J Am Vet Med Assoc 1988;193:1075–9.
3. Elmore RG. Food-animal regional anesthesia: bovine blocks: internal pudendal (pubic) nerve block. Vet Med Small Anim Clin 1980;75(9):1432–8.
4. Mickelsen WD, Weber JA, Memon MA. Use of transrectal ultrasound for the detection of seminal vesiculitis in a bull. Vet Rec 1994;135:14–5.
5. Anderson DE, St Jean G, Desrochers A, et al. Use of Doppler ultrasonography and positive-contrast corpus cavernosography to evaluate a persistent penile hematoma in a bull. J Am Vet Med Assoc 1996;209:1611–4.
6. Moll HD, Wolfe DF, Hathcock JT. Cavernosography for diagnosis of erection failure in bulls. Compend Contin Educ 1983;15:1160–4.
7. Wolfe DF, Moll HD. Examination and special diagnostic procedures of the penis and prepuce. In: Wolfe DF, Moll HD, editors. Large animal urogenital surgery. 2nd edition. Philadelphia: Williams and Wilkins; 1998. p. 226.
8. Linhart RD, Parker WG. Seminal vesiculitis in bulls. Compend Contin Educ Pract Vet 1988;10:1427–32.
9. Cavalieri J, Van Camp SD. Bovine seminal vesiculitis. A review and update. Vet Clin North Am Food Anim Pract 1997;13:233–41.
10. Morgan G. Surgical correction of abnormalities of the reproductive organs of bulls and preparation of teaser animals. In: Youngquist RB, Threlfall WR, editors. Current therapy in large animal theriogenology. 2nd edition. St Louis (MO): Saunders Elsevier; 2007. p. 243–52.
11. Anderson DE. Surgery of the prepuce and penis. Vet Clin North Am Food Anim Pract 2008;24:245–51.
12. Kasari TR, McGrann JM, Hooper RN. Cost-effectiveness analysis of treatment alternatives for beef bulls with preputial prolapse. J Am Vet Med Assoc 1997; 211:856–9.

13. Memon MA, Dawson LJ, Usenik EA, et al. Preputial injuries in beef bulls: 172 cases (1980–1985). J Am Vet Med Assoc 1988;193:481–5.
14. Chenoweth PJ, Osborne HG. Breed differences in abnormalities of the reproductive organs of young beef bulls. Aust Vet J 1978;54:463–8.
15. Hardin DK, Bierschwal CJ. Management of preputial injuries in the bull. Bovine Clin 1984;4:7–8.
16. Desrochers A, St Jean G, Anderson DE. Surgical management of preputial injuries in bulls: 51 cases (1986-1994). Can Vet J 1995;36:553–6.
17. Baxter GM, Allen D, Wallace CE. Breeding soundness of beef bulls after circumcision: 33 cases (1980–1986). J Am Vet Med Assoc 1989;194:948–52.
18. Armstrong CL, Wolfe DW, Koziol JH, et al. Preputial stoma: a novel surgical approach for semen collection in bulls with phimosis due to preputial stenosis; three cases (2007–2014). Clin Theriogenol 2015;7:419–23.
19. Hopkins FM. Diseases of the reproductive system of the bull. In: Youngquist RS, Threlfall WR, editors. Current therapy in large animal theriogenology. 2nd edition. St Louis (MO): Saunders Elsevier; 2007. p. 240–3.
20. Gilbert RO. Penile surgery. In: Fubinl SL, Ducharme NG, editors. Farm animal surgery. St Louis (MO): Saunders; 2004. p. 366–74.
21. Ashdown RR, Glossop CE. Impotence in the bull: (3) rupture of the corpus cavernosum penis proximal to the sigmoid flexure. Vet Rec 1983;113:30–7.
22. Wolfe DF, Mysinger PW, Hudson RS, et al. Ventral rupture of the penile tunica albuginea and urethra distal to the sigmoid flexure in a bull. J Am Vet Med Assoc 1987;190:1313–4.
23. Pearson H. Surgery of the male genital tract in cattle: a review of 121 cases. Vet Rec 1972;91:498–509.
24. Walker DF. Penile surgery in the bovine: part II. Mod Vet Pract 1979;60:931–4.
25. Musser JMB, St Jean G, Vestweber JG, et al. Penile hematoma in bulls: 60 cases (1979-1990). J Am Vet Med Assoc 1992;201:1416–8.
26. Wolfe DF, Beckett SD, Carson RL. Acquired conditions of the penis and prepuce. In: Wolfe DF, Moll HD, editors. Large animal urogenital surgery. 2nd edition. Baltimore (MD): Williams and Williams; 1998. p. 237–72.
27. Walker DF, Young SL. The fascia lata implant technique for correcting bovine penile deviations. Proc Soc Theriogenol 1979;99–102.
28. Mobile S, Walker DF, Crowley RR. An experimental evaluation of the response of the bull penis to carbon fiber implants. Cornell Vet 1982;72:350–60.
29. Young SL, Hudson RS, Walker DF. Impotence in bulls due to vascular shunts from the corpus cavernosum penis. J Am Vet Med Assoc 1977;171:643–8.
30. Ashdown RR, David JSE, Gibbs C. Impotence in the bull: (1) abnormal venous drainage of the corpus cavernosum penis. Vet Rec 1979;104:423.
31. Wolfe DF, Hudson RS, Walker DF. Failure of penile erection due to vascular shunt from corpus cavernosum penis to the corpus spongiosum penis in a bull. J Am Vet Med Assoc 1984;184:1511–2.
32. O'Connor ML. Estrus detection. In: Youngquist RS, Threlfall WR, editors. Current therapy in large animal theriogenology. 2nd edition. St Louis (MO): Saunders; 2007. p. 270–8.
33. Smith DR. Estrus detection. In: Morrow DA, editor. Current therapy in theriogenology. 2nd edition. St Louis (MO): Saunders; 1986. p. 153–8.
34. Claxton MS. Methods of surgical preparation of teaser bulls. Compend Contin Educ Pract Vet 1989;11:974–81.
35. Morgan GL, Dawson LJ. Development of teaser bulls under field conditions. Vet Clin North Am Food Anim Pract 2008;24:443–53.

36. Riddell MG. Prevention of intromission by estrus-detector males. In: Wolfe DF, Moll HD, editors. Large animal urogenital surgery. 2nd edition. Baltimore (MD): Williams and Williams; 1998. p. 335–43.
37. Hendrickson DA. Techniques in large animal surgery. 3rd edition. Ames (IA): Blackwell Publishing; 2007.
38. Gill MS. Surgical techniques for preparation of teaser bulls. Vet Clin North Am Food Anim Pract 2008;24:123–35.
39. Riddell MG. Developmental anomalies of the scrotum and testis. In: Wolfe DF, Moll HD, editors. Large animal urogenital surgery. 2nd edition. Baltimore (MD): Williams and Williams; 1998. p. 283–94.
40. Brinsko SP, Blanchard TL, Varner DD, et al. Manual of equine reproduction. 3rd edition. Maryland Heights (MO): Mosby Elsevier; 2011.
41. Gilbert RO. Surgery of the male reproductive tract. In: Fubini SL, Ducharme NG, editors. Farm animal surgery. St Louis (MO): Saunders; 2004. p. 351–9.
42. Ewoldt JM. Surgery of the scrotum. Vet Clin North Am Food Anim Pract 2008;24: 253–66.
43. Wolfe DF. Accessory sex gland. In: Wolfe DF, Moll HD, editors. Large animal urogenital surgery. 2nd edition. Baltimore (MD): Williams and Williams; 1998. p. 321–5.

Surgical Procedures of the Genital Organs of Cows

Tulio M. Prado, DVM, MS[a],*, Jim Schumacher, DVM, MS[a], Lionel J. Dawson, BVSc, MS[b]

KEYWORDS

- Bovine • Cow • Surgery • Genitalia • Fertility

KEY POINTS

- Injuries affecting the reproductive tract of cows can cause pathologic changes that result in substantial economic and genetic losses to beef or dairy producers.
- Cows with conformational abnormality of the genitalia are candidates for reproductive surgery if the results of a breeding soundness examination indicate that the procedure is likely to restore fertility.
- Different surgical techniques are commonly used by practitioners/clinicians of theriogenology to treat and restore fertility, which preserves genetic potential and economic productivity for the owner.

PRESURGICAL CONSIDERATIONS
History

Most abnormalities of the reproductive tract causing infertility are easily diagnosed from the cow's history and physical examination. The history should include the cow's current reproductive status, prior drug therapy, behavioral changes, conception rates, duration of the condition, previous injuries or illnesses, and prior treatments and urogenital surgery performed. Information may also include any incidence of abortion, twinning, dystocia, and neonatal death.

Examination of the Genital Organs of the Cow

Findings during physical examination are the most helpful indicators for surgically correcting abnormalities of the reproductive tract causing infertility. The general conformation of the perineum, vulvar seal integrity, and shape of the perineal body should be evaluated visually.

Disclosure: The authors have nothing to disclose.
[a] Department of Large Animal Clinical Sciences, College of Veterinary Medicine, University of Tennessee, 2407 River Drive, Knoxville, TN 37996, USA; [b] Veterinary Clinical Sciences, Center for Veterinary Health Sciences, Oklahoma State University, 2065 West Farm Road, Stillwater, OK 74078, USA
* Corresponding author.
E-mail address: tprado@utk.edu

Vet Clin Food Anim 32 (2016) 727–752
http://dx.doi.org/10.1016/j.cvfa.2016.05.016   vetfood.theclinics.com
0749-0720/16/$ – see front matter © 2016 Elsevier Inc. All rights reserved.

Vaginal examinations are performed with a speculum with a light source. The perineum should be washed before the speculum is inserted, and an epidural anesthesia is indicated. The vulvar lips are parted, and the lubricated speculum is introduced into the vestibule and directed dorsocranially, avoiding the external urethral orifice. It is passed through the vestibule and redirected horizontally into the vaginal vault (**Fig. 1**).

Digital palpation of the vagina and cervix is an important part of the genital examination (**Fig. 2**). Palpation and ultrasonographic examination of the reproductive organs are important means of evaluating the reproductive tract (**Fig. 3**).

Other tools to evaluate the reproductive tract include vaginoscopy, endometrial cytology, hysteroscopy, and reproductive hormonal profile. Karyotyping is indicated when infertility cannot be explained.

Abnormalities that can be corrected by reconstructive surgery to restore fertility include the following:

- Pneumovagina: accumulation of air in the vagina
- Urovagina: pooling of the urine in the cranial vagina
- Perineal injury: caused by fetal malposture during calving
- Cervical lacerations: caused by insufficient dilation of the cervix during parturition

Surgical procedures on the reproductive tract (with the exceptions of cesarean section, uterine torsion, vaginal and uterine eversions, and ovariectomy) are performed to correct urogenital abnormalities. This article discusses the most common surgical procedures performed to correct vulvar and vestibular abnormalities, as well as vaginal and uterine eversions and ovariectomy. Readers should refer to veterinary surgical texts for more detailed descriptions of these and other surgical procedures involving the reproductive tract of the cow.[1,2]

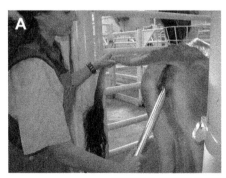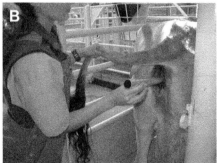

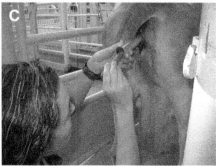

Fig. 1. (*A*) Inserting a vaginal speculum through the labia. (*B*) The speculum is repositioned horizontally to enter the vagina. (*C*) The vagina and cervix are observed through the speculum.

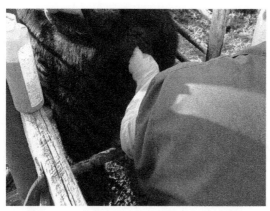

Fig. 2. A digital vaginal examination.

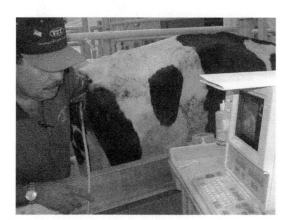

Fig. 3. Transrectal palpation and ultrasonographic examination.

Surgery of the Vestibule, Vagina, and Cervix

Episiotomy

Episiotomy is indicated to prevent tearing of the dorsal commissure of the vulva and of the vestibule when there is an oversized fetus or inadequate relaxation/stenosis of the caudal aspect of the birth canal. Using a scalpel, an incision is made at the 2 or 10 o'clock position of the labia. This location is chosen to avoid extending the incision into the rectum. The incision begins on the skin at the mucocutaneous edge of the labia and extends dorsolaterally; 8 to 10 cm should be sufficient to allow delivery of the fetus without tearing of the vestibule (**Fig. 4**). Desensitizing the perineum before performing an episiotomy is not necessary because the vulva is insensitive during the second stage of labor. However, to close the wound after delivery, the site of episiotomy must be desensitized by administering epidural anesthesia. The incision is closed after the fetus has been delivered using an absorbable suture material to eliminate the need for suture removal (**Fig. 5**).[3,4] The mucosal portion of the incision is left to heal by second intention.

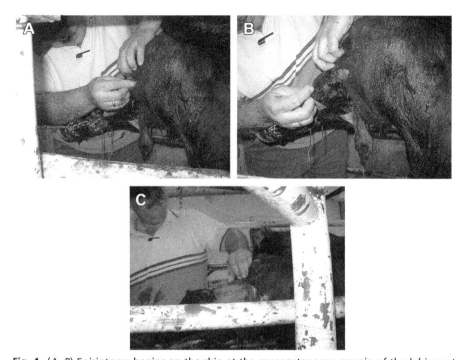

Fig. 4. (*A, B*) Episiotomy begins on the skin at the mucocutaneous margin of the labium at the 2:00 or 10:00 o'clock position. Length and depth should be sufficient to allow delivery of the fetus. (*C*) Delivery of the calf after episiotomy.

Pneumovagina

The surgical procedure used most commonly to correct pneumovagina is the Caslick vulvoplasty, in which the labia are sutured together from the dorsal commissure to slightly below the floor of the ischium after a strip of tissue has been excised from the mucocutaneous margin of each labium. The procedure in the cow is identical to that in the mare (**Fig. 6**).[5]

A Caslick vulvoplasty may be insufficient to correct pneumovagina when the vulva has deviated far cranially and dorsally.

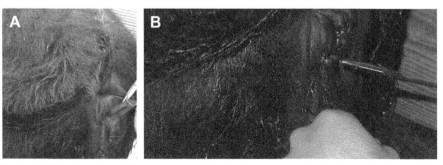

Fig. 5. (*A*) Suturing the episiotomy, using absorbable suture, after the fetus has been delivered. (*B*) The episiotomy has been closed completely with sutures.

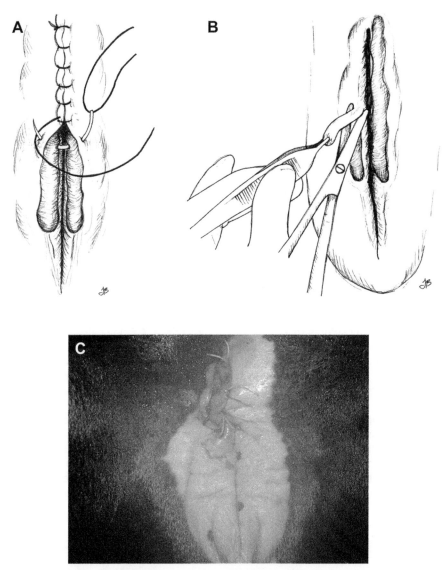

Fig. 6. (A) Trimming the mucocutaneous margins of the labia in preparation for Caslick vulvoplasty. (B) Caslick vulvoplasty using an interlocking Ford suture pattern. (C) A completed Caslick vulvoplasty. (From Dawson LJ, Peter AT. An update on vaginal and uterine eversions in cattle. Clin Theriogenol 2012;4:115; with permission.)

Urovagina

Urine pooling is less commonly observed in the cow than in the mare, perhaps because, when a cow becomes infertile for any reason, including urovagina, the cow is usually culled without investigation of the problem causing the infertility.[6,7]

Urine pooling in cows can often be resolved with urethral extension surgery. A procedure in mares has been modified and adapted for use in cows.[8,9] Feed and hay are

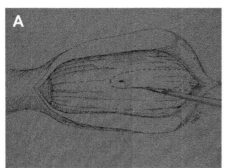
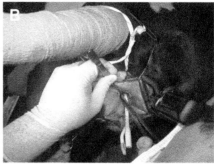

Fig. 7. (*A*) U-shaped mucosal dissection for creating a urethral extension. (*B*) Mucosal dissection for creating a urethral extension. (*From* St Jean G, Hull BL, Robertson JT, et al. Urethral extension for correction of urovagina in cattle. A review of 14 cases. Vet Surg 1988;17:258–62; with permission.)

withheld for 30 hours, and water for 12 hours. The cow should stand in a squeeze chute and caudal epidural is administered. The tail is wrapped and tied dorsally to the crossbar of the chute, and feces are removed from the rectum. A tampon made from a 75-mm (3-inch) stockinet filled with cotton gauze is placed into the rectum to prevent defecation. The perineal area is prepared for surgery and the vulvar lips retracted with stay sutures to expose the urethral orifice. A Foley catheter is inserted into the bladder and the cuff inflated. A U-shaped mucosal incision is made on the floor and sides of the vestibule with the apex centered 1 cm cranial to the urethral orifice (**Fig. 7**). The branches of the U are extended caudally to a point approximately 2 cm cranial to the labia; on the labia, the arms of the incision are aimed to a point midway between the dorsal ventral commissure of the labia. The right and left ventral edges of the mucosal incision are dissected ventrally, and the right and left dorsal edges of the incision are dissected dorsally until right and left dorsal and ventral shelves are created that are of sufficient width to allow apposition separately over the urinary catheter without tension. The right and left ventral shelves are apposed using 2-0 absorbable suture in a continuous Lembert suture pattern (**Fig. 8**). The dorsal shelves are apposed with the same suture in a continuous horizontal mattress pattern (**Fig. 9**). These

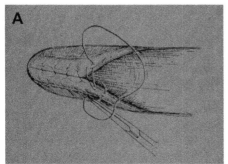
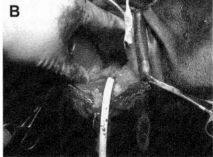

Fig. 8. (*A*) Suturing the right and left ventral shelves to create a urethral extension. (*B*) The first layer of a urethral extension has been completed. (*From* St Jean G, Hull BL, Robertson JT, et al. Urethral extension for correction of urovagina in cattle. A review of 14 cases. Vet Surg 1988;17:258–62; with permission.)

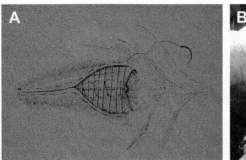 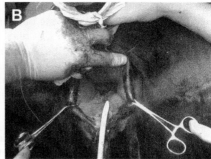

Fig. 9. (*A*) Apposition of the dorsal shelves to complete the urethral extension. (*B*) The completed urethral extension. Dorsal and ventral shelves have been apposed. (*From* St Jean G, Hull BL, Robertson JT, et al. Urethral extension for correction of urovagina in cattle. A review of 14 cases. Vet Surg 1988;17:258–62; with permission.)

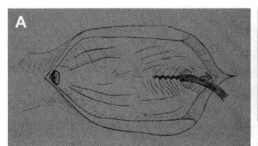 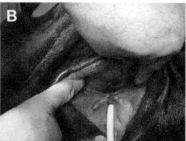

Fig. 10. (*A*) The urethral extension extending from the urethral orifice to near the labia. (*B*) The completed urethral extension. (*From* St Jean G, Hull BL, Robertson JT, et al. Urethral extension for correction of urovagina in cattle. A review of 14 cases. Vet Surg 1988;17:258–62; with permission.)

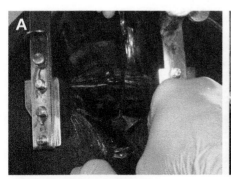 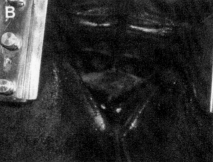

Fig. 11. (*A*) Dyeing the vestibular mucosa with methylene blue. (*B*) Staining the vestibular mucosa helps distinguish between vestibular mucosa and submucosal tissue.

shelves create a tube of vaginal mucosa extending from the urethral orifice to the labia (**Fig. 10**). The same technique has been used in a llama with urine pooling.[10]

To differentiate between mucosa and submucosa, the authors dye the mucosa of the vestibule by dispersing a small amount of 1% new methylene blue dye throughout the vestibule (**Fig. 11**).[11] A Foley catheter is left in situ for 24 hours, and the cow is observed to ensure that it is able to void urine. A modified surgical technique to correct urine pooling in the cow has also been reported.[8]

Rectovestibular laceration and fistula

A perineal laceration or fistula occurs at parturition when the calf's foot or nose catches the annular fold of the hymen at the vaginovestibular junction.[12]

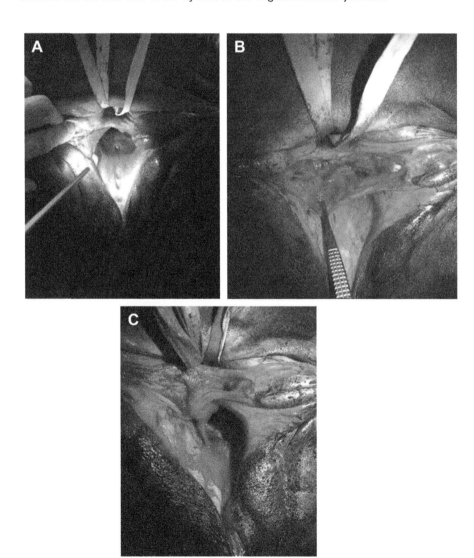

Fig. 12. (*A*) Third-degree perineal laceration of a cow. (*B*) Rectovestibular stage of third-degree perineal body repair. (*C*) Anoperineal stage of third-degree perineal body repair.

A first-degree perineal laceration involves only the skin and mucous membrane of the dorsum of the vestibule. A second-degree perineal laceration is characterized by disruption of the constrictor vulvae muscle, compromising the ability of the perineal musculature to constrict the vestibule. A third-degree perineal laceration is characterized by a complete disruption of tissue between the rectum and vestibule, resulting in a common rectal and vestibular vault. A rectovestibular fistula occurs when the tissue between the rectum and vestibule is perforated by the calf, but the malposture of the calf is corrected before the calf is delivered, allowing at least a portion of the perineal body to remain intact. Cows with a first-degree perineal laceration can be treated with a Caslick vulvoplasty, but cows with a second-degree perineal laceration require a vestibuloplasty because the constrictor vulvae muscle is disrupted, causing the perineum to sink, predisposing the cow to pneumovagina and urovagina. An attempt to repair a perineal laceration immediately after injury is unsuccessful because the lacerated tissue soon becomes inflamed and contaminated with feces and other debris.

A third-degree perineal laceration is performed in a manner similar to that described for mares with a laceration and is composed of 2 stages: rectovestibular reconstruction and anoperineal reconstruction using a 6-bite suture pattern.[13] When performing the rectovestibular stage of repair, the authors prefer that the dissection between the rectal and the vaginal submucosa is extended for several centimeters cranial to the tear to enable placement of sutures that invert vaginal submucosa and mucosa into the vaginal lumen and rectal submucosa into the rectal lumen, thereby relieving tension on more caudally placed sutures that oppose the rectal and vestibular shelves; this, in turn, decreases the likelihood of a fistula forming at the cranial aspect of the repair (**Fig. 12**).

Vaginal eversion

Prepartum vaginal or cervical eversion should be replaced and secured promptly before contamination, laceration, sepsis, fibrosis, and necrosis ensue.[14] Producers should be educated to seek veterinary assistance. Many techniques of preventing vaginal or cervical eversion after the eversion has been corrected have proved to be effective, and the technique chosen depends on the condition of the everted tissue. However, better techniques for resolving chronic vaginal eversion are still needed.[15,16]

Some treatments prevent recurrence by narrowing the birth canal by creating adhesions between the retroperitoneal surface of the vagina and adjacent structures.[17,18] Considering the suffering the cow may endure because of the eversion and

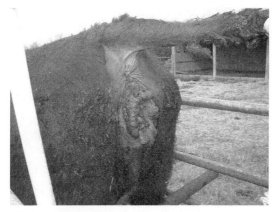

Fig. 13. Grade 1 vaginal eversion.

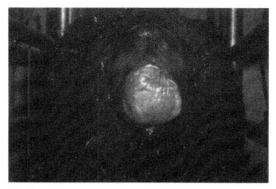

Fig. 14. Grade 2 vaginal eversion.

subsequent eversions, and considering the hereditary nature of the problem, veterinarians should strongly suggest removing affected cows from the herd.

Vaginal eversions are classified into 4 grades, according to the severity of eversion and the extent of injury[15,19–23]:

- Grade 1 eversion (**Fig. 13**): a small area of the vaginal mucosa protrudes intermittently through the vulvar lips when the cow lies down. Often, this tissue becomes dehydrated and traumatized, leading to other grades of severity.

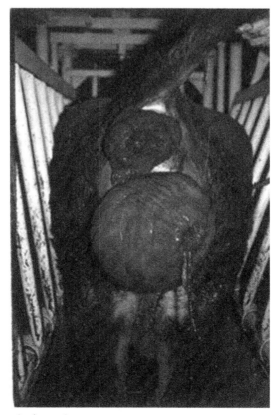

Fig. 15. Grade 3 vaginal eversion.

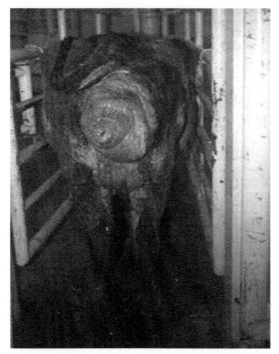

Fig. 16. Grade 4a vaginal eversion.

- Grade 2 eversion (**Fig. 14**): the vaginal mucosa protrudes through the vulvar lips continuously, and occasionally the urinary bladder becomes trapped within the everted vagina. If left untreated, grade 2 eversion quickly progresses to a grade 3 eversion.
- Grade 3 eversion (**Fig. 15**): the entire vaginal mucosa and cervix protrude continuously through the vulvar lips, and the urinary bladder is entrapped within the everted tissue. The exposed cervical seal may liquefy, allowing bacterial contamination of the uterus, placentitis, and death of the fetus.
- Grade 4a eversion (**Fig. 16**): often referred to as cervical eversion or cervicovaginal eversion. This terminology distinguishes it from eversion of the cervix alone, as is observed in *Bos indicus* breeds (**Fig. 17**). In eversion of the cervix alone, only the cervix everts as a pedunculated mass through the vulva.

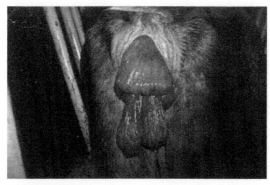

Fig. 17. Eversion of the cervix alone.

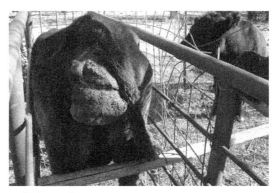

Fig. 18. Grade 4b vaginal eversion.

- Grade 4b eversion (**Fig. 18**): the cervicovaginal eversion persists for such a duration that the entire vaginal mucosa appears necrotic and fibrotic. Infection may become so extensive that the urinary bladder becomes necrotic and septic peritonitis may ensue.[21,22]

The primary objectives of treatment of a pregnant cow for vaginal eversion are to replace and retain the vagina within the pelvic canal and to deliver and wean a live calf. The management and treatment options can be placed in 2 general categories: those designed to supply only a temporary solution and those designed to achieve permanent reduction or treatment. Permanent treatment such as Minchey or modified Minchey vaginopexy, and Winkler cervicopexy are rarely performed by practitioners. However, a commercial kit (JorVet Prolapse Kit; Jorgenson Labs, Loveland, CO) is available to simplify the Minchey and modified Minchey vaginopexy.

The treatment selected may need to be abandoned if a complication to that treatment, such as tenesmus, develops. If the cow is close to parturition, the most sensible treatment may be to induce parturition.

Short-term options

Caslick vulvoplasty A Caslick vulvoplasty should be reserved only for cows with a nonirritated, grade 1 vaginal eversion that are close to parturition and not expected to develop tenesmus (**Fig. 19**). Caslick vulvoplasty, in many cases, is insufficient to retain the vaginal mucosa within the pelvic canal. The cow may develop tenesmus, causing disruption of the sutured tissue and protrusion of vaginal mucosa ventral to

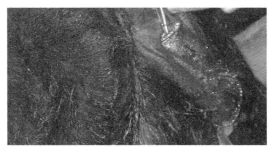

Fig. 19. Caslick suture being applied to a nonpregnant cow with grade 1 eversion.

the sutured portion of the labia. Embryo donor cows, which are frequently superstimulated with hormones, are the best candidates for Caslick vulvoplasty as a treatment of vaginal eversion.[24]

Insertion of a perivulvar retention stitch (Buhner stitch) Insertion of a perivulvar retention stitch (ie, Buhner stitch) is an effective treatment of cows with an eversion more advanced than grade 1.[25–27] The incisions must be deep so that the suture is placed as cranial to the labia as possible. The disadvantage of the Buhner stitch is that the cow needs assistance at parturition, or the vulva may be traumatized, or the cow may be unable to deliver the calf.

To insert a perivulvar retention suture, the perineum is desensitized by administering epidural anesthesia, the vulva is washed with an antiseptic soap, and a 1-cm vertical stab incision is made on the perineal raphe distal to the vulva. A second incision is made midway between the anus and dorsal commissure of the vulva. A long straight needle, such as the Buhner needle, is inserted deeply at the ventral incision and directed dorsally around one side of the vulva and through the dorsal incision. Tape, such as umbilical tape or nonwicking nylon tape, is passed through the eye of the needle, and the needle is retracted through the ventral incision, along with the tape.

The procedure is repeated on the contralateral side of the vulva, and the 2 exposed ends of the suture encircling the vulva are tied together, leaving about a 2-finger-sized opening in the ventral aspect vulva for escape of urine. The strands of suture should be tied in such a manner that the knot can be undone (**Fig. 20**). The knot

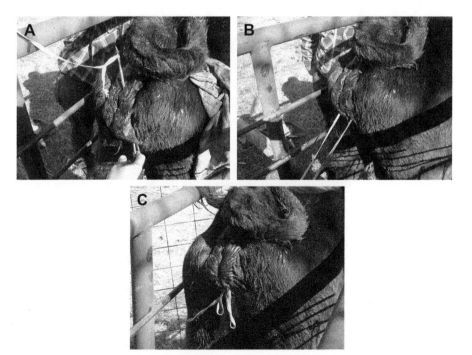

Fig. 20. (*A*) Insertion of a Buhner needle to treat a cow for vaginal eversion. (*B*) The Buhner tape encircles the labia. (*C*) Complete Buhner suture.

can be undone in anticipation of parturition but can be retied if the cow reprolapses before parturition.[28]

Bootlace technique This technique is more likely to result in retention of the vagina than is a Caslick vulvoplasty. To perform the bootlace technique, the perineum is desensitized by administering epidural anesthesia, the vulva is cleansed with an antiseptic soap, and 4 to 5 small eyelets composed of umbilical tape or hog nose rings are inserted along each side of the vulva at the junction of the haired and hairless margin of the perineum.[15] Umbilical or Buhner tape is laced through the eyelets, much like shoelaces are laced in a boot. As the tape is tightened, the labia tend to invert into the vulva, disrupting the labial seal. As when using a perivaginal suture, the tape must be untied before the cow calves to avoid serious trauma to the cow's vulva (**Fig. 21**).

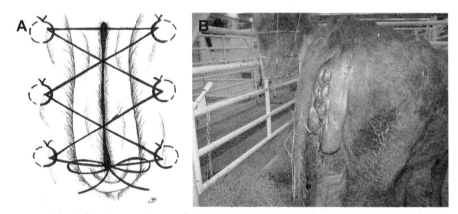

Fig. 21. (*A*) The bootlace technique for retaining a vaginal prolapse. (*B*) Bootlace technique applied to cow to retain a prolapsed vagina. (*From* Dawson LJ, Peter AT. An update on vaginal and uterine eversions in cattle. Clin Theriogenol 2012;4:115; with permission.)

Horizontal mattress suture (Halstead) technique For this technique, a suture needle and suture are passed deeply through the base of the dorsal aspect of the labium across the vulvar cleft and through the base of the contralateral labium. The needle is then passed back through the labia, in the same plane, about 2 to 3 cm ventral to the first strand. The size of the vulvar opening is decreased by inserting more interrupted horizontal mattress sutures ventral to the first suture, leaving a 2-finger-sized opening in the ventral aspect of the vulva for escape of urine.

The disadvantage of this technique is that vulvar edema frequently develops even when the sutures are tightened only moderately. Dispersing tension with stents helps avoid excessive edema. Two 13-mm (half-inch) pieces of polyvinyl chloride (PVC) tubing or wooden dowels, each cut the length of the vulva and containing holes drilled 2 to 3 cm apart, can be used as stents.[28] A piece is placed on each side of the vulva, and the horizontal mattress sutures are passed through the holes

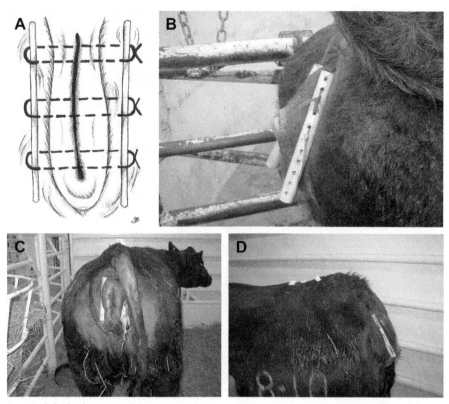

Fig. 22. (*A*) The horizontal mattress technique to retain a vaginal prolapse. Note the location of the stents. They are applied to disperse pressure exerted by the suture. (*B*) Horizontal mattress sutures to retain a prolapsed vagina. By placing sutures through a PVC pipe, pressure exerted by the sutures is dispersed. (*C*) Horizontal mattress sutures to retain a prolapsed vagina. By placing sutures through PVC pipe, pressure exerted by the sutures is dispersed. (*D*) Horizontal mattress sutures to retain a prolapsed vagina. By placing sutures through PVC pipe, pressure exerted by the sutures is dispersed. (*From* Dawson LJ, Peter AT. An update on vaginal and uterine eversions in cattle. Clin Theriogenol 2012;4:115; with permission.)

before being passed through tissue (**Fig. 22**). Latex tubing can also be used as stents. As with other methods of retaining the vagina within the pelvic canal, the sutures must be untied before the cow calves to avoid serious trauma to the cow's vulva.

Deep vertical mattress suture technique This technique is similar to the horizontal mattress suture technique described earlier and differs only in that vertical mattress sutures, rather than horizontal mattress sutures, are used to decrease the size of the vulvar opening. Stents, as described earlier for use with horizontal mattress sutures, can be used to disperse tension on the vulva (**Fig. 23**).

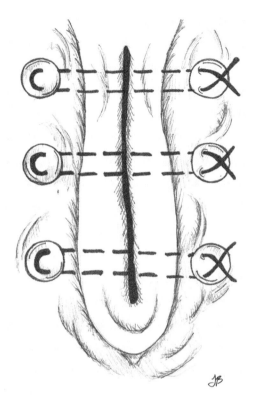

Fig. 23. The deep vertical mattress technique to retain a prolapsed vagina. Buttons are used as a stent instead of PVC pipe. (*From* Dawson LJ, Peter AT. An update on vaginal and uterine eversions in cattle. Clin Theriogenol 2012;4:115; with permission.)

Surgery of the Uterus and Ovaries

Uterine eversion

The incidence of mortality from uterine eversion has been reported to range from 18% to 20%.[19] The genetic propensity of cows for developing uterine eversion and the likelihood of increased susceptibility to uterine eversion after subsequent parturitions are unknown, but genetic predisposition to uterine eversion has not been identified. A cow that has had uterine eversion seems to be at no increased risk of having a recurrence at subsequent parturitions.[29–31]

Uterine eversion usually occurs within 24 hours after parturition, with most eversions occurring within a few hours after parturition.[32] Although the condition is uncommon (<1%), it is one of the true emergency situations encountered in farm animal practice. The uterus rapidly becomes edematous and hemorrhagic and may evert to the extent that the uterine artery ruptures (**Fig. 24**), leading rapidly to shock and death.

Owners should be instructed not to transport the cow. Many affected cows are unable to rise because they are hypocalcemic, have obturator nerve paralysis, or are exhausted.

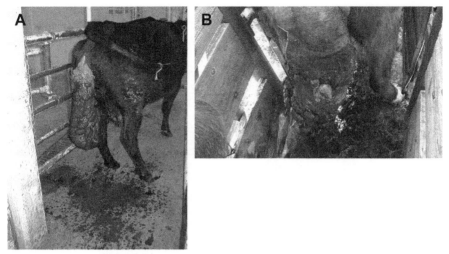

Fig. 24. (*A, B*) A contaminated, edematous, and hemorrhagic everted uterus.

Many factors contribute to uterine eversion, including reduced uterine contractility caused by primary or secondary uterine inertia.[17,19,24] Other causes of uterine eversion besides uterine inertia include persistent tenesmus associated with dystocia, forced extraction of calf, retained fetal membranes, delayed cervical involution, and laceration of the vagina or vestibule.[30] However, hypocalcemia may be the result, rather than a cause, of uterine eversion. The roles of parity and hypocalcemia in the cause of uterine eversion remain an enigma.[33–35] Nonanimal factors include extreme weather conditions and the dietary composition of the pasture.

Practical tips for reducing uterine eversions have been described.[21,24,30,31,36–50] The everted uterus can be replaced with the cow standing or recumbent (**Fig. 25**). Replacing the uterus with the cow recumbent is greatly facilitated by positioning the cow in sternal recumbency with both hind limbs extended caudally, thereby tilting

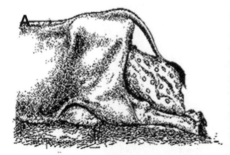 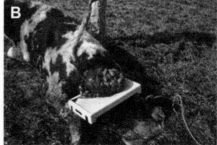

Fig. 25. (*A*) An everted uterus can be replaced with the cow recumbent. (*B*) The tray is used to elevate the uterus and to keep it clean. (*From* Dawson LJ, Peter AT. An update on vaginal and uterine eversions in cattle. Clin Theriogenol 2012;4:115; with permission.)

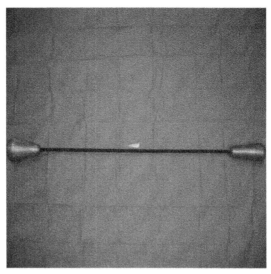

Fig. 26. A probang used to fully invert the uterine horns. Note that the ends of the probang are rounded.

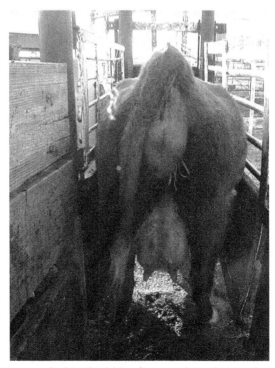

Fig. 27. Buhner suture applied to the labia after a prolapsed uterus has been replaced.

its pelvis cranially.[24] If the cow is standing, it can be cast and rolled into sternal recumbency. Some clinicians prefer to replace the uterus with the cow standing, provided that the cow can be adequately restrained and help is available to lift the uterus with a towel or bed sheet. The chance of immediate recurrence can be eliminated if the eversion is reduced completely. A probe with rounded edges (**Fig. 26**) is commonly used to ensure that the tip of the uterine horn is fully inverted and to prevent tears.

The need for placing a suture in the vulva for 24 to 48 hours after the uterus has been replaced is controversial (**Fig. 27**). Reeversion is highly unlikely, unless the cow is unable to rise or if tenesmus commences.

Uterine amputation

Uterine amputation is a salvage procedure used when the uterus is necrotic or severely traumatized. The uterus can be amputated using an open or closed approach.[19,22,51,52] In the open approach, the uterine body is incised, and the uterine vessels in the stretched broad ligament are identified, double ligated, and severed, along with the mesometrium before the uterus is amputated. The advantage of the open approach is that viscera contained within the everted uterus can be returned to the abdomen before amputation. With this approach, the lumen of the uterus and its contents, including the mesometrium and its vessels, are exposed through an incision that extends cranially from the cervix to the bifurcation of the uterine horn. Slightly overlapping mattress sutures are then placed across the uterine body adjacent to the cervix, the uterus is amputated 2 to 3 cm distal to these sutures, and the uterine stump is sutured using a simple continuous suture pattern. Postoperative treatment should include administration of tetanus toxoid, a nonsteroidal antiinflammatory, and antibiotics.

Using the closed approach (**Fig. 28**) to amputate the uterus, the entire uterus is encircled with 1 or more strangulating sutures, composed of surgical tubing, bungee cord, or the bloodless castrating unit used for castrating large bulls (Callicrate Bander, No-Bull Enterprises, St Francis, KS), causing the uterus to slough in 10 to 14 days. With this approach, viscera within the everted uterus can be unintentionally included in the sutures, causing the death of the cow.

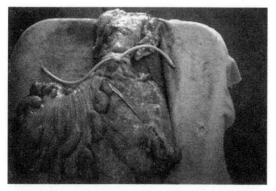

Fig. 28. A closed approach for uterine amputation. Note the location of the ligature.

Ovariectomy

Bilateral ovariectomy is performed on the following 3 distinct populations of cows:

1. Feedlot heifers to suppress estrus, which decreases injuries, enhances feed consumption and daily gain, and prevents pregnancy.
2. Cows in the US Department of Agriculture's brucellosis control program.
3. Research cows, in which the entire ovaries are needed for evaluation of follicles, follicular fluids, and hormones produced within the ovary.

Unilateral ovariectomy may be indicated for removal of a diseased ovary.[53–55]

Ovariectomy is usually performed with the cow standing in a squeeze chute. Withholding feed for 24 hours reduces abdominal fill, and decreases contact between the large intestine and the reproductive tract. If the ovaries are to be removed through a vaginal approach, epidural anesthesia should be administered to desensitize the perineum and vagina. If the ovaries are to be removed through a flank approach, the flank should be desensitized with a field block or with paravertebral anesthesia.

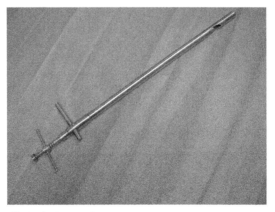

Fig. 29. Kimberling-Rupp instrument.

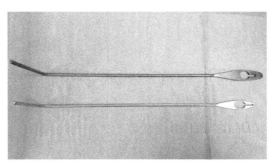

Fig. 30. Willis instrument.

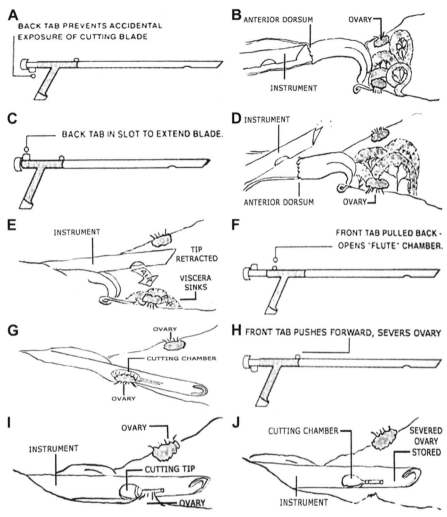

Fig. 31. The use of the Meagher ovary flute, as described in the text. (*Courtesy of* Harry Disney, DVM.)

Vaginal approach

The most common approach for spaying heifers is the vaginal approach because the ovaries of heifers are small enough to be removed in this manner.[56] The instruments available in the United States for removing ovaries using the vaginal approach are the Kimberling-Rupp instrument (**Fig. 29**), the Willis instrument (**Fig. 30**), and the new Meagher ovary flute (made by Harry Disney, DVM, Libby, MT), which is the spay instrument preferred by the authors (**Fig. 31**).[57–60]

The Meagher ovary flute instrument is introduced into the vagina with its cutting head retracted. The cutting tip is then exposed to penetrate the vaginal wall. The cutting blade is retracted after the instrument enters the abdomen, and air flows into the peritoneal cavity, causing the viscera to retract from the abdominal wall, thus reducing the likelihood of damaging the viscera with the instrument. The shaft of the instrument is retracted, opening the cutting chamber, and an ovary is placed into the cutting chamber using a hand placed per rectum. The operator inserts the ovary into the cutting chamber with fingers and thumb placed around the instrument and the ovary per rectum. A shallow groove milled into the tube identifies the position of the aperture. The palpating hand and rectal tissue should not feel stuck to the instrument, nor should the operator feel a mass of tissue funneling into the aperture. Pressure to sever the ovarian pedicle is minimal, and so resistance to transection indicates that more than the ovary has entered the cutting chamber. After the second ovary is cut from its attachment, the instrument is withdrawn.[60]

Flank approach

The heifer is restrained in a squeeze chute, and the left paralumbar fossa is prepared for sterile surgery. A 15-cm incision is made in the fossa through the skin, musculature,

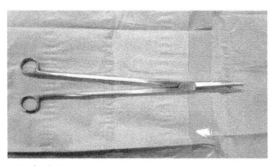

Fig. 32. Curved, serrated scissors.

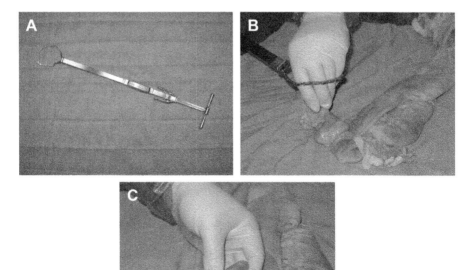

Fig. 33. (*A*) A chain écraseur. (*B* and *C*) Applying the chain of a chain écraseur to the pedicle of an ovary.

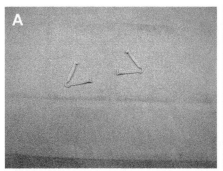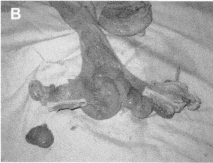

Fig. 34. (*A*) Umbilical clamps for ovariectomy. (*B*) Umbilical clamps applied to the ovarian pedicles.

and peritoneum. The right ovary is identified and separated from its bursa. With the ovary held in the left hand, the ovarian pedicle is transected with curved serrated scissors (**Fig. 32**) inserted through the flank incision. The left ovarian pedicle is transected similarly. The Willis spay instrument can also be used, depending on the size of the ovaries. The ovaries of an adult cow and diseased ovaries are too big to fit the spay instruments described earlier.

Laparoscopy ovariectomy in a standing cow, as well as an écraseur (**Fig. 33**) or umbilical cord clamps (**Fig. 34**), can be used to prevent uncontrolled hemorrhage when removing a diseased ovary or ovaries from an adult cow.[61–63] The flank incision is closed in 3 or 4 layers. The cow receives antibiotic treatment for 3 to 5 days after surgery.

REFERENCES

1. Youngquist RS, Braun WF Jr. Abnormalities of the tubular genital organs. Vet Clin North Am Food Anim Pract 1993;9:309–22.
2. Bostedt H. Surgical treatment of injuries and positional changes in the vulvoperineal region of cows. Tierarztl Prax Suppl 1985;1:26–32 [in German].
3. Wolfe DF, Baird AN. Female urogenital surgery in cattle. Vet Clin North Am Food Anim Pract 1993;9:369–88.
4. Gilbert RO. Dystocia cause by stenosis or constriction of the vulva and vestibule. In: Fubini SL, Ducharme NG, editors. Farm animal surgery. Philadelphia: Saunders Elsevier; 2004. p. 395.
5. Goncagul G, Seyrek Intas K, Kumru IH, et al. Prevalence and accompanying signs of pneumovagina and urovagina in dairy cows in the Southern Marmara region. Tierarztl Prax Ausg G Grosstiere Nutztiere 2012;40:359–66.
6. Gautam G, Nakao T. Prevalence of urovagina and its effects on reproductive performance in Holstein cows. Theriogenology 2009;71:1451–61.
7. Slusher S. Modified perineoplasty. Paper presented at: Western States Veterinary Conference. Las Vegas (NV), February 17–18, 1986.
8. Prado TM, Schumacher J, Hayden SS, et al. Evaluation of a modified surgical technique to correct urine pooling in cows. Theriogenology 2007;67:1512–7.
9. St Jean G, Hull BL, Robertson JT, et al. Urethral extension for correction of urovagina in cattle: a review of 14 cases. Vet Surg 1988;17:258–62.
10. Prado TM, Morgan GL, Prado ME, et al. Urethrovaginal fistula in a llama. Bov Pract 2002;36:22–6.

11. Prado TM, Schumacher J, Kelly GM, et al. Evaluation of a modification of the McKinnon technique to correct urine pooling in mares. Vet Rec 2012;170:621.

12. Dreyfuss DJ, Tulleners EP, Donawick WJ, et al. Third-degree perineal lacerations and rectovestibular fistulae in cattle: 20 cases (1981–1988). J Am Vet Med Assoc 1990;196:768–70.

13. Walker DR, Vaughan JT. Bovine and equine urogenital surgery. Philadelphia: Lea & Febiger; 1980. p. 80–3.

14. Wolfe DF. Theriogenology to enhance animal well-being. Clin Theriogenol 2011;3: 180–4.

15. Johansen RD. Repair of prolapsed vagina in the cow. Vet Med Small Anim Clin 1968;63:252–6.

16. Pierson RE. A review of surgical procedures for correction of vaginal prolapses in cattle. J Am Vet Med Assoc 1961;139:352–6.

17. Dawson LJ, Peter AT. An update on vaginal and uterine eversions in cattle. Clin Theriogenol 2012;4:115–31.

18. Hattangady SR, Deshphande KS. Case reports on "through and through" stay suture technique for retention of vaginal prolapse. Indian Vet J 1967;44:528–30.

19. Roberts SJ. Veterinary obstetrics and genital diseases (Theriogenology). 2nd edition. Ithaca (NY): Edwards Bros; 1971.

20. Hopper RM. Surgical correction of abnormalities of genital organs of cows. In: Youngquist RS, Threlfall WR, editors. Current therapy in large animal theriogenology. 2nd edition. St Louis (MO): WB Saunders; 2007. p. 463–72.

21. Miesner MD, Anderson DE. Management of uterine and vaginal prolapse in the bovine. Vet Clin North Am Food Anim Pract 2008;24:409–19.

22. Youngquist RS. Surgical correction of abnormalities of genital organs of cows. In: Youngquist RS, editor. Current therapy in large animal theriogenology. 1st edition. Philadelphia: WB Saunders; 1997. p. 429–40.

23. Arthur GH. Recent advances in bovine obstetrics. Vet Rec 1966;79:638–9.

24. Barker CA. The modified Caslick operation in the handling of chronic prolapse of the vagina. Can J Comp Med Vet Sci 1950;14:380–2.

25. Buhner F. Simple surgical treatment of uterine and vaginal prolapse. Tierdraztl Umsch 1958;13:183–8 [in German].

26. Bierschwal CJ, DeBois CHW. The Buhner method for control of chronic vaginal prolapse in the cow (review and evaluation). Vet Med Small Anim Clin 1971;66: 230–6.

27. Pittman T. Practice tips. Can Vet J 2010;51:1347–8.

28. Lamp JH, Lamp TM. A method for correcting vaginal prolapse in a cow. Vet Med Small Anim Clin 1981;76:395–6.

29. Plenderleith B. Prolapse of the uterus in the cow. In Pract 1986;1:14–5.

30. Odegaard SA. Uterine prolapse in dairy cows. A clinical study with special reference to incidence, recovery and subsequent fertility. Acta Vet Scand Suppl 1977; 63:1–124.

31. Gardner IA, Reynolds JP, Risco CA, et al. Patterns of uterine prolapse in dairy cows and prognosis after treatment. J Am Vet Med Assoc 1990;197:1021–4.

32. Richardson GF, Klemmer AD, Knudsen DB. Observations on uterine prolapse in beef cattle. Can Vet J 1981;22:189–91.

33. Markusfeld O. Periparturient traits in seven high dairy herds, incidence rates, association with parity, and interrelationships among traits. J Dairy Sci 1987;70: 158–66.

34. Risco CA, Reynolds JP, Hird D. Uterine prolapse and hypocalcemia in dairy cows. J Am Vet Med Assoc 1984;185:1517–9.

35. Patterson DJ, Bellows RA, Burfening PJ. Effects of caesarean section, retained placenta and vaginal or uterine prolapse on subsequent fertility in beef cattle. J Anim Sci 1981;53:916–21.
36. Caldwell HS. Eversion of uterus in a maiden heifer. Vet Rec 1933;29:688–9.
37. Baxter K. Replacing the prolapsed bovine uterus [comment]. Vet Rec 2004; 155:344.
38. Biggs A, Osborne R. Uterine prolapse and mid-pregnancy uterine torsion in cows. Vet Rec 2003;152:91–2.
39. Bullard JF. A case of uterine prolapse in a Hereford with unusual lay treatment. J Am Vet Med Assoc 1946;109:462.
40. Foster SJ. A pneumatic appliance for the replacement of the prolapsed uterus of the cow. Vet Rec 1972;91:418.
41. Hibberd RC. Replacing the prolapsed bovine uterus [comment]. Vet Rec 2004; 155:96.
42. Johnston RW. Uterine prolapse in the cow [letter]. Vet Rec 1986;118:252.
43. Levine HD. Partial uterine prolapse associated with uterine foreign body in a cow. J Am Vet Med Assoc 1990;197:759–60.
44. Lyons AR. Uterine prolapse in the cow. Vet Rec 1986;118(17):492.
45. Garcia-Saco E, Gill MS, Paccamonti DL. Theriogenology question of the month: laparoscopy to assist replacement of the uterus. J Am Vet Med Assoc 2001; 219:443–4.
46. Abdullahi US, Kumi-Diaka J. Prolapse of the nongravid horn in a cow with a seven-month pregnancy: a case report. Theriogenology 1986;26:353–6.
47. White A. Clinical: uterine prolapse in the cow. Livestock 2007;12:21–3.
48. Wilson PJ. A pneumatic appliance for the replacement of the prolapsed uterus of the cow. Vet Rec 1972;90:729–30.
49. Munro IB. Replacing the prolapsed bovine uterus. Vet Rec 2004;155:344.
50. Narasimhan KS, Thangaraj TM, Subramanyam R. A method of retention of recurrent prolapse of the uterus in bovines. Indian Vet J 1967;44:67–73.
51. Wenzel JG, Baird AN, Wolfe DF, et al. Surgery of the uterus. In: Wolfe DF, Moll HD, editors. Large animal urogenital surgery. 2nd edition. Philadelphia: Williams and Wilkins; 1998. p. 423.
52. Roberts SJ. Amputation of the prolapsed uterus. Cornell Vet 1949;39:438–9.
53. Garber MJ, Roeder RA, Combs JJ, et al. Efficacy of vaginal spaying and anabolic implants on growth and carcass characteristics in beef heifers. J Anim Sci 1990; 68:1469–75.
54. Roberts TW, Peck DE, Ritten JP. Cattle producers' economic incentives for preventing bovine brucellosis under uncertainty. Prev Vet Med 2012;107:187–203.
55. Spicer LJ, Alvares P, Prado TM, et al. Effects of intraovarian infusion of insulin-like growth factor-I on ovarian follicular function in cattle. Domest Anim Endocrinol 2000;18:265–78.
56. Drost M, Savio JD, Barros CM, et al. Ovariectomy by colpotomy in cows. J Am Vet Med Assoc 1992;200:337–9.
57. Rupp PG, Kimberling CV. A new approach for spaying heifers. Vet Med Small Anim Clin 1982;77:561–5.
58. Habermehl NL. Heifer ovariectomy using the Willis spay instrument: Technique, morbidity and mortality. Can Vet J 1993;34:664–7.
59. Meyer D. Spaying pays. Beef Magazine. 2005. Available at: http://beefmagazine. com/mag/beef_spaying_pays. Accessed February 1, 2016.
60. Disney H. The Meagher ovary flute. Available at: http://spaytool.com/index.html. Accessed February 1, 2016.

61. Bleul U, Hollenstein K, Kähn W. Laparoscopic ovariectomy in standing cows. Anim Reprod Sci 2005;90:193–200.
62. Boileau MJ, Jann HW, Confer AW. Use of a chain écraseur for excision of a pharyngeal granuloma in a cow. J Am Vet Med Assoc 2009;234:935–7.
63. Youngquist RS, Garverick HA, Keisler DH. Use of umbilical cord clamps for ovariectomy in cows. J Am Vet Med Assoc 1995;207:474–5.

Surgery of the Distal Limb

Karl Nuss, Prof Dr med vet

KEYWORDS

- Lameness • Digits • Injury • Infection • Resection • Amputation • Fractures
- Luxations

KEY POINTS

- Diseases of the bovine digit remain the major cause of painful lameness in cattle and commonly constitute a diagnostic and therapeutic challenge for clinicians.
- Prompt wound revision and early treatment of sole ulcers is critical; otherwise, purulent infection of the wound can be expected.
- Deep infections of the distal limb may be treated by digit salvage techniques.
- Postoperative care is more involved, lameness persists longer, and cost of treatment is higher after salvage techniques than after amputation.
- Luxations and fractures of the digits often are amenable to conservative treatment, but may be treated surgically if indicated.

INTRODUCTION

Lameness is now recognized as the most common impairment of the health status and well-being of the modern dairy cow.[1–5] Several studies found that severe lameness with scores of 3 of 3 and 4 to 5 of 5 occurred in 26.6%[6] and 18.3%[7] of examined cows, respectively. The majority of painful lameness disorders affect the claws, and sole ulcer and white line disease are most common.[8–10] When recognized and treated early, these lesions generally have a good prognosis and respond well to treatment.[11] Uncomplicated sole ulcers become keratinized and heal after a mean duration of 14 ± 8.7 days after treatment that included paring, a bandage, and a wooden block glued to the unaffected partner claw, whereas affected claws treated in a similar way but without a block on the other claw require an average of 28 ± 19 days to heal.[12,13] However, even successfully treated, uncomplicated sole ulcers are often prone to recurrence and a high (40%) cull rate.

There have been several comprehensive reviews over the last few years of the surgical treatment of distal limb disorders in cattle. Various resection and amputation techniques have been described and discussed in detail.[14–20] The surgeon must

---

The author has nothing to disclose.
Farm Animal Department, Vetsuisse Faculty University of Zurich, Winterthurerstrasse 260, CH-8057 Zurich, Switzerland
E-mail address: karl.nuss@uzh.ch

have an excellent anatomic knowledge of the bovine lower limb for a successful outcome.[15] Sound anatomic understanding also is required for the interpretation of ultrasound and radiographic images of the bovine limb.[21,22] Relevant structures of the bovine digit are shown in **Fig. 1**.

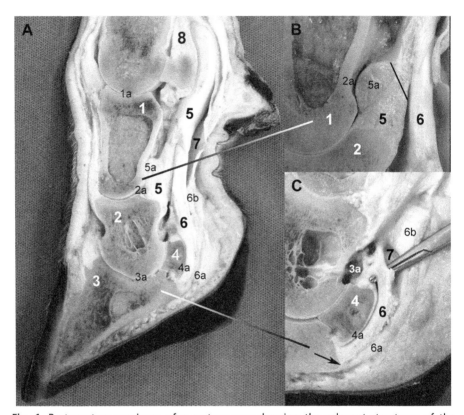

Fig. 1. Post-mortem specimen of a mature cow showing the relevant structures of the bovine digit. The dotted lines point to close-up images. (*A*) Sagittal overview of the digit. 1 = first phalanx; 1a = metacarpophalangeal joint; 2 = second phalanx; 2a = proximal interphalangeal joint; 3 = third phalanx/pedal bone; 3a = distal interphalangeal joint; 4 = distal sesamoid bone; 4a = podotrochlear bursa; 5 = superficial flexor tendon; 5a = section of the palmar/plantar ligament of the second interphalangeal joint; 6 = deep digital flexor tendon; 6a = deep digital flexor retinaculum/distal annular ligament of the digits inserting at the flexor tubercle; 6b = origin of the distal cruciate ligament of the digits; 7 = common digital flexor tendon sheath; 8 = suspensory ligament of the interosseus muscle. (*B*) Enlargement of the area of the proximal interphalangeal joint from (*A*) numbers according to (*A*); the solid oblique black line across the superficial digital flexor tendon (5) indicates the tenotomy site in cases with purulent tenosynovitis and flexor tendon infection. (*C*) Enlargement of the area of the distal sesamoid bone from (*A*), numbers according to (*A*); arrow indicates fibers of the distal flexor retinaculum that insert at the flexor tubercle. Above, a hemostat penetrates the synovial lining of the digital flexor tendon sheath into the navicular bursa to illustrate the close relationship between pedal joint, bursa, and tendon sheath. The close anatomic relationship between the distal sesamoid bone (4) and the common digital flexor tendon sheath (7) explains the considerable risk of entering the latter during removal of the distal sesamoid bone.

INDICATIONS

Surgery of the distal limb is required commonly for the treatment of acute deep injuries (eg, cuts, perforations, contusions, compound phalangeal fractures, infection of the tip of the claw) or deep complicated infections resulting from chronic local lesions (eg, sole ulcer, white line disease). The attributes 'deep' and 'complicated' indicate that the corium or the subcutis has been breached and that 1 or more of the anatomic structures shown in **Fig. 1**, namely, tendons, ligaments, bones, bursae, tendon sheaths, or joints, are affected. So-called non-healing claw lesions were mentioned recently as an indication for open amputation.[23,24] Non-healing claw lesions include toe ulcers, white line disease, and sometimes sole ulcers that are complicated by secondary infection with treponemes in bovine digital dermatitis (strawberry foot rot) and fail to respond to standard methods of treatment. However, despite the terminology used for this disease complex, many of these lesions respond favorably to proper surgical wound treatment consisting of paring defective claw tissue under local anesthesia, application of a bandage, gluing a block to the healthy partner claw, and regular follow-up examination.[25] These lesions also can be treated strategically using open amputation, which has a good prognosis, is less involved than conventional treatment, and has been shown to extend the productive lifespan of the cow.[26]

Surgical treatment usually is not indicated when both claws of a foot are severely affected or when 2 claws of different limbs have deep infections. Ascending or phlegmonous thrombophlebitis has a poor prognosis and affected cows often are ill and the skin of the affected foot is infected, hyperemic, and very painful. Thrombophlebitis is readily diagnosed ultrasonographically.[27] In addition, acute generalized and chronic recurring laminitis usually is a contraindication for surgical treatment. The prognosis is affected adversely by accompanying organ diseases including hepatic lipidosis, abomasal displacement, or metritis. Economic considerations such as replacement costs or the sentimental value of a cow to the owner also must be considered when making a treatment decision regarding surgery.

INSTRUMENTS

Good fixation of the foot or the leg is an important requirement for successful surgery of the distal limbs. This is afforded by height-adjustable claw trimming chutes, which provide good access to the distal limb with the exception of the dorsal part of the foot. The disadvantage of a foot trimming chute is that the surgical field is more prone to contamination and the cow has much more freedom of movement than when a horizontal tilt table is used.[28] Aseptic conditions usually can be provided and maintained throughout the procedure in cows fixed on a tilt table (**Fig. 2**), especially when sedation and fixation of multiple body parts are used.[29] The surgeon works in a standing position and the claws can be accessed from all sides. The surgery itself, including bandaging and blocking the healthy partner claw, are more easily achieved with the cow in lateral recumbency rather than in a standing position.

In addition to standard surgical instruments, a self-retaining sharp Weitlaner wound spreader, tenaculum forceps, a strong double-edged knife or a strong raspatory instrument, and a drill with a cutting drill bit[30] are helpful. For closed[31] and open[32] digit amputation at the level of the distal metaphysis of the first phalanx, Gigli wire with handles (and a Buhner needle to feed the wire between the toes for closed amputation) also are needed.

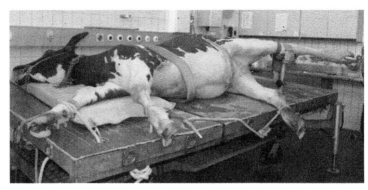

Fig. 2. Sedated cow on a tilt table prepared for surgical treatment of septic tenosynovitis of the lateral digit of the left hind foot. All 4 feet have been trimmed and a tourniquet has been applied above the left hock in preparation for intravenous regional anesthesia.

SURGICAL PREPARATION

Ideally, cows to be operated in lateral recumbency are fasted for at least 12 hours to avoid regurgitation and respiratory impairment caused by ruminal tympany. Emergency treatment can be given to cows in a chute without fasting. General anesthesia usually is required for tenosynovioscopy and arthroscopy,[33,34] in which case the cow should be fasted for at least 24 hours with no access to water for 4 to 6 hours before the procedure.

Claw trimming is recommended before foot surgery to examine the claws for lesions of the corium and also to prevent postoperative overload of the healthy digit or claw. Cattle referred for digit surgery often have a long history of on-farm treatments and many already have a block on the healthy claw. However, early lesions of the corium under these blocks are not uncommon and should be ruled out first by removing the block because they would preclude surgery.

Transient iatrogenic nerve damage is a concern both for cattle treated in a chute or on a table. This damage can be minimized by padding exposed body parts (see **Fig. 2**) and by keeping the surgical time as brief as possible by optimal planning. Transient radial nerve paresis after lateral recumbency is common and, when it occurs, the standing cow is supported until the condition resolves on its own, which usually is rapid. If paresis is more severe, a splint bandage is applied to the affected limb and the cow given supportive treatment, including antiinflammatory drugs.

Sedation using xylazine or a multimodal sedation (eg, K-stun) is ideal for claw surgery in cattle in lateral recumbency[29] and is discussed elsewhere in this issue. Sedation reduces anxiety and stress, and the animals are less likely to defecate. However, high sedative doses provide only temporary suppression of struggling in cows. Standing cattle restrained in a chute are only lightly sedated because otherwise they may go down. Heavily pregnant cows should be given a tocolytic before sedation with an alpha agonist. After recovery from lateral recumbency, pregnant cows should be examined for uterine torsion.

Antibiotics and analgesics are given parenterally before the operation. Penicillin and other broad-spectrum beta-lactam antibiotics, and ketoprofen or meloxicam, are appropriate for this purpose.[35,36] The affected digit is cleaned, clipped to the level of the proximal part of the metacarpus or metatarsus, and prepared aseptically.[37] If the procedure includes intravenous regional anesthesia (IVRA) or a proximal 4-point nerve block, this is carried out at the proximal end of the metacarpus/metatarsus after aseptic preparation of the area.

Although IVRA has been used for many years in human[38] and veterinary medicine,[39] it not a risk-free procedure. Adverse effects of IVRA in cattle include thrombosis and thromboembolism.[27,40] Moreover, IVRA of an infected foot often is followed by bacteremia,[41,42] which is why this type of anesthesia should be accompanied by parenteral antibiotic treatment. When local anesthesia—nerve blocks or IVRA—was used for sequestrectomy, cattle were more likely to undergo 2 or more surgical procedures than cattle in which the sequestrum was removed with the aid of general anesthesia.[43] However, general anesthesia is not usually indicated for claw surgery. An alternative to IVRA is the use of a 4-point nerve block at the level of the metacarpus/metatarsus. A tourniquet is then applied to the anesthetized limb to control hemorrhage during surgery. This eliminates venipuncture and the risk of thrombosis is reduced. An additional advantage is that the pain associated with the application of the tourniquet and congestion[44] is reduced or eliminated. More studies of potential adverse effects of IVRA on healing and on the occurrence of postoperative complications are needed.

Antibiotic intravenous regional perfusion ensures high antibiotic concentrations in the tissue and has been used mainly in horses and cattle with deep septic disease processes in a limb.[45,46] Empirically, this form of antibiotic treatment seems to have a positive impact on infections of the foot, although it was not superior to other forms of antibiotic administration for the treatment of digital dermatitis.[44] In any case, the antibiotic concentration should be kept low enough to minimize the risk of vascular irritation, thrombosis, and soft tissue necrosis (eg, penicillin G, 100,000 to a maximum of 10^6 IU per foot).[27,40]

In case of resection surgery through the sole–heel area, the claw horn is removed using a disc until only a paper-thin horn layer remains. This technique facilitates excision of the infected tissue with a scalpel. After thinning of the horn, the entire claw is cleaned again, dried, and prepared aseptically.

AFTERCARE

The surgical principles of perioperative and postoperative wound management after claw surgery have been described in detail elsewhere.[16,19,47,48] Lactated Ringer's solution and solutions containing antiseptic chemicals such as povidone iodine or chlorhexidine are popular flush solutions. It is important that the latter be used at the correct concentrations (povidone iodine concentration of <0.2% and chlorhexidine concentration of <0.05%), because higher concentrations can induce significant synovitis and may exacerbate intrathecal disease.[19] Flush solutions containing antibiotics also are commonly used, but standardized protocols do not exist; their use is based largely on personal preference and experience of the surgeon. However, locally applied antiseptic and antibiotic solutions may delay wound healing.[49] When flushing and cleaning a wound cavity, only mild curettage should be used to avoid disturbing the granulation process. Depending on the type of surgery and healing progress, systemic antibiotic treatment for 5 to 10 days after surgery is recommended.

After completion of surgical treatment, severely contaminated or infected wounds are best left to heal by secondary intention. The wound may be left open or partially sutured; good drainage is essential. A variety of wound draining systems are available, and sometimes polyurethane foam wound dressings used in human medicine are recommended to aid in drainage.[50] A well-padded bandage that extends about 10 cm (4 inches) proximal to the dewclaws is applied to protect the wound; sometimes, a splint bandage or a fiberglass cast is indicated.[51] The first bandage change should be done 3 to 5 days postoperatively under sterile conditions. If a gauze tampo-nade or gauze drainage was left in place, it is removed, ideally using distal nerve blocks. Lavage or curettage of the wound is usually not indicated at this stage. The wound is then redressed and rebandaged. A second bandage change is done 5 days later and, if healing is normal, further bandage changes are done every 2 to 3 weeks, depending on wound healing or the surgeon's preference. Most wounds heal completely within about 8 weeks. The degree of lameness is expected to decrease to about 2/5 within 7 to 10 days of surgery. If possible, the block should be left in place for 10 to 12 weeks and then removed from the partner claw to avoid overloading the corium.

After resection of the deep digital flexor tendon or the pedal joint or after extirpation of the sesamoid bone, the claw is usually stabilized using a fixation device of the sur-geon's preference. Fixation can be achieved using a piece of metal attached to the block on the healthy claw and bent over the operated claw, a wire looped through a hole in the tips of both claws, a bandage, or a bridge made from methyl methacry-late.[17,30] Correct positioning of both claws usually can be obtained,[52] provided that the fixation is kept in place long enough. When it is not feasible to apply a block to the healthy claw or when there are reasons to remove the block soon after the oper-ation, healing may be compromised and 'tipping' of the claw (defined as upward tilting of the claw) occurs.[53] Bandage material used for fixation, even heavy material and ad-hesive tape, quickly loses stability after application. Fixation of the operated claw after granulation is complete can be prolonged by attaching a horseshoe-shaped piece of wood to the bottom of the claw using methyl methacrylate. A dry and clean environ-ment, for instance in a tie stall or a straw-bedded box stall, is critical for healing.[54] The aftercare of a cow that underwent claw surgery requires considerable effort and expense for 2 to 3 months, and this should be discussed with the owner beforehand.

COMPLICATIONS

Complications characterized by delayed healing may occur after resection or ampu-tation procedures, but are more common after resection because removal of all infected tissues is more difficult.[17,55] Delayed healing manifests by persistence of local inflammation, reluctance to bear weight, moderate to severe lameness beyond 7 to 10 days postoperatively, recurrence of purulent discharge, abscess formation, and sequestra. These complications require extensive wound revision and possibly a change in antibiotics. A sole ulcer in the healthy claw caused by the block is another possible complication, which sometimes can be overcome by using a padded bandage that involves both claws and stabilizes the operated claw in the correct po-sition. Obviously, a healthy partner claw is absolutely essential when a claw is ampu-tated.[53,56] Healing may be delayed when cutaneous abscesses are present, and suturing the skin in such cases may cause problems that are not encountered with open amputation.[57] Osteitis of the stump of the first phalanx is an occasional compli-cation and is treated by removing the affected bone with a ronguer or burr. Infection of adjacent joints or the common digital flexor tendon sheath is rare but can occur.

Almost one-half of the cows undergoing digit or claw amputation or resection are culled within a year of surgery,[26,52,53,58,59] most of them because of other claw disor-ders. The remaining cows can be productive and remain in the herd for several years.

MANAGEMENT OF INJURIES

Injuries to the distal limb are not uncommon in cattle housed in tie stall or free stall op-erations. All parts of the digit may be affected and in most cases vital structures including ligaments, tendon sheaths, tendons, and joints are injured because of the relative paucity of soft tissue in the lower limb. The injuries are not always accompanied by severe hemorrhage or large wounds and therefore may be missed in the early stages. Furthermore, the feet are often soiled with feces, and lameness can be surprisingly mild initially, even when vital structures are injured. Caretakers must be trained in recognizing cattle with foot injuries so that they can be removed from the herd and treated in a timely fashion.[60] Contaminated and neglected foot wounds rapidly undergo severe purulent infection and are then very difficult or impossible to treat, and the only way to save the cow may be amputation of the affected digit (**Fig. 3**).

The surgical treatment of such injuries (**Fig. 4**) is elaborate and complex, and includes the removal of loose claw horn, curettage of tendons, ligaments, and bones, wound irrigation, puncture and flushing of joints and tendon sheaths, installation of drains, suturing the different tissue layers, and bandaging. If possible, a block is glued to the sole of the healthy claw to ease the pressure on the injured claw. Extensive wounds, particularly those associated with wound dehiscence and other complications, require several weeks for healing and, accordingly, intensive aftercare and regular monitoring of the healing process.

RESECTION OF THE APEX OF THE PEDAL BONE

Resection of the tip of the pedal bone is indicated for treatment of infection caused during foot trimming, by excessive abrasion on rough flooring, or by fracture of the horn capsule, including the tip of the pedal bone (**Fig. 5A**). Because of the etiology of these traumatic injuries, multiple claws are often affected,[61–63] which adversely affects the prognosis, as well as the indication for resection.

The extent of the infection is best assessed radiographically (**Fig. 5B**). The infected osteolytic bone is accessed from the apex of the sole and removed using a drill, held

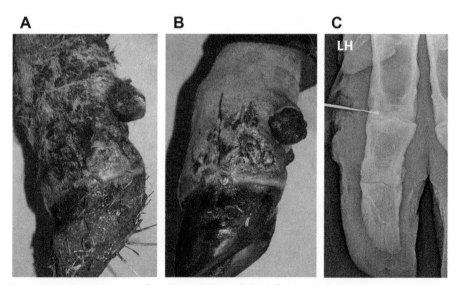

Fig. 3. Four-day-old injury of the lateral digit of the left hind limb in a 3-year-old cow. (*A*) View of the injury on admission and (*B*) after cleaning the foot. (*C*) Plantarodorsal radiographic view with a probe inserted into the proximal interphalangeal joint. The lateral claw was amputated, and the cow remained in the herd for at least 3 years.

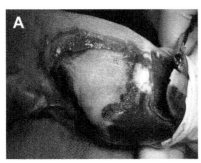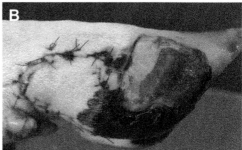

Fig. 4. Laceration in the lateral digit of the right forelimb in a cow. (A) View of the cuts about 5 hours after the injury. The common digital flexor tendon sheath, parts of the superficial and deep flexor tendons, both interphalangeal joints, the abaxial claw capsule, and the pedal bone were affected. (B) Wound healing without complications 12 days after surgery; the pedal bone is covered by granulation tissue. Bandaging was continued and a wooden block was attached to the other claw. The cow was still in the herd 4 years postoperatively.

parallel to the dorsal wall of the claw, until only healthy bone is visible. A Forstner drill[30] can be used to remove the tip of the pedal bone quickly and under continuous flushing with Ringer's solution. Drilling is discontinued when all infected bone has been removed and only whitish, well-vascularized bone substance is visible. When in doubt, 1 to 2 mm of healthy bone is removed to reduce the risk of recurrence.[18] Future deformation of the horn capsule should be expected when more than one-third of the pedal bone requires removal because of the diminished shaping effect of the bone.

The simplest alternative to bone removal by drilling is resection of the entire tip of the bone using a wire saw.[64] Angle grinders that are also used for regular foot care are strongly discouraged because of the risk of contamination of the bone and because of the likelihood that the procedure would be imitated by lay people.[65] Cornification of the defect usually requires 5 to 6 weeks, but can take more than 8 weeks after an extensive resection. Bandages are applied during the entire healing period and the block on the healthy claw is left in place until cornification is complete.

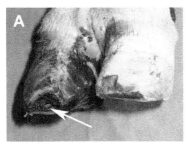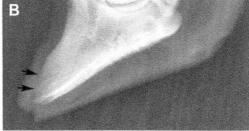

Fig. 5. Right hind foot of a dairy cow with infection of the tip of the pedal bone caused by excessive use of a grinder on the claw wall during foot trimming exposing the white line. (A) A defect is visible in the lateral claw between the sole and the wall, exposing necrotic corium (arrow). (B) Radiograph of the affected lateral digit (abaxioaxial view). The tip of the pedal bone is less radiodense indicating osteomyelitis (black arrows) and spread of the infection deeper into the bone.

SEQUESTRA OF THE PEDAL BONE

Infection of the tip or rim of the pedal bone does not always lead to osteomyelitis, but can lead to the formation of a sequestrum.[43,55] Pedal bone sequestra often occur in association with other pathologic conditions, such as sole ulcer, white line disease, toe ulcer, double sole, and sole trauma associated with foreign body penetration. Lameness usually is less pronounced with a sequestrum than with osteomyelitis. In 1 study,[43] 9 of 16 sequestra of the pedal bone were in a lateral claw of a hind limb.

Sequestra can be diagnosed clinically by a fistulous tract, but when in doubt the diagnosis should be confirmed radiographically (**Fig. 6**). Most sequestra are extracted readily after removal of the corium. If the bed of the sequestrum consists of granulation tissue, no debridement is needed because the granulation delimits the sequestrum and protects the underlying bone. Complications after removal of a sequestrum generally are rare, but recurrence necessitating a second surgical intervention is possible.[43]

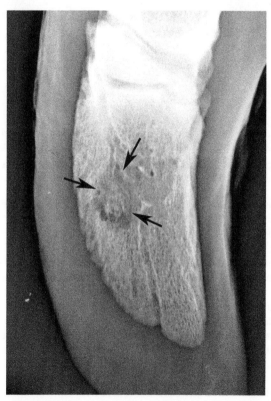

Fig. 6. Palmarodorsal radiographic view of the pedal bone of the lateral claw of the right thoracic limb in a 7-year-old cow with a sequestrum (*arrows*). The sequestrum was removed under local anesthesia (distal nerve block), the empty sequestrum bed flushed, a block was attached to the partner claw, and a bandage was applied. Healing was prolonged but ultimately successful, and the cow remained in the herd for at least 7 months.

NON-HEALING CLAW LESIONS

Lesions of the corium with secondary infection by treponemes may occur at any location in the claw but are most commonly associated with white line lesions (wall ulcers) or toe necrosis.[24,25,66,67] Non-healing claw lesions also can occur at the dorsal aspect of the claw, originating at the coronet and undermining full-thickness vertical fissures (**Fig. 7**A).

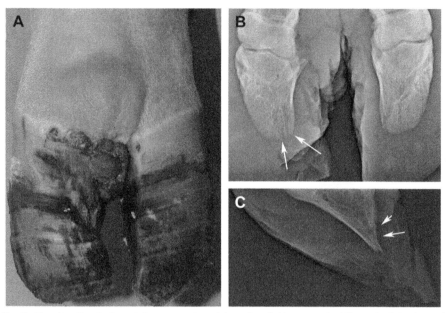

Fig. 7. Non-healing lesion at the coronet and dorsal wall (deep vertical fissure) of the lateral claw of the right hind limb. (*A*) Clinical appearance before treatment. (*B, C*) Plantarodorsal and abaxioaxial radiographic views of the lateral claw. The tip of the pedal bone is atrophic (*arrows*), but not osteolytic; therefore, resection of the tip of the pedal bone or claw amputation was not indicated. Removal of horn and necrotic corium, bandaging, and a block on the other claw resulted in complete healing.

There is hypergranulation of the corium and the adjacent horn is widely undermined, often accompanied by foul-smelling necrosis. The pedal bone may be atrophied, but is not necessarily infected (**Fig. 7**B, C). Whether removal of the tip of the pedal bone is indicated or not is based mainly on the clinical findings, which include degree of lameness and of localized infection, and, last but not least, the appearance of the lesion after trimming. Pedal bones from non-healing hoof lesions sometimes have conspicuous sharp sole spicules and exostoses.[67,68] Non-healing claw lesions are considered indications for claw amputation by some clinicians.[24,26,69]

RESECTION OF THE DISTAL INTERPHALANGEAL JOINT

The goal of resection of the distal interphalangeal joint is the preservation of the affected claw despite the presence of deep extensive damage to the joint. Cartilaginous as well as bony parts of the joint are removed with the intention of achieving ankylosis of the joint in the medium term (7–12 months). Complicated sole ulcers, severe white line disease, deep heel injuries, localized interdigital necrosis, and septic hematogenous arthritis are indications for joint resection. Resection of the joint also may preserve the claw in cases with acute open infected fracture of the pedal bone with joint involvement.[18,70] Osteoarthritis and deformity of the joint are other indications for resection.[71,72]

There are different surgical approaches that depend on the localization of the lesion or the fistulous tract and include the abaxial approach[73,74] and dorsal, axial, and palmar/plantar approaches.[16,17] When a palmar/plantar approach is chosen, the insertion of the deep flexor tendon can be accessed through the sole,[53,75] the combined sole–heel area,[76–78] or the heel.[72,79] Parts of the coronet and heel pad should be preserved if possible to facilitate postoperative tissue regeneration and weight bearing. All infected tissue surrounding a fistulous tract in the sole is generously excised down to the pedal bone. When the combined sole–heel access is used, a wound spreader in the fetlock area provides optimum visibility of the surgical field (**Fig. 8**A). The deep flexor tendon and the distal sesamoid bone can be removed under visual control, abscesses can be identified, and contamination of proximal structures avoided.

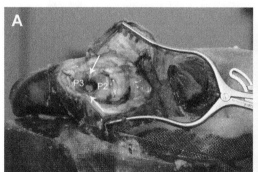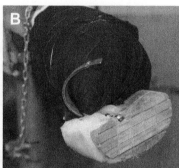

Fig. 8. Plantar approach for resection of the distal interphalangeal joint in a cow with complicated white line disease. (*A*) The wound spreader provides good visibility; the deep flexor tendon and the distal sesamoid bone have been removed and the joint (*arrows* between *P2* and *P3*) has been partly drilled out. (*B*) A wooden block on the partner claw reduces pressure in the operated claw, and a piece of metal attached to the block and bent into a loop over the operated claw prevents overextension of the latter. The metal is finally covered with tape to avoid injuries.

The distal interphalangeal joint can be resected using a special drill[30,52,80] and fixation achieved using a strut of metal attached to the block on the healthy claw and bent over the operated claw (**Fig. 8**B). Provided that optimal healing and successful ankylosis occurs, the weight-bearing function and cosmetic appearance of the foot after joint resection is better than after amputation.[52,81,82] However, the prognosis of resection—and amputation—in terms of healing and extension of the productive life of the cow strongly depends on the nature of the original problem.[18,26] Joint resection because of infection limited to the heel and the caudal one-third of the claw capsule has a better prognosis than with other indications. Furthermore, the synovia of the joint should have sufficient fluidity to drain easily from the joint. Fibrinopurulent or purulent inflammation of the distal interphalangeal joint accompanied by abscess formation along the joint capsule near the coronet is less amenable to resection because complete removal of multiple cartilage and bone necroses is difficult. Ankylosis may fail when all articular components of both the second and third phalanges are drilled out,[52] and amputation may be a better option.

RESECTION OF BOTH FLEXOR TENDONS WITHIN THE COMMON DIGITAL FLEXOR TENDON SHEATH

A clinical diagnosis of infection of the tendon sheath can be confirmed by centesis and ultrasonography[22,83,84] (**Fig. 9**A–C). In addition to systemic antibiotic treatment, lavage

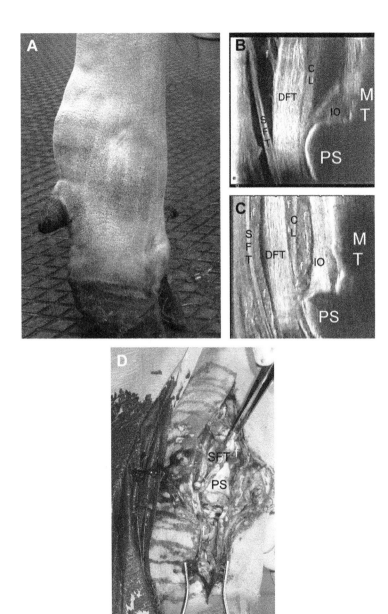

Fig. 9. Tenosynovitis of the common digital flexor tendon sheath. (*A*) Typical clinical appearance of tenosynovitis with swelling of the lateral digit of the right hind limb. The swelling is most prominent proximal to the dewclaws. (*B*) Ultrasonographic image of serofibrinous tenosynovitis viewed from the plantar aspect of the foot; this is an indication for lavage of the tendon sheath using needles or tenosynovioscopy. CL, check ligament between the interosseus muscle and the SFT (to form the manica flexoria); DFT, deep digital flexor tendon; f, fibrin; IO, branches of suspensory ligament of interosseus muscle to the proximal sesamoid bone = PS; MT, metatarsal bone; SFT, superficial flexor tendon. (*C*) Ultrasonographic image of fibrinopurulent tenosynovitis; key as in (*B*); fibrin deposits are an indication for treatment using tenosynoviotomy. (*D*) Resection of the deep and superficial flexor tendons. PS, proximal sesamoid bone; SFT, stump of the superficial digital flexor tendon and check ligament after removal of the distal part of the tendon at the second phalanx (see **Fig. 1B**).

of the tendon sheath using hypodermic or spinal needles or tenosynovioscopy, and placement of a drain, are indicated in acute inflammation of the tendon sheath; these measures have a fair to good prognosis.[19,34,85] Drains also have been used successfully with infection of both tendon sheaths.[86]

Resection of the flexor tendons is indicated for the treatment of purulent tenosynovitis or tendinitis, which may arise from a puncture wound—for instance from a pitch fork—or from ascending infection from a sole ulcer, or rarely from hematogenous spread of bacteria. This procedure is recommended particularly for purulent tenosynovitis and tendinitis. When the proximal interphalangeal joint also is affected, it is opened from the palmar/plantar aspect, flushed, and drained.[50]

Anatomic orientation is often difficult upon initial opening of the tendon sheath because of the presence of fibrin, pus, and adhesions (**Fig. 9**C, D). The first step of the resection is longitudinal incision of the superficial flexor tendon. This allows the surgeon to exteriorize the deep flexor tendon and to identify the proximal end of the tendon sheath, to cut the deep flexor tendon below the bifurcation, and to prepare it distally. The deep flexor tendon is severed at the distal end of the tendon sheath under visual control to avoid opening the podotrochlear bursa or the distal interphalangeal joint. In cases with a sole ulcer, the tendon is cut at the flexor tubercle. Tenotomy of the superficial flexor tendon begins at the distal end about 2 to 3 cm above the flexor tuberosity of the middle phalanx (see **Fig. 1**B) to spare the proximal interphalangeal joint. Proximally, the superficial flexor tendon is adjacent to the palmar/plantar pouches of the proximal interphalangeal joint, which also must be spared. The superficial flexor tendons of both digits unite at the level of the proximal border of the proximal sesamoid to form a single tendon. The affected tendon is prepared carefully distal to the level of the merging tendons. Transection of the superficial flexor tendon and of the check ligament is achieved by cutting in an oblique axial to proximoabaxial direction to ensure complete removal of all diseased tendon tissue.[18,19]

To prevent hypergranulation (proud flesh), the dorsal part of the wound may be sutured to just below the dewclaws; the foot is bandaged to just below the hock. A block with a fixation device is glued to the partner claw. Cattle with fibrinous or purulent infection in both tendon sheaths of the same leg should be culled.[16,19] In cases of severe claw infection, resection of the flexor tendons occasionally must be combined with claw amputation or resection techniques.

CLAW AMPUTATION

Claw or digit amputation can have an absolute medical indication or a relative economic indication.[58] The former relates to cases in which salvage of the claw or toe is no longer possible and the latter relates to cows in which salvage would be feasible from a surgical standpoint but not indicated from an economic standpoint (beef cattle). Resection surgery is more demanding than amputation and lameness usually resolves more rapidly after amputation. So-called high amputation at the level of the distal epiphysis of the first phalanx is the preferred technique and can be done with wound closure and primary healing, or the wound can be left open to heal by secondary intention. When amputation with primary wound healing is chosen (**Fig. 10**A), a lateral and a medial skin flap are created, which are sutured closed after thorough removal of all infected tissue.[31] This technique allows for primary wound healing in a large proportion of cases.[87] Packing of the wound with gauze or other absorbent material and wound drainage are recommended in cases with extensive tissue necrosis.

For open amputation at the level of the first phalanx,[32] a Gigli wire is placed in the interdigital space and the affected claw is severed in an oblique proximoabaxial

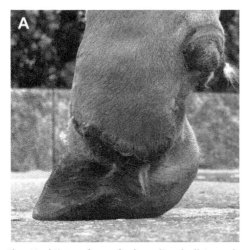
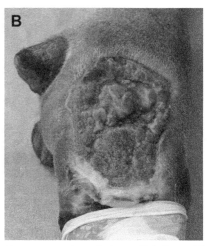

Fig. 10. (*A*) Forefoot of a breeding bull 3 weeks after amputation of the medial claw with primary wound healing. (*B*) Three weeks after open amputation in a hind foot of a cow, the wound is still large but healing without complications, and granulation and epithelialization are progressing normally.

direction. This creates a large wound and exposes the distal part of the first phalanx. The wound is bandaged with bandage changes 2 to 4 days later and again 10 to 14 days later, after which time the wound is left open.[26,32] A layer of granulation tissue forms by about 2 weeks after amputation (**Fig. 10**B) and skin closure is achieved after about 8 to 10 weeks. Open amputation is much less demanding surgically, ensures optimum wound drainage, and requires little instrumentation. Open amputation also is the technique of choice when there are large abaxial skin defects or abscesses.

With the primary focus on non-healing claw lesions, a recent study found that, after open amputation of a hind claw, cows remained in the herd for a mean duration of 22 months and after amputation of a forelimb claw, for a mean duration of 36 months.[26] These results are better than those of older studies that found that cows remained in the herd for a mean of 20 months after amputation and 18 months after resection of the distal interphalangeal joint.[52,56] The results of the more recent studies were likely better because surgery was done during the early stages of the disease process. Bulls that underwent claw amputation or resection and had a good recovery (15 of /21 bulls) remained in the herd for a mean duration of 24.6 months (range, 7–84).[88]

Protection of the wound with a block on the healthy claw is possible but usually not necessary after "high" digit amputation because there is little stress on the wound. Provided that there are no complications, weight-bearing in the affected limb returns to near-normal within a few days of amputation, and pain seems to subside quickly. The general health status and appetite were shown to improve faster after amputation than after distal sesamoid bone extirpation or resection of the distal interphalangeal joint.[53]

FRACTURES AND LUXATIONS

Pedal bone fracture is the most common digital fracture in cattle and is a typical injury of medial forelimb claws of pastured cattle.[70,89] Most of these fractures are closed, whereas pedal bone fractures that are sometimes seen in cattle on slatted floors typically affect the lateral hind claws and tend to be open. Closed fractures are best

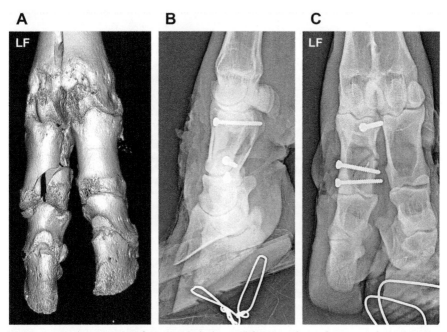

Fig. 11. Surgical treatment of proximal phalangeal fracture through open reduction and internal fixation in a 40-month-old cow. (*A*) A 3-dimensional (3D) computed tomography (CT) image of a multifragment fracture of the first phalanx with involvement of the metacarpophalangeal and proximal interphalangeal joints. A series of 3D image reconstructions was generated from the CT scan for the planning of optimal screw placement. (*B, C*) Intraoperative radiographic views of the operated digit (a block was glued to the healthy claw preoperatively and wires through the block were used to fix the foot under tension to a ring in the wall so that the operated digit was freely suspended and accessible from all sides). Internal fixation with three 4.5-mm cortical screws in lag fashion for adaption of the fracture fragments to the main abaxial fragment. In addition to the block, a fiberglass cast was applied. The cow was still in the herd 9 months after surgery.

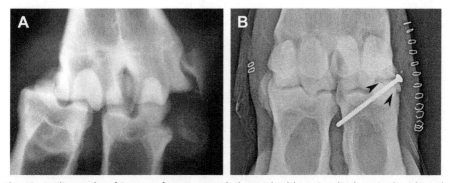

Fig. 12. Radiographs of 2 cases of metacarpophalangeal subluxation (P1 luxation) with avulsion fracture of P1 in 2 cattle. (*A*) This cow had skin abrasions and claw injuries; no treatment was instituted and the cow was culled. (*B*) In this case, the luxation was reduced surgically under general anesthesia. Fixation of the avulsion fracture (*arrowheads*) of the lateral P1 was achieved using a lag screw and a transfixation pin cast; this cow remained in the herd for at least 30 months postoperatively.

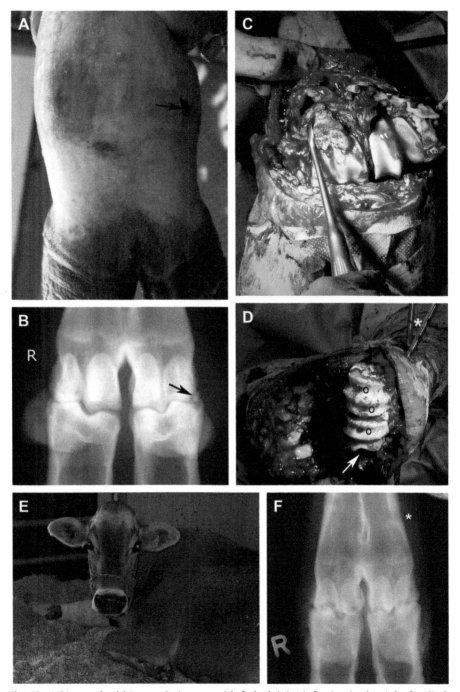

Fig. 13. A 39-month-old Brown Swiss cow with fetlock joint infection in the right forelimb. (*A*) The cause of the infection was a puncture injury (*arrow*). (*B*) Dorsopalmar radiographic view of the fetlock showing an avulsed piece of bone (*arrow*) in the region of the port of entry near the collateral ligament. (*C*) Dorsal arthrotomy. The extensor tendons and collateral ligaments have been severed and fibrin deposits removed, and (*D*) after complete

treated with a wooden block glued to the partner claw for 8 to 10 weeks. This is usually sufficient for clinical healing, whereas radiographic resolution of the fracture is slower and takes 6 to 8 months. Open pedal bone fractures may respond to conservative treatment but usually require pedal joint resection,[70] or amputation of the digit, especially in neglected cases.

Closed or open fracture of the middle phalanx is very rare and fracture of the first phalanx is an occasional occurrence. Closed fractures or unilateral phalangeal luxation can be treated by relieving the strain on the digit with a block glued to the healthy partner claw or by applying a cast for 6 to 8 weeks. The animal should be kept in a box stall for another 2 to 3 weeks after cast removal. Surgical treatment of proximal phalangeal fracture with joint involvement (**Fig. 11**) reduces the risk of subsequent arthrosis.

Luxation of the middle phalanx also is very rare and only 1 case in a heifer has been described in detail. Bilateral luxation of the middle phalanges of a hind limb was treated by arthrodesis; however, although ankylosis was achieved, pain relief was not attained and the cow did not remain in the herd.[90]

Metacarpophalangeal luxation or subluxation, also referred to as P1 luxation (**Fig. 12**A), in contrast, is relatively common and case reports of these conditions have been published.[91,92] Closed luxations and subluxations of P1 are preferably treated by means of reposition and application of a fiberglass cast. Surgical fixation of a fragment can be used in avulsion fractures (**Fig. 12**B). There is also a report of the treatment of chronic subluxation of the metatarsophalangeal joint using collateral ligament prosthesis in a cow.[92] In compound luxations, surgical arthrodesis is recommended because it is preferable (less pain, shorter recovery) to spontaneous ankylosis of the joint that is very like to occur.[92]

RESECTION OF THE PROXIMAL INTERPHALANGEAL JOINT OR THE FETLOCK JOINT

Infection of the proximal interphalangeal joint may be caused directly by a perforating injury or result from cellulitis or hematogenous spread of bacteria. If interdigital cellulitis is the primary cause, other synovial structures such as extensor/flexor tendon sheaths also may be affected, and treatment becomes more demanding. If infection is limited to the proximal interphalangeal joint, resection of the joint is the treatment of choice.[16] An existing wound or draining tract is used to access the joint, and arthrotomy usually is carried out from the abaxial or dorsal aspect to avoid the flexor tendons and major blood vessels. The joint is debrided with a curette or a drill until solid bone is felt. Postoperative treatment is analogous to that described for resection of the distal interphalangeal joint. The prognosis is considered good.[16,88,93]

As a last resort, the fetlock joint can be reamed out (**Fig. 13**). For complete arthrotomy and forced ankylosis, the fetlock joint is opened dorsally by making a semicircular incision at the level of the articular surface of the proximal phalanx[94,95] (see **Fig. 13**C). The incision is extended through the collateral ligaments to gain complete access to the palmar/plantar joint cavities and the proximal sesamoid bones. The joint is flexed maximally and all of the articular cartilage and infected subchondral bone is removed;

---

exposure of the joint, damaged cartilage and bone particularly at the port of entry (*arrow*) have been removed with a drill with osteostixis (*o*) for promotion of ankylosis and transfixation pins (*asterisk*). (*E*) The cow was kept at the clinic for 2 months; pins were removed after 5 weeks and cast was removed after 2 months. (*F*) Radiographic view at cast removal and change to splint bandage; there is osseous proliferation at the metacarpophalangeal interphase, and the pin hole in the metacarpal bone (*asterisk*) is still visible. The cow remained in the herd for at least 8 years postoperatively.

osteostixis may be used to enhance ankylosis. The skin is closed, and a full limb cast or a transfixation pin cast is applied (see **Fig 13**E). The prognosis after this procedure is fair.

SUMMARY

The animal suffering and financial cost incurred by disorders of the distal limbs in cattle are enormous, and the treatment of lame cows therefore is a socially relevant veterinary responsibility.[1,64] Injuries, fractures, luxations, and particularly deep chronic septic processes pose major diagnostic and therapeutic challenges, often exacerbated by the necessity for immediate on-farm treatment. On a positive note, the diagnostic possibilities in distal limb lesions of cattle have improved considerably because of the ubiquitous availability of ultrasonography; with practice, fractures, sequestra, bone and joint infections, abscesses, and thrombosis can be visualized quickly and reliably.[16] This allows the clinician to make a sound prognosis and aids in deciding whether a surgical salvage technique, amputation, or culling is indicated. The therapeutic dogma that alternatives to digital amputation are "by no means 100% successful" still holds true.[55] In contrast, digit amputation is not suitable for all lesions, and by no means is complication free. Although open amputation reliably eliminates non-healing lesions,[26] it should not, in principle, replace the more involved surgical treatment options.[25]

REFERENCES

1. Huxley JN. Lameness in cattle: an ongoing concern. Vet J 2012;193(3):610–1.
2. Chapinal N, Barrientos AK, von Keyserlingk MA, et al. Herd-level risk factors for lameness in freestall farms in the northeastern United States and California. J Dairy Sci 2013;96(1):318–28.
3. Cook NB. Prevalence of lameness among dairy cattle in Wisconsin as a function of housing type and stall surface. J Am Vet Med Assoc 2003;223(9):1324–8.
4. Sarjokari K, Kaustell KO, Hurme T, et al. Prevalence and risk factors for lameness in insulated free stall barns in Finland. Livest Sci 2013;156(1–3):44–52.
5. Solano L, Barkema HW, Pajor EA, et al. Prevalence of lameness and associated risk factors in Canadian Holstein-Friesian cows housed in freestall barns. J Dairy Sci 2015;98(10):6978–91.
6. Archer SC, Green MJ, Huxley JN. Association between milk yield and serial locomotion score assessments in UK dairy cows. J Dairy Sci 2010;93(9):4045–53.
7. Tadich N, Flor E, Green L. Associations between hoof lesions and locomotion score in 1098 unsound dairy cows. Vet J 2010;184(1):60–5.
8. Bicalho RC, Cheong SH, Cramer G, et al. Association between a visual and an automated locomotion score in lactating Holstein cows. J Dairy Sci 2007;90(7):3294–300.
9. Blackie N, Bleach EC, Amory JR, et al. Associations between locomotion score and kinematic measures in dairy cows with varying hoof lesion types. J Dairy Sci 2013;96(6):3564–72.
10. Cramer G, Lissemore KD, Guard CL, et al. Herd-level risk factors for seven different foot lesions in Ontario Holstein cattle housed in tie stalls or free stalls. J Dairy Sci 2009;92(4):1404–11.
11. Thomas HJ, Miguel-Pacheco GG, Bollard NJ, et al. Evaluation of treatments for claw horn lesions in dairy cows in a randomized controlled trial. J Dairy Sci 2015;98(7):4477–86.

12. Lischer CJ, Dietrich-Hunkeler A, Geyer H, et al. Healing process of uncomplicated sole ulcers in dairy cows kept in tie stalls: clinical description and blood chemical investigations. Schweiz Arch Tierheilkd 2001;143(3):125–33 [in German].

13. Lischer CJ, Wehrle M, Geyer H, et al. Healing process of claw lesions in dairy cows in alpine mountain pastures. Dtsch Tierarztl Wochenschr 2000;107(7): 255–61 [in German].

14. Anderson DE, Miesner MD. Surgical management of orthopedic and musculoskeletal diseases of feedlot calves. Vet Clin North Am Food Anim Pract 2015; 31(3):425–39, vii.

15. Desrochers A, Anderson DE. Anatomy of the distal limb. Vet Clin North Am Food Anim Pract 2001;17(1):25–38, v.

16. Desrochers A, Anderson DE, St Jean G. Surgical diseases and techniques of the digit. Vet Clin North Am Food Anim Pract 2008;24(3):535–50, vii.

17. Heppelmann M, Kofler J, Meyer H, et al. Advances in surgical treatment of septic arthritis of the distal interphalangeal joint in cattle: a review. Vet J 2009;182(2): 162–75.

18. Nuss K. Surgery of the bovine digit. In: Anderson DE, Rings DM, editors. Current veterinary therapy food animal practice. 5th edition. St Louis (MO): Saunders Elsevier; 2009. p. 242–50.

19. Steiner A, Anderson DE, Desrochers A. Diseases of the tendons and tendon sheaths. Vet Clin North Am Food Anim Pract 2014;30(1):157–75, vi.

20. Van Amstel S, Shearer J. Manual for treatment and control of lameness in cattle. Hoboken (NJ): Blackwell Publishing; 2006.

21. Steiner A, Geissbuhler U, Stoffel M, et al. Bovine radiology - digital diagnostic atlas. Berne (Switzerland): Vetsuisse Faculty University of Berne; 2010.

22. Kofler J, Geissbuhler U, Steiner A. Diagnostic imaging in bovine orthopedics. Vet Clin North Am Food Anim Pract 2014;30(1):11–53.

23. Blowey R. Non-healing hoof lesions in dairy cows. Vet Rec 2011;169(20):534.

24. Atkinson O. Non-healing hoof lesions in dairy cows. Vet Rec 2011;169(21):561–2.

25. Kofler J, Glonegger-Reichert J, Dietrich J, et al. A simple surgical treatment for bovine digital dermatitis-associated white line lesions and sole ulcers. Vet J 2015;204(2):229–31.

26. Pedersen SL. Digit amputation - getting it right for a productive future. Paper presented at: Proceedings of the Cattle Lameness Conference 2012. Sixways, Worcester, May 2, 2012.

27. Kofler J, Martinek B, Kubber-Heiss A, et al. Generalised distal limb vessel thrombosis in two cows with digital and inner organ infections. Vet J 2004;167(1): 107–10.

28. Sixt A, Stanek C, Möstl E. Der Einfluß verschiedener Methoden der Klauenkorrektur auf den Plasmakortisolspiegel bei der Milchkuh. Wien Tierarztl Monatsschr 1997;84(7):181–8.

29. Rizk A, Herdtweck S, Offinger J, et al. The use of xylazine hydrochloride in an analgesic protocol for claw treatment of lame dairy cows in lateral recumbency on a surgical tipping table. Vet J 2012;192(2):193–8.

30. Clemente C. Chirurgie am Fuß des Rindes. 1st edition. Hengersberg (Germany): Schober; 1989.

31. Pfeiffer W. Operationskursus für Tierärzte und Studierende. 5th edition. Berlin: Richard Schoetz Verlagbuchhandlung; 1912.

32. Greenough PR, MacCallum F, Weaver AD. Method of digital amputation above the coronet. In: Greenough PR, MacCallum F, Weaver AD, editors. Lameness in cattle. Philadelphia: J.B. Lippincott; 1972. p. 235–7.
33. Blaser M, Bertagnoli A, Raber M, et al. Arthroscopic approaches to the fetlock joint of adult cattle: a cadaver study. Vet J 2012;193(3):701–6.
34. Bertagnoli A, Raber M, Morandi N, et al. Tenovaginoscopic approach to the common digital flexor tendon sheath of adult cattle: technique, normal findings and preliminary results in four clinical cases. Vet J 2012;191(1):121–7.
35. Feist M, Köstlin R, Nuss K. Untersuchung des Schmerzausdruckverhaltens von Kühen nach Klauenoperationen. Tierarztl Prax Ausg G Grosstiere Nutztiere 2008;36(G):367–76.
36. Offinger J, Herdtweck S, Rizk A, et al. Postoperative analgesic efficacy of meloxicam in lame dairy cows undergoing resection of the distal interphalangeal joint. J Dairy Sci 2013;96(2):866–76.
37. Desrochers A, St-Jean G, Anderson DE, et al. Comparative evaluation of two surgical scrub preparations in cattle. Vet Surg 1996;25(4):336–41.
38. Bier A. Über einen neuen Weg Localanästhesie an den Gliedmassen zu erzeugen. Arch Klin Chir 1908;86:1007–16.
39. Antalovsky A. Technika mistni nitrozilni anestesie na distalnich castech koncetin un skotu. Vet Med (Praha) 1965;7:413–20.
40. Steiner A, Ossent P, Mathis GA. Intravenous congestion anesthesia/-antibiotic administration in cattle–indications, technics, complications. Schweiz Arch Tierheilkd 1990;132(5):227–37 [in German].
41. Simpson KM, Streeter RN, Taylor JD, et al. Bacteremia in the pedal circulation following regional intravenous perfusion of a 2% lidocaine solution in cattle with deep digital sepsis. J Am Vet Med Assoc 2014;245(5):565–70.
42. Simpson KM, Streeter RN, Cramer S, et al. Caudal vena caval thrombosis following treatment of deep digital sepsis. Can Vet J 2012;53(2):182–6.
43. Valentino LW, St Jean G, Anderson DE, et al. Osseous sequestration in cattle: 110 cases (1987-1997). J Am Vet Med Assoc 2000;217(3):376–83.
44. Rodrigues CA, Hussni CA, Nascimento ES, et al. Pharmacokinetics of tetracycline in plasma, synovial fluid and milk using single intravenous and single intravenous regional doses in dairy cattle with papillomatous digital dermatitis. J Vet Pharmacol Ther 2010;33(4):363–70.
45. Rubio-Martínez LM, Elmas CR, Black B, et al. Clinical use of antimicrobial regional limb perfusion in horses: 174 cases (1999–2009). J Am Vet Med Assoc 2012;241(12):1650–8.
46. Varasano V, Mortellaro CM, Argentieri V, et al. Clinical efficacy of a single intravenous regional limb perfusion (IVRLP) with Marbofloxacin for treating acute interdigital phlegmon in thirty dairy cows. Paper presented at: 18th International Symposium & 10th International Conference on Lameness in Ruminants. Valdivia, Chile, November 22–25, 2015.
47. Desrochers A. General principles of surgery applied to cattle. Vet Clin North Am Food Anim Pract 2005;21(1):1–17.
48. Anderson DE, Desrochers A, St Jean G. Management of tendon disorders in cattle. Vet Clin North Am Food Anim Pract 2008;24(3):551–66, viii.
49. Shearer J, Plummer P, Schleining J, et al. Effect of topical treatment with oxytetracycline soluble powder or copper sulfate powder on healing of claw lesions. Paper presented at: 18th International Symposium & 10th International Conference on Lameness in Ruminants. Valdivia, Chile, November 22–25, 2015.

50. Kofler J, Martinek B. New surgical approach to the plantar fetlock joint through the digital flexor tendon sheath wall and suspensory ligament apparatus in cases of concurrent septic synovitis in two cattle. Vet J 2005;169(3):370–5.
51. Mulon PY, Desrochers A. Indications and limitations of splints and casts. Vet Clin North Am Food Anim Pract 2014;30(1):55–76.
52. Nuss K. Zur Klauengelenksresektion beim Rind. Eine Analyse von 281 Fällen [Inaugural-Dissertation]. München (Germany): Chirurgische Tierklinik der Tierärztlichen Fakultät; Ludwig-Maximilians-Universität; 1988.
53. Starke A, Heppelmann M, Beyerbach M, et al. Septic arthritis of the distal interphalangeal joint in cattle: comparison of digital amputation and joint resection by solar approach. Vet Surg 2007;36(4):350–9.
54. Raundal PM, Forkman B, Andersen PH, et al. Lame cows benefit from being housed in recovery pens. Paper presented at: 18th International Symposium & 10th International Conference on Lameness in Ruminants. Valdivia, Chile, November 22–25, 2015.
55. Baxter GM, Lakritz J, Wallace CE, et al. Alternatives to digit amputation in cattle. Comp Cont Educ Pract 1991;13(6):1022–35.
56. Pejsa TG, St Jean G, Hoffsis GF, et al. Digit amputation in cattle: 85 cases (1971-1990). J Am Vet Med Assoc 1993;202(6):981–4.
57. Weaver AD. Performing amputation of the bovine digit. Vet Med 1991;12:1230–3.
58. Funk KA. Late results after toe and claw amputation in cattle. Berl Munch Tierarztl Wochenschr 1977;90(8):152–6 [in German].
59. Guller K, Martig J. Follow-up examinations after toe amputation in cattle. Schweiz Arch Tierheilkd 1977;119(12):501–10 [in German].
60. Leach KA, Paul ES, Whay HR, et al. Reducing lameness in dairy herds–overcoming some barriers. Res Vet Sci 2013;94(3):820–5.
61. Nuss K, Kostlin RG, Bohmer H, et al. The significance of ungulocoriitis septica (traumatic) in the toe of the bovine claw. Tierarztl Prax 1990;18(6):567–75 [in German].
62. Kofler J. Clinical study of toe ulcer and necrosis of the apex of the distal phalanx in 53 cattle. Vet J 1999;157(2):139–47.
63. van Amstel SR, Shearer JK, Palin FL. Moisture content, thickness, and lesions of sole horn associated with thin soles in dairy cattle. J Dairy Sci 2004;87(3):757–63.
64. Dirksen G. Pflegemassnahmen und Operationen an den Zehen. In: Dirksen G, Gründer H, Stöber M, editors. Innere Medizin und Chirurgie des Rindes. 4th edition. Berlin: Wien Parey-Blackwell; 2002. p. 978–95.
65. Burnell M, Reader J. Digit amputation by lay foot trimmers. Vet Rec 2010;167(25): 985.
66. Gomez A, Dopfer D, Cook NB, et al. Non-healing hoof lesions in dairy cows. Vet Rec 2011;169(24):642.
67. Blowey R, Chesterton N. Non-healing hoof lesions in dairy cows in Chile. Vet Rec 2012;170(7):187–8.
68. Blowey R. Non-healing hoof lesions in dairy cows. Vet Rec 2012;170(1):26–7.
69. Blowey R. Changing indications for digit amputation in cattle. Vet Rec 2011; 169(9):236–U272.
70. Köstlin RG, Petzoldt F-J. Zur Klauenbeinfraktur beim Rind. Tierärztl Umsch 1985; 40(11):864–74.
71. Lewis AJ, Sod GA, Gill MS, et al. Distal interphalangeal joint arthrodesis in seven cattle using the Acutrak Plus screw. Vet Surg 2009;38(5):659–63.

72. Mulon PY, Babkine M, d'Anjou MA, et al. Degenerative disease of the distal inter-phalangeal joint and sesamoid bone in calves: 9 cases (1995-2004). J Am Vet Med Assoc 2009;234(6):794–9.

73. Fritsch R. Therapie von Klauenkrankheiten beim Rind. In: Knezevic P, editor. Int Tagung Orthopädie bei Huf- und Klauentieren. Hannover (Germany): Schaper; 1985. p. 105–13.

74. Zulauf M, Jordan P, Steiner A. Fenestration of the abaxial hoof wall and implanta-tion of gentamicin-impregnated collagen sponges for the treatment of septic arthritis of the distal interphalangeal joint in cattle. Vet Rec 2001;149(17):516–8.

75. Assmus G. Erfahrungen mit der Resektion des Klauensesambeines beim Rind. Nord Vet Med 1964;16(Suppl 1):326–34.

76. Westhues M, Breuer D. Klauengelenksresektion und Sehnenresektion beim Klauengeschwür des Rindes. Nord Vet Med 1964;(Suppl I):335–43.

77. Clemente C. Beitrag zur Weiterentwicklung der Sehnenresektion und der Klauen-gelenksresektion beim Rind. Tierärztl Umsch 1965;20:108–10.

78. Nuss K, Weaver MP. Resection of the distal interphalangeal joint in cattle: an alter-native to amputation. Vet Rec 1991;128(23):540–3.

79. Greenough PR, Ferguson JG. Alternatives to amputation. Vet Clin North Am Food Anim Pract 1985;1(1):195–203.

80. Kersjes AW, Németh F, Rutgers L, et al, editors. A colour atlas of large animal sur-gery. St Louis (MO): Mosby; 1985.

81. Bicalho RC, Cheong SH, Guard CL. Field technique for the resection of the distal interphalangeal joint and proximal resection of the deep digital flexor tendon in cows. Vet Rec 2007;160(13):435–9.

82. Merkens HW. Radical surgery (amputation) or conservative treatment (drainage) in cases of septic pedal arthritis and navicular bursitis in cattle. Tijdschr Dierge-neeskd 1977;102(5):326–9 [in Dutch].

83. Kofler J. Ultrasonographic imaging of pathology of the digital flexor tendon sheath in cattle. Vet Rec 1996;139(2):36–41.

84. Kofler J. Ultrasonographic examination of the musculoskeletal system in cattle. Tierarztl Prax Ausg G Grosstiere Nutztiere 2011;39(5):299–313 [in German].

85. Morandi N, Bertagnoli A, Steiner A. Tenovaginoscopic lavage for treatment of septic tenosynovitis in a breeding bull. Vet Rec 2009;165(14):415–6.

86. Kofler J. New possibilities for the diagnosis of septic tenosynovitis of the digital flexor tendon sheath in cattle using sonography–therapy and long-term results. Dtsch Tierarztl Wochenschr 1994;101(6):215–22 [in German].

87. Vertenten G, Gasthuys F, Muylle S, et al. Bovine digit amputation with primary closure: surgical technique and follow-up of 45 cases. Paper presented at: 15th International Symposium and 7th Conference on Lameness in Ruminants. Kuopio, Finland, June 9–13, 2008.

88. Kofler J, Feist M, Starke A, et al. Resection of the distal/proximal interphalangeal joint and digit amputation in 21 breeding bulls–indications, clinical findings and longterm outcome. Berl Munch Tierarztl Wochenschr 2007;120(3–4):156–64 [in German].

89. Numans S, Wintzer HJ. Gedeckte Klauenbeinfrakturen während des Weidegangs beim Rind. Dtsch Tierarztl Wochenschr 1958;65:201–4.

90. Muggli E, Weidmann E, Bruderer A, et al. Arthrodesis of the proximal interphalan-geal joints of a hindlimb in a heifer. Vet Comp Orthop Traumatol 2015;28(1): 67–72.

91. Greenough PR, McCallum FJ, Weaver AD. Luxation and subluxation of the fetlock joint. In: Greenough PR, McCallum FJ, Weaver AD, editors. Lameness in cattle. 1st edition. Philadelphia: J.B. Lippincott Company; 1972. p. 208.

92. Rothlisberger J, Schawalder P, Kircher P, et al. Collateral ligament prosthesis for the repair of subluxation of the metatarsophalangeal joint in a jersey cow. Vet Rec 2000;146(22):640–3.

93. Kofler J. Die septische Arthritis des Krongelenkes beim Rind - Klinische, röntgenologische sowie sonographische Befunde und Behandlung. Berl Munch Tierarztl Wochenschr 1995;108(8):281–9.

94. Van Huffel X. Surgical treatment of joint and tendon disease in calves and cattle. Cattle Pract 1996;4(2):187–92.

95. Verschooten F, De Moor A, Steenhaut M, et al. Surgical and conservative treatment of infectious arthritis in cattle. J Am Vet Med Assoc 1974;165(3):271–5.

Surgical Management of Septic Arthritis

Pierre-Yves Mulon, Dr Vet[a],*, André Desrochers, DMV, MS[b],
David Francoz, Dr Vet, MSc[b]

KEYWORDS

• Septic arthritis • Cattle • Joint lavage • Arthrotomy • Arthroscopy

KEY POINTS

• Diagnostic tests used to diagnose joint sepsis include radiographic studies, ultrasonography of the joint, and synovial fluid analysis.
• Treatment should be prompt and aggressive; long-term administration of antibiotics, pain management, and joint lavages are often necessary treatment.
• Joint lavage techniques include tidal irrigation, through-and-through lavage, arthroscopy, and arthrotomy.
• Commonly infected joints include the fetlock, carpus, tarsus, and stifle.

 Video content accompanies this article at http://www.vetfood.theclinics.com.

Septic arthritis is a common cause of bovine lameness. In a study reporting incidence of lameness in dairy herds, Bargai and Levin[1] reported that arthritis represented 13.8% of the cases. Consequences may be dramatic if not treated adequately, resulting in chronic pain, decreased range of motion, and decreased joint function. Septic arthritis is very painful, causing alteration of normal joint physiology and leading to rapid and permanent destruction of the cartilage or bone. An early diagnosis as well as a prompt and effective treatment are essential to restoring normal function of the infected joint. In severe cases, septic arthritis may lead to culling of the animal or humane euthanasia.

ETIOLOGY

Bacteria colonize the joint in 3 different ways: (1) through a wound directly invading the joint, (2) by close proximity of a primary infection site to the joint and migration the bacteria within the inflamed tissue into the joint, and (3) by crossing the synovial

The authors have nothing to disclose.
[a] Large Animal Clinical Science Department, College of Veterinary Medicine, University of Tennessee, 2407 River Drive, Knoxville, TN 37996, USA; [b] Faculté de Médecine Vétérinaire, Université de Montréal, St-Hyacinthe, Quebec, Canada
* Corresponding author.
E-mail address: pymulon@gmail.com

membrane from the capillary vessels during bacteremia. In this manner, joints can become infected remotely from the primary source of infection.[2]

Adult cows tend to suffer more from the first 2 etiologies of septic arthritis and therefore a single joint is usually infected (**Fig. 1**). Calves, especially those suffering from lack of transfer of passive immunity, are more likely to have multiple joints infected owing to the bacteria present in the bloodstream. The primary sources of infection for septic arthritis in calves are commonly umbilical infection, pneumonia, otitis media/interna, and/or enteritis.[3–5] In a study of 39 cases of calves suffering of omphalophlebitis, septic arthritis was diagnosed on 11.[3] However, remote septic arthritis has also been described in adults owing to chronic endocarditis and severe mastitis.[6,7] Knowing the history of the calf helps the veterinarian to determine a therapeutic plan, because bacteria may differ depending on the primary disease.

PATHOPHYSIOLOGY

Immediately after bacterial colonization within a joint, proliferation ensues and initiates an acute inflammatory response. This fast reaction of the joint against pathogens produces a cascade of events that leads to the increased concentration of proinflammatory mediators. A rapid recruitment of polymorphonuclear granulocytes and activated macrophages follows the bacterial proliferation, leading to the substantial release of proinflammatory cytokines such as tumor necrosis factor-α, and interleukins 1 and 6.[8] All these molecules promote osteoclast differentiation and bone reabsorption.

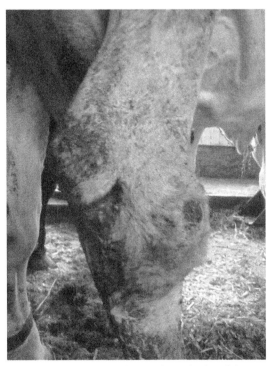

Fig. 1. Chronic, deep laceration over the plantarolateral side of the tarsocrural joint in an adult Holstein cow. The infection ultimately reached the plantarolateral recess of the tarsocrural joint. The swelling on the lateral aspect of the hock is a hygroma owing to repeated external trauma and should not be misinterpreted as joint distension.

Matrix metalloproteinase release leads to subsequent bone and cartilage degradation. Cartilage proteoglycan production decreases over time and leads to loss of biometrical properties of the cartilage. Fibrin covers both cartilage and synovial structures and creates bacterial reservoirs within the joint, as well as barriers that reduce the cartilage nutrition through the synovial fluid. The presence of a joint effusion secondary to increased synovial fluid production increases intraarticular pressure, which mechanically impedes blood and nutrient supply to the joint and further exacerbates cellular damage. In severely affected joints, the fibrin will create a pannus covering the entire joint. Ultimately, the immune response to the infection leads to the destruction of the cartilage and the synovial tissues.

DIAGNOSIS
Clinical Presentation

Usually, lameness is the first clinical sign observed by the owner. Onset of clinical signs may vary from progressive swelling or a sudden non–weight-bearing lameness. In experimentally induced septic arthritis, clinical signs appeared within 4 to 8 hours after intraarticular bacterial inoculation.[9] Joint distension is variable, but will always provoke intense pain with the animal toe touching or walking on 3 legs. Fever is rarely present in adults contrary to young calves owing to concomitant diseases like pneumonia, otitis, or umbilical infection. Joint distension, increased heat over the affected joint, and pain on palpation and manipulation of the joint are other common clinical signs (**Fig. 2**). Palpation of all other joints is mandatory especially in young calves where polyarthritis is more frequent.

Lameness is obvious in most cases (Video 1). However, it may remain discreet in some cases and careful attention to the stance and protection of the affected limb

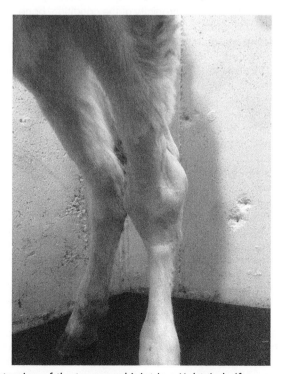

Fig. 2. Severe distension of the tarsocrural joint in a Holstein heifer.

may be necessary during the examination. Distal interphalangeal joint aside (discussed elsewhere in this issue), the most common joints affected are the fetlock, carpus, tarsus, and stifle. Shoulder, elbow, and hip can also be infected and the diagnosis is more challenging[10] in these joints.

Careful examination of any wound in close proximity of a joint should be made. The area over the wound and the joint should be clipped and surgically prepared. Sterile water-soluble gel in the wound bed will prevent hair from becoming trapped within the wound. A needle is then inserted aseptically in the joint away from the wound and sterile saline can be injected into the joint. Observation of saline flowing through the wound confirms the communication between the wound and the joint.

Differential diagnosis should include degenerative joint disease,[11] such as osteochondrosis,[12] luxation, ligament injury, hemarthrosis, intraarticular fracture, and idiopathic arthritis.[13] Eventually, septic tenosynovitis or physitis induces a severe lameness that may mimic clinical presentation of septic arthritis. Palpation and manipulation of the affected area is painful and periarticular soft tissue swelling may render joint distension more difficult to palpate.

Specific attention should be given to the known sources of primary infection. A thorough evaluation of the umbilicus as well as the lungs is indicated. Ultrasonography can be a very useful diagnostic tool to evaluate other structures like the lungs and umbilicus.[14]

Medical Imaging

Radiography is useful to identify bony lesions. Subchondral bone radiolucency takes time to appear and the delay between the lesion and its radiographic appearance is 2 weeks on average. In acute conditions, only soft tissue periarticular swelling is observed on radiographs. With the chronicity of the condition, bone lysis may become visible starting with small circular lesions surrounded by sclerosis evolving to major destruction of the bone and architecture of the joint (**Fig. 3**).

If radiography is not readily available, ultrasonography is a useful tool to evaluate the synovial cavity.[15] A 7.5- to 10-MHz linear probe allows the examination of superficial structures and can be use on the entire forelimb and the distal aspect of the hindlimb; the stifle and hip are best evaluated using a 3.5- to 5-mHz convex probe. The joint distension allows a clear evaluation of the joint. Joint fluids appears hypoechoic and tends to become more hyperechoic as the fibrin clots invade the joints as the arthritis turns chronic and purulent. The cartilage appears also hypoechoic and the subchondral bone is identified as the highly hyperechoic line underlying the cartilage (**Fig. 4**A). Becoming more familiar with the joint structure, bone lysis can be identified using ultrasonography by a defect within the subchondral bone. Compressing the synovial cavity with the transducer may create turbulences within the cavity if the distension is mostly from liquid effusion; however, the absence of turbulence within the joint suggests a solid content compatible with clotted fibrin. Visualization of large coalescent fibrin clots floating within the synovial fluid, or absence of flow phenomena is an indication for an open arthrotomy rather than performing a through-and-through needle lavage of the joint. Ultrasonography also allows to detect subchondral lysis at an early stage because the ultrasound waves are not reflected by the bone surface if altered. If lameness is suspected to originate from the hip, ultrasonography will be very useful to image the joint (**Fig. 4**B). Ultrasonographic images of the hip are obtained using a 3.5-MHz transducer positioned longitudinally along the femoral neck. In adults, ultrasonographic examination of the coxofemoral joint is more appropriate considering the technical difficulties to obtain good quality radiographic views.

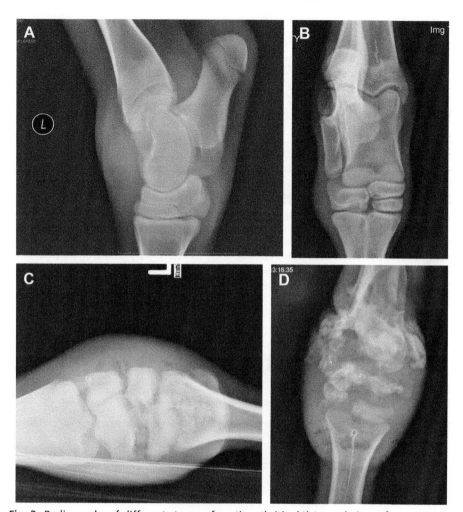

Fig. 3. Radiographs of different stages of septic arthritis. (*A*) Lateral view of a tarsus in a Holstein heifer. A soft tissue swelling is present over the joint; however, no bone lesions are noticed. (*B*) Dorsoplantar view of the tarsus in a 6-week-old Holstein heifer. Moderate soft tissue swelling is present on the lateral aspect of the tarsometatarsal joint, a circular radiolucent area is observed on the tarsal bone. (*C*) Dorsopalmar view of a carpus of a 3-month-old Holstein heifer. Multiple radiolucent areas (gas opacities) are visible within the intercarpal and carpometacarpal joint as a result of a chronic pressure sores communicating with the joint. A significant soft tissue swelling is present and the distal row of carpal bones have lost their normal anatomic appearance. (*D*) Dorsopalmar view of a 5-month-old angus calf. The carpal bone lysis is extremely severe associated with bone destruction of the radius and peripheral bone reaction to the infection.

CLINICAL PATHOLOGY

Arthrocentesis (**Fig. 5**) allows cytologic evaluation and bacteriologic culture. Cytologic analysis allows the clinician to differentiate arthropathies. Arthrocentesis can be performed on standing or recumbent animals. Regardless of the technique used, proper restraint is necessary. Light sedation may be given before attempting joint puncture because it will limit the limb withdrawal reflex commonly observed.

A

B

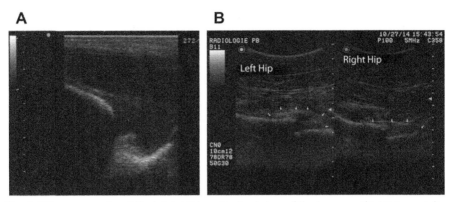

Fig. 4. Ultrasonography of the joint. (*A*) Longitudinal view of the tarsocrural joint in a moderately distended joint. The subchondral bone appears hyperechoic. The synovial fluid appears hypoechoic. (*B*) Ultrasonographic evaluation of the hip in a young Holstein heifer. The joint capsule (*arrowhead*) appears distended on the left side, it appears completely normal on the right side. *Arrows* delineate the synovial membrane of both coxo-femoral joint underlying the distension of the affected one (*left*) with the control in the normal one (*right*).

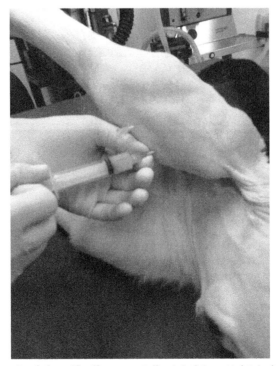

Fig. 5. Arthrocentesis of the stifle (femoropatellar joint) in a Holstein heifer aspirating a yellow-colored, opaque synovial fluid. The area has been clipped and aseptically prepared. The spinal needle is inserted between the medial and median patellar ligament in a torso-caudal direction to slide it underneath the patella.

The area over the joint should be aseptically prepared to limit the risk of contamination of the joint by commensal skin organisms. Hair clipping has been questioned in horses in the past years for arthrocentesis[16]; however, it is the authors' opinion that it should be performed in ruminants owing to the usual gross contamination of the hair. Anatomic landmarks for needle positioning for each joint are described in **Table 1**. Synovial fluid can be analyzed for cytology (purple top tube with EDTA), specific enzymes, and glucose (red top tubes) or bacteriology (sterile dry tube or specific transport media). Examination of the viscosity and turbidity of the synovial fluid is often diagnostic (**Fig. 6**). Cytologic evaluation can be used to confirm joint sepsis (**Fig. 7**). Rohde and colleagues[17] investigated the cytologic analysis of 130 cases of joint diseases in cattle and found that odds of having a septic arthritis were 4 times greater than suffering from a nonseptic arthropathy if synovial joint analysis indicated a total protein concentration of greater than 4.5 g/dL. This group also found that the odds of having a septic joint were 17.5 times greater if synovial joint analysis indicated a nuclear cell count of more than 25,000 cells/mL, 15.4 times greater if the polymorphonuclear cell count was more than 20,000 cells/mL, and 30 times greater if the percentage of polymorphonuclear neutrophils was more than 80%. In a model of induced septic arthritis in calves with a treatment started 24 hours after the inoculation, the mean percentage of polymorphonuclear neutrophils cells remained at more than 80% for up to 2 weeks after inoculation, even if the animals had resolved clinical septic arthritis.[9]

Synovial fluid collected aseptically after surgical preparation of the joint should be submitted for bacteriologic analysis, aerobic and anaerobic culture. A negative result does not guarantee the absence of bacteria within the joint. In a study of 172 cases of septic arthritis, positive bacterial culture was obtained in 60% of the cases.[18] *Truepurella pyogenes* was identified as the most common bacteria, followed by streptococci, enterobactariaceae, and pasteurellaceae.[18] Despite being less commonly isolated, Pseudomonas,[18] *Lactococcus lactis,*[19] *Erysipelothrix rhusiopathiae,*[20] *Salmonella typhymurium,*[21] and even *Borrelia burgdorferi*[22] have also been identified as potential intraarticular pathogens. To maximize the growth of the bacteria, the synovial fluids should be placed in a specific transport culture media, such as Port-a-Cul (Becton Dickinson, Franklin Lakes, NJ). Blood culture systems may also be used; however, their choice is important as some may inhibit growth of *Mycoplasma*.

Mycoplasma spp. is an increasingly recognized organism responsible for various systemic infections including septic arthritis.[23,24] Culture of these pathogens is fastidious and is not routinely performed. It is the author's opinion that specific request for *Mycoplasma spp* and *Histophilus somni* should be performed whenever possible to better evaluate the incidence of their involvement in septic arthritis.

Polymerase chain reaction has been developed for several pathogens in many diagnostic laboratories as an alternative to bacterial culture. Polymerase chain reaction is usually associated with a faster result and a greater sensitivity. However, limitations of a positive result are the inability to determine whether the bacteria was alive in the sample, and its antimicrobial sensitivity. Moreover, the polymerase chain reactions actually available are developed for a particular bacterium and specific tests need to be requested for each pathogen of concern.

MEDICAL MANAGEMENT OF SEPTIC ARTHRITIS

Both medical and surgical management of septic arthritis target the reduction of the bacterial load, the diminution of the concentration of inflammatory mediators, and pain management.

Table 1
Landmarks for arthrocentesis in cattle

Articulations	Compartment(s)	Arthrocentesis Sites	Needle Length	Communication in Compound Joints	Difficulty
Distal interphalangeal joint	(1)	Proximal to the coronary band, lateral to the extensor process, aiming the needle with an 60° angle in a distopalmar/plantar direction	1″ or 1.5″		++
Fetlock	(2) Lateral and medial	In flexion, needle inserted dorsally with an angle of 45° in a distal position	1″ or 1.5″	100% between lateral and medial compartment	+
		Between the proximal sesamoid bone and metacarpus or metatarsus	1″		0
		If distended, proximal to the proximal sesamoid bone, and just palmar/plantar to the metacarpus/tarsus	1″		0
Carpus	(3) a. Antebrachiocarpal	Lateral and medial to extensor carpi radialis (a and b)	1″ or 1.5″	Antebrachiocarpal and midcarpal: 13%	0
	b. Midcarpal	Lateral and medial to the common digital extensor (all 3 compartments)	1″ or 1.5″	Midcarpal and carpometacarpal: 100%	0
	c. Carpometacarpal	Medial to the lateral digital extensor (c)	1″		+
Tarsus	(4) • Tarsocrural	Proximal, dorsal and lateral or medial to the digital extensor (a and b)	1″ or 1.5″	Tarsocrural and proximal intertarsal: 100%	0
	• Proximal intertarsal	Lateral and medial plantar pouch for joint lavage and arthrotomy (a)	1″ or 1.5″		0
	• Distal intertarsal	Medial aspect, between the fused second and third tarsal bone and the fused central and fourth tarsal bone	3/4″ or 1″	Distal intertarsal and tarsometatarsal: 30%	++++
	• Tarsometatarsal				

Joint		Landmarks	Needle	Size	Communication	Grade
Stifle	(3)					
	a. Lateral femorotibial	Cranial or caudal to the collateral ligament (a and b)	Spinal needle	1.5″	No direct communication between the 2 femorotibial joints	+
	b. Medial femorotibial					
	c. Femoropatellar	Between the medial and middle patellar ligaments with a spinal needle aiming under the patella (c)			Medial femorotibial and femoropatellar: 100% Lateral femorotibial and femoropatellar: 60%	++
Elbow	(1)	Cranial to the collateral ligament; if distended, cranial and lateral to the lateral humeral epicondyle In the angle formed by the lateral humeral epicondyle and the olecranon with the needle in a craniodistal direction		1″		+
Shoulder	(1)	Cranial approach: needle inserted caudomedially in the notch between the cranial and caudal portion of the lateral tuberosity Lateral approach: cranial to the infraspinatus muscle tendon, 1 cm to the caudal portion of the lateral tuberosity	Spinal needle		No direct communication between the joint and the infraspinatus tendon bursa, attention should be paid not to enter it when performing the arthrocentesis	++ +++
Hip	(1)	Cranial to the greater trochanter of the femur, aiming caudomedially with an angle of 45° in the horizontal plane. Addition of ultrasonography may facilitate the arthrocentesis	Spinal needle			++++

Levels of difficulty of each arthrocentesis are graded from 0 to ++++ from the easiest to the most difficult.
Adapted from Desrochers A, Francoz D. Clinical management of septic arthritis in cattle. Vet Clin North Am Food Anim Pract 2014;30(1):184–85; with permission.

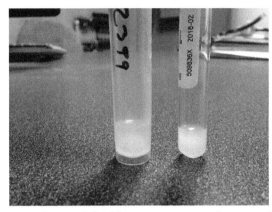

Fig. 6. Gross evaluation of synovial fluid from a septic joint. The synovial fluid appears very cloudy.

ANTIMICROBIAL THERAPY

Antimicrobial therapy is the central point in the management of septic arthritis. However, to date, there is no evidence in human or veterinary medicine on the ideal or best antimicrobial treatment regimen. A systematic review and metaanalysis in human medicine failed to identify any evidence on the advantage of 1 treatment regimen over another.[25] Additionally, these investigators concluded that there was a paucity of high-quality evidence on antimicrobial treatment of septic arthritis. To our knowledge, evidence of treatment efficacy in food animal species remains scarce and no randomized clinical trials are available.

Antimicrobial therapy should be instituted at the earliest time after establishing the diagnosis. Empirical antimicrobial therapy should be instituted first and then switched if bacterial culture or results become available and support changing the antimicrobial

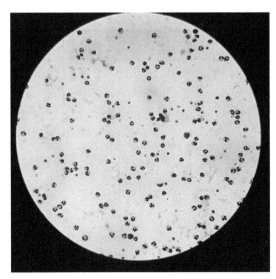

Fig. 7. Cytologic evaluation of the synovial fluid, stained with diff-quick. A large predominance of polymorphonuclear cells (neutrophils) on the smear confirms the diagnosis of septic joint in this animal.

therapy. The choice of empirical antimicrobial therapy should be based on host consideration (age of the animal, production), the clinical presentation (ie, acute or chronic; hematogenous or extension of local infection or direct trauma to into the joint), knowledge of local prevalence of drug resistance to particular pathogens, and legality. Broad spectrum and bactericidal antimicrobials are often recommended as initial therapy.[26] Additionally, an antimicrobial drug targeting mycoplasma should be used in first intent in calves, particularly in those suffering from bovine respiratory disease or otitis media/interna.

In a recent study, Jones and colleagues[27] demonstrated that the synovial fluid concentration of tulathromycin, gamithromycin, and florfenicol in the hindlimb fetlock joint were higher for a longer period of time compared with plasma values. Intraarticular diffusion of trimethoprim–sulfadiazine, penicillin, cefapirin, and oxytetracycline have proven to be sufficient to treat cases of septic arthritis in calves.[28–30] Ceftiofur has also been used successfully to treat experimentally induced septic arthritis in calves.[9] Fluoroquinolones have a broad spectrum of activity including *Mycoplasma spp*, making their use attractive. However, they are not labelled for treatment of septic arthritis, and off-label use of these antimicrobials is illegal in cattle in the United States. Additionally, chondrotoxicity has been a concern for this class of antibiotimicrobial. Administration of twice daily of ciprofloxacine at 15 mg/kg for 14 consecutive days in 6- to 8-week-old lambs failed to produce hyaline chondrotoxicity, nor did it alter the growth velocity at the growth plate.[31] A 10-day treatment regimen of marbofloxacin has been reported to be successful in calves without any adverse effects reported.[32] However, the use of quinolones is limited to countries where they are permitted and in respect of judicious use of antimicrobial drugs. They should not be used as primary treatment.

As recommended in human medicine, the intravenous (IV) route of administration is favored at first. After that, treatment may be continued via intramuscular or subcutaneous administration. However, one should consider the patient and feasibility of the treatment; it is not always possible to administer medication on a daily basis in many circumstances, making long-acting antibiotics attractive. It is the author's opinion that ideally medications are administered via the IV route in young calves to spare the underdeveloped muscles. An IV catheter may be placed in the jugular vein and changed regularly to avoid catheter-related complications; alternatively, placement of long-term catheters decreases the need for catheter changes.

Local delivery of antibiotics has been advocated to increase the intraarticular concentration. Regional limb perfusion has proven to be a simple and effective technique for the treatment of synovial sepsis in the distal portion of the limbs in large animal.[33] Tourniquet selection is important. Levine and colleagues[34] demonstrated that a narrow rubber tourniquet placed above the carpus was ineffective to achieve adequate concentration of antibiotics in the distal limb and recommended the used of either wide rubber or a pneumatic tourniquet. Interestingly, synovial concentrations of antibiotics were not statistically different using 3 different volumes (10, 30, and 60 mL) of perfusate in horses[35]; no difference was found in a recent study comparing the tourniquet application times (20 vs 30 minutes) in standing horses.[36] Most studies on regional limb perfusion in large animals have investigated aminoglycoside regional limb perfusion in horses. In a recent study evaluating the synovial concentration in the metacarpophalangeal joint after 1.5 g of combined ampicillin–sulbactam for regional limb perfusion in adult cattle, Depenbrock and colleagues[37] found that the concentration remained above the minimum inhibitory concentration for a mean of 18.9 hours after infusion.

The ideal duration of antimicrobial therapy is unknown. Several weeks ($\geq$3 weeks) are commonly recommended. However, clinical trials in human medicine have shown that, in cases of uncomplicated septic arthritis owing to methicillin-sensitive *Staphylococcus aureus*, 10 days of therapy is sufficient.[38,39] In an experimental model of acute

Escherichia coli septic arthritis in calves, 20 days of antimicrobial treatment was instituted. However, rapid recovery (clinical signs and negative bacterial detection in synovial fluid) occurred within 1 week, suggesting a shorter duration of treatment.[9] As mentioned, a 10-day treatment duration has been demonstrated efficacious in calves with naturally occurring septic arthritis.[32] Complementary examination, such as blood work and inflammatory biomarkers as well as synovial fluid analysis, could be used to help the veterinary practitioner decide on the duration of antimicrobial treatment.

CONTROL OF THE INFLAMMATORY PROCESS

Joint destruction occurs secondary to the inflammatory process that develops in response to invading bacteria. Steroids and nonsteroidal drugs can be used to control the inflammatory process. The use of corticosteroids is controversial. Steroids can induce an immunosuppression, which could enhance the infectious process. However, experimental models of septic arthritis in mice and rabbits have demonstrated that simultaneous administration of corticosteroids and antimicrobial drugs reduced the severity of the synovial inflammation and no evidence of worsening of infection was reported.[40,41] Additionally, 2 clinical trials in children have demonstrated that the combination of systemic administration of corticosteroids (dexamethasone for 4 days) and antimicrobial drugs shorten the duration of illness.[42–45] Actual consensus about corticosteroid used based on a metaanalysis is a reduction of the duration of both symptoms and inflammatory markers.[46] Unfortunately, no data are available in cattle on the potential beneficial effect of systemic corticosteroid administration in association with antimicrobial therapy in cases of septic arthritis.

PAIN MANAGEMENT

Pain management is an important element of the treatment plan of septic arthritis. Septic arthritis induces a high intensity nociceptive stimulus. Nonsteroidal antiinflammatory drugs have been used for decades to lower the swelling and to reduce pain associated with infection. Ketoprofen (3 mg/kg IV) and flunixin (1.1 mg/kg) are used on a regular basis. Meloxicam is a more selective cyclooxygenase-2 inhibitor approved in Europe and Canada (0.5 mg/kg IV or subcutaneously [SC]). Its use has gained popularity among veterinarians in Canada for the treatment of orthopedic infection. Coetzee and colleagues[47] found that lameness scores improved after oral administration of meloxicam (0.5 mg/kg orally) once daily for 4 consecutive days after induction of a transitory articular inflammation with amphotericin B. No side effect regarding appetite based on the average daily weight gain was reported.

If pain is refractory to administration of nonsteroidal anti-inflammatory drugs, multimodal pain management should be attempted to allow the animal to be more comfortable, but also to allow the joint to be mobilized with the maximal range of motion. Gabapentin (10 mg/kg orally, every 12 hours) has been advocated for this purpose for deep orthopedic sepsis.[48] Acupuncture has been shown to be an effective treatment for knee pain in osteoarthritis in human medicine.[49] Acupuncture can also be added to the pain management plan of cattle suffering from severe lameness.

Opioids can be used for multimodal pain management. Butorphanol (0.02 mg/kg IV or SC, 4–6 times a day), Morphine (0.05–1 mg/kg SC, 2–6 times a day) and buprenorphine (0.005–0.01 mg/kg SC, 2–4 times a day) have been described for use in orthopedic infection.[48] Recently, opioid-induced adverse effects (agitation, altered consciousness, hyperthermia, mydriasis and nystagmus, vocalization, and hyperresponsiveness to stimulation) were described after the combined use of morphine epidural (0.1 mg/kg) and fentanyl patch (100 µg/hour) to treat a persistent lameness after the surgical and medical management of stifle septic arthritis. Side effects were alleviated with the administration of naloxone (5 μg/kg) diluted and given slowly IV over 3 minutes.[48,50]

SURGICAL TREATMENT OPTIONS

Surgical treatment is complementary to medical management and aims to reduce the synovial pressure and bacterial load. Inflammation of the joint induces distension of the synovial membrane and is responsible for the pain associated with septic arthritis. Alleviating the synovial pressure by joint aspiration will increase the comfort of the animal. Through and through needle lavage, performing arthrotomies, or flushing the joint under arthroscopic guidance are possible ways to relieve synovial pressure. Eventually, if the cartilage and bone are severely impaired and joint viability condemned, arthrodesis may be attempted for some joints as a salvage procedure.

Joint interventions are painful. Animals must be sedated and appropriate analgesia used. Locoregional anesthesia of the forelimb can be achieved by performing a brachial plexus block using either electrostimulation or ultrasound guidance to ascertain the accurate position of the needle before injecting the anesthetic solution.[51–55] The hindlimb can easily be anesthetized with an epidural block. Alternatively, IV infusion of anesthetic solution distal to a tourniquet provides an additional level of anesthesia. It is important to practice strict aseptic principles to avoid contamination. The joint is, therefore, surgically prepared and sterile gloves are worn throughout the procedure.

Tidal Irrigation

Tidal irrigation is performed by inserting a single needle in the joint at a specific location (see **Table 1**) and injecting fresh isotonic solution in several aliquots that are subsequently withdrawn. Polyionic solutions such as Ringers solution and plasmalyte are recommended. However, in the case of septic arthritis, the use of isotonic saline (0.9% NaCl) remains suitable owing to extreme changes of the synovial environment. The volume of fluid injected varies by joint. The diameter of the needle should be large enough to allow thick, purulent synovial fluid to be drained. This type of irrigation is generally used for proximal joint infection such as the hip or shoulder for which establishing a lavage system with 2 portals is challenging.[10]

Through-and-through Lavage

In a field situation, 2 to 4 hypodermic needles (18–14 G) are inserted into the joints at specific anatomic landmarks (**Fig. 8**; see **Table 1**). One needle serves as ingress point and the remaining allow the evacuation of the lavage solution (egress). In a hospital setting, portals can be made using 3.2- to 5.0-mm arthroscopic egress cannulas (**Fig. 9**). Through-and-though joint lavage is indicated for acute infection when fibrin deposits and clots are minimal within the joint. The volume of solution administered is an important consideration and the author recommends to administer a minimum of 1 liter per joint.

During a joint lavage, care should be taken to avoid subcutaneous fluid extravasation. Turbulences facilitating evacuation of fibrin clots can be generated by temporarily obstructing 1 egress needle to increases the intraarticular pressure. This also facilitates the fluid to reach more distant recesses within the joint. After the joint lavage, the needles are removed and the punctures sites are protected with a sterile bandage for 12 hours.

Joint lavages may be repeated over the course of the treatment and their frequency varies depending on the severity of lesions and the clinical improvement after the

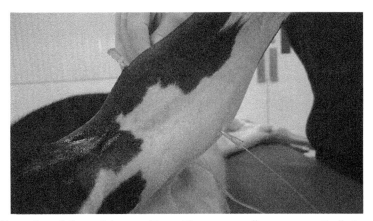

Fig. 8. Through and through lavage. Three 18-gauge needles were aseptically inserted on the elbow of this Holstein Heifer. The ingress needle is held by the hand of the surgeon and fluid exits the joint by the foremost needles. The flow is adequate for the medial needle, and positioning of the lateral needle should be readjusted.

lavage. Up to 3 washes at 24-hour intervals may be required. Too many of these procedures (>3) can induce harmful reactive synovitis deterring the healing process.

Arthrotomy

Arthrotomy is used for chronic conditions in which fibrin clots quickly obscure needles. Arthrotomy sites are identical to the sites of arthrocentesis. Arthrotomies permit lavage of the joints directly with a syringe and an isotonic, polyionic solution. The animal should be heavily sedated or anesthetized and positioned in lateral recumbency with the affected limb uppermost. The swollen joint is clipped and surgically prepared. The needles are inserted in the distended joint and a #11 scalpel blade is inserted along the needle to create an incision between 0.5 and 1 cm. The introduction of forceps (eg, Magill forceps) in the wound then allows removal of fibrin clots. The same procedure is performed on the opposite side of the joint, then a communication

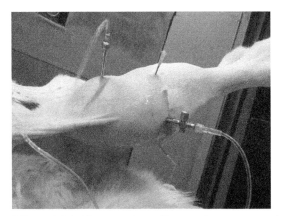

Fig. 9. Through and through joint lavage using arthroscopic egress cannula. The egress cannulas are inserted at the same location as that for arthrocentesis. They allow larger fibrin clots to be flushed out and a larger flow rate of lavage solution.

between the 2 openings is established and lavage can be performed using sterile isotonic solution directly with a 60-mL catheter tip syringe. The wounds heal by secondary intention. They should remain protected with a nonadhesive sterile dressing that can absorb exudative fluid flowing through the wound for several days. Wounds over the stifle joints (femorotibial and femoropatellar) are best protected with a roll of gauze sutured to the skin because of the difficulty to apply a bandage to the proximal limb. A daily bandage change is required to assess the progress of wound healing.

Joint lavage should be repeated over the next few days following the same rules as for fine needle lavages.

Arthroscopy

Arthroscopy is arguably the best treatment option for septic joint. This technique provides superior articular lavage because of the large volumes that can be flushed through the joint. In addition, it allows direct visualization of articular cartilage and can dislodge debris in the joint recesses with more precision than for the 2 previous techniques (Video 2).

The main disadvantages of this technique are the associated costs. This surgery preferentially uses inhalation anesthesia with endotracheal intubation. The equipment is expensive and represents a major investment, especially for infrequent use. Technique is extremely important, and there is a steep learning curve, which may require additional training.

By following the known landmarks for arthrocentesis, a needle is inserted into the joint. An arthroscopic portal is made by stab incision with a #11 scalpel blade. The arthroscopic sleeve of the arthroscope is coupled to a mandrel to aid in introducing the sleeve through the synovial membrane. The mandrel is exchanged for an atraumatic mandrel to penetrate further into the joint without damaging hyaline cartilage. The arthroscope is inserted and a full evaluation of the joint is initiated. A second port is then created on the opposite side to allow proper triangulation when using instruments. A large-diameter cannula is inserted in place of the instrument and provides for fluid egress with minimal subcutaneous extravasation.

Arthroscopy wounds should then be protected under a sterile dressing, and are left to heal by secondary intention. Chronic septic arthritis in cattle can be quite fibrinous and purulent making arthroscopy tedious for newcomers. In this situation, arthrotomy is more efficient at debriding the infected joint.

ARTHRODESIS/FACILITATED ANKYLOSIS

Arthrodesis of high-motion joints have been reported in the literature.[10,56] However, this treatment solution applies more to septic arthritis of the distal interphalangeal joint (please see Nuss K: Surgery of the Distal Limb, in this issue). Arthrodesis should be considered as a salvage procedure to treat a nonresponsive joint infection. Owners should be warned on the invasiveness of the procedure and the expected long convalescence time. Other considerations should be taken into account during the decision making process such as the housing or facilities at the farm, the value of the animal and its intended use afterwards.

PROGNOSIS

Owing to the delay between the initial contamination of the joint and patient presentation, prognosis should be kept guarded for most cases. Despite adequate and aggressive treatment, pannus formation can always occur, turning into a vicious cycle that may end up with the euthanasia of the animal (**Fig. 10**). Fair prognosis may be given

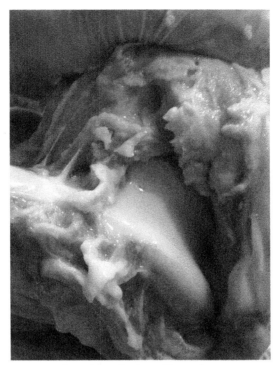

Fig. 10. Post mortem image of a Holstein heifer suffering from unresponsive septic arthritis. A fibrinous exudate is present on the entire joint covering all the synovial membrane.

to animals with acute onset of signs that are treated immediately and aggressively if no boney lesions are seen on radiographs or ultrasonography.

Severe debilitating concomitant diseases such as omphalophlebitis or pneumonia in calves and endocarditis in adults worsen the prognosis. It is the authors' opinion that a poor prognosis should be given to animals with more than 2 joints affected.

SUMMARY

Treatment of septic arthritis can be successful, but requires early intervention for a favorable outcome. The prognosis associated with septic arthritis must be made in consideration of the severity and chronicity of disease. The feasibility of joint lavage and arthrotomies in farm situations is limited by available facilities. Although sterility may be more challenging to achieve, these procedures may still be possible in a farm environment, although ideally these interventions are performed in a hospital setting. Arthroscopy is generally reserved for hospital environments. Hospitalization at the clinic can be easily limited to 3 initial joint lavages, and then the animal can be returned to the farm to finish medical treatment.

SUPPLEMENTARY DATA

Supplementary data related to this article can be found at http://dx.doi.org/10.1016/j.cvfa.2016.05.014.

REFERENCES

1. Bargai U, Levin D. Lameness in the Israeli dairy herd - a national survey of incidence, types, distribution and estimated cost (first report). Isr J Vet Med 1993; 48(2):88–91.
2. Desrochers A. Septic arthritis. In: Fubini SL, Ducharme NG, editors. Farm animal surgery. St Louis (MO): Saunders; 2004. p. 494–7.
3. Marchionatti E, Nichols S, Babkine M, et al. Surgical Management of omphalophlebitis and long term outcome in calves: 39 cases (2008-2013). Vet Surg 2016;45:194–200.
4. Gagea MI, Bateman KG, Shanahan RA, et al. Naturally occurring Mycoplasma bovis- associated pneumonia and polyarthritis in feedlot beef calves. J Vet Diagn Invest 2006;18(1):20–40.
5. Bernier Gosselin V, Francoz D, Babkine M, et al. A retrospective study of 29 cases of otitis media/interna in dairy calves. Can Vet J 2012;53:957–62.
6. Power HT, Rebhun WC. Bacterial endocarditis in adult dairy cattle. J Am Vet Med Assoc 1983;182(8):806–8.
7. Wilson DJ, Skirpstunas RT, Trujillo JD, et al. Unusual history and initial clinical signs of Mycoplasma bovid mastitis and arthritis in first-lactation cows in a closed commercial dairy herd. J Am Vet Med Assoc 2007;230(10):1519–23.
8. Colavite PM, Sartori A. Septic arthritis: immunopathogenesis, experimental models and therapy. J Venom Anim Toxins Incl Trop Dis 2014;20:19.
9. Francoz D, Desrochers A, Fecteau G, et al. Synovial fluid changes in induced infectious arthritis in calves. J Vet Intern Med 2005;19:336–43.
10. Desrochers A. Surgical management of septic arthritis in the proximal limb of ruminants. Proceedings of the American College of Veterinary Surgeons Surgery Summit. Nashville (TN): American College of Veterinary Surgeons; 2015.
11. Mulon PY, Babkine M, d'Anjou MA, et al. Degenerative disease of the distal interphalangeal joint and sesamoid bone in calves: 9 cases (1995-2004). J Am Vet Med Assoc 2009;234(6):794–9.
12. Mulon PY. Osteochondrosis. In: Anderson DE, Rings DM, editors. Current veterinary therapy 5 – food animal practice. Philadelphia: Saunders; 2009.
13. Desrochers A, Francoz D. Clinical management of septic arthritis in cattle. Vet Clin North Am Food Anim Pract 2014;30(1):177–203.
14. Buczinski S, Forté G, Bélanger AM. Short communication: ultrasonographic assessment of the thorax as a fast technique to assess pulmonary lesions in dairy calves with bovine respiratory disease. J Dairy Sci 2013;96(7):4523–8.
15. Kofler J, Geissbühler U, Steiner A. Diagnostic imaging in bovine Orthopaedics. Vet Clin North Am Food Anim Pract 2014;30:11–53.
16. Wahl K, Adams SB, Moore GE. Contamination of joints with tissue debris and hair after arthrocentesis: the effect of needle insertion angle, spinal needle gauge, and insertion of spinal needles with and without stylet. Vet Surg 2012;41(3): 391–8.
17. Rohde C, Anderson DE, Desrochers A, et al. Synovial fluid analysis in cattle: a review of 130 cases. Vet Surg 2000;29(4):341–6.
18. Francoz D, Desrochers A, Fecteau G, et al. A retrospective study of joint bacterial culture in 172 cases septic arthritis in cattle. Paper presented at: 20th ACVIM forum. Dallas, May 29–June 1, 2002.
19. Witchel ME, Fenwick SG, Hunter J, et al. Septicaemia and septic arthritis in a neonatal calf caused by *Lactococcus lactis*. Vet Rec 2003;153(1):22–3.

20. Dreyfuss DJ, Stephens PR. *Erysipelothrix rhusiopathiae*-induced septic arthritis in a calf. J Am Vet Med Assoc 1990;197(10):1361–2.
21. Blake N, Scott PR, Munroe GA. Septic phisitis, arthritis and osteomyelitis probably caused by *Salmonella typhimurium* DT104 in beef suckler calves. Cattle Practice 1997;5(4):345–6.
22. Boulouis HJ, Maillard R, Haddad MA. Lyme borreliosis in cattle. XXIV World Buiatrics Congress. Nice (France), 2006. p. 527–31.
23. Maunsell FP, Woolums AR, Francoz D, et al. Mycoplasma bovis infections in cattle. J Vet Intern Med 2011;25:772–83.
24. Adegboye DS, Halbur PG, Nutsch RG, et al. Mycoplasma bovis-associated pneumonia and arthritis complicated with pyogranulomatous tenosynovitis in calves. J Am Vet Med Assoc 1996;209:647–9.
25. Stengel D, Bauwens K, Sehouli J, et al. Systematic review and meta-analysis of antibiotic therapy for bone and joint infections. Lancet Infect Dis 2001;1(3):175–88.
26. Constable PD, Pyörälä S, Smith GW. Guidelines for antimicrobial use in cattle. In: Guardabassi L, Jensen LB, Kruse H, editors. Guide to antimicrobial use in animals. Ames (IA): Blackwell; 2008. p. 143–60.
27. Jones ML, Washburn KE, Fajt VR, et al. Synovial fluid pharmacokinetics of tulathromycin, gamithromycin and florfenicol after a single subcutaneous dose in cattle. BMC Vet Res 2015;11:26.
28. Brown MP, Gronwall RR, Pattio N, et al. Pharmacokinetics and synovial fluid concentrations of cephapirin in calves with suppurative arthritis. Am J Vet Res 1991; 52(9):1438–40.
29. Shoaf SE, Schwark WS, Guard CL, et al. Pharmacokinetics of trimethoprim/sulfadiazine in neonatal calves: influence of synovitis. J Vet Pharmacol Ther 1986;9:446.
30. Guard CL, Byman KW, Schwark WS. Effect of experimental synovitis on disposition of penicillin and oxytetracycline in neonatal calves. Cornell Vet 1989;79:161.
31. Sansone JM, Wilsman NJ, Leiderman EM, et al. The effect of fluoroquinolone antibiotics on growing cartilage in the lamb model. J Pediatr Orthop 2009;29(2): 189–95.
32. Grandemange E, Gunst S, Woehrle F, et al. Field evaluation of the efficacy of Marbocyl(R) 2% in the treatment of infectious arthritis of calves. Ir Vet J 2002;55:237–40.
33. Lallemand M, Francoz D. Antibiotics regional intravenous perfusion. Point Vet 2015;46:34 [in French].
34. Levine DG, Epstein KL, Ahern BJ, et al. Efficacy of three tourniquets for intravenous antimicrobial perfusion in standing horses. Vet Surg 2010;39(8):1021–4.
35. Hyde RM, Lynch TM, Clarck CK, et al. The influence of perfusate volume on antimicrobial concentration in synovial fluid following intravenous regional limb perfusion in the standing horse. Can Vet J 2013;54:363–7.
36. Aristizabal FA, Nieto JE, Guedes AG, et al. Comparison of two tourniquet application times for regional intravenous perfusions with amikacin in sedated or anesthetized horses. Vet J 2016;208:50–4.
37. Depenbrock SM. Pharmacokinetics of ampicillin-sulbactam in serum and synovial fluid samples following regional intravenous administration in the distal hind limb of adult cattle [Thesis]. The Ohio State University; 2015.
38. à Peltola H, Pääkkönen M, Kallio P, et al. Prospective, randomized trial of 10 days versus 30 days of antimicrobial treatment, including a short-term course of parenteral therapy, for childhood septic arthritis. Clin Infect Dis 2009;48:1201–10.
39. Peltola H, Pääkkönen M, Kallio P, et al. Clindamycin vs. first-generation cephalosporins for acute osteoarticular infections of childhood—a prospective quasi-randomized controlled trial. Clin Microbiol Infect 2012;18:582–9.

40. Sakiniene E, Bremell T, Tarkowski A. Addition of corticosteroids to antibiotic treatment ameliorates the course of experimental Staphylococcus aureus arthritis. Arthritis Rheum 1996;39(9):1596–605.
41. Wysenbeek AJ, Volchek J, Amit M, et al. Treatment of staphylococcal septic arthritis in rabbits by systemic antibiotics and intra-articular corticosteroids. Ann Rheum Dis 1998;57(11):687–90.
42. Odio CM, Ramirez T, Arias G, et al. Double blind, randomized, placebo-controlled study of dexamethasone therapy for hematogenous septic arthritis in children. Pediatr Infect Dis J 2003;22(10):883–8.
43. Harel L, Prais D, Bar-On E, et al. Dexamethasone therapy for septic arthritis in children: results of a randomized double-blind placebo-controlled study. J Pediatr Orthop 2011;31(2):211–5.
44. Meijer MC, van Weeren PR, Lijkenhuizen AB. Clinical experiences of treating septic arthritis in the equine by repeated joint lavage: a series of 39 cases. J Vet Med A Physiol Pathol Clin Med 2000;47(6):351–65.
45. Madison JB, Tulliers EP, Ducharme NG, et al. Idiopathic gonitis in heifers: 34 cases (1976-1986). J Am Vet Med Assoc 1989;194(2):273–7.
46. Farrow L. A systematic review and meta-analysis regarding the use of corticosteroids in septic arthritis. Musculoskeletal Disorders 2015;16:241–8.
47. Coetzee JF, Mosher RA, Anderson DE, et al. Impact of oral meloxicam administered alone or in combination with gabapentin on experimentally induced lameness in beef calves. J Anim Sci 2014;92:816–29.
48. Anderson DE, Edmondson MA. Prevention and management of surgical pain in cattle. Vet Clin North Am Food Anim Pract 2013;29(1):157–84.
49. Selfe TK, Taylor AG. Acupuncture and osteoarthritis of the knee: a review of randomized, controlled trials. Sam. Community Health 2008;31(3):247–54.
50. Marchionatti E, Lardé H, Steagall PVM. Opioid-induced adverse effects in a Holstein calf. Vet Anaesth Analg 2015;42:229–30.
51. Lardé H, Nichols S, Bussières G. Use of neurostimulation to localize and anesthetize the brachial plexus of calves undergoing metacarpal surgery. American College of Veterinary Surgeons Veterinary Symposium November 3–5, Chicago, Illinois. Vet Surg 2011;40:E17–42.
52. Iwamoto J, Yamagishi N, Sasaki K, et al. A novel technique of ultrasound-guided brachial plexus block in calves. Res Vet Sci 2012;93:1467–71.
53. Re M, Blanco J, Gómez de Segura IA. Ultrasound-guided nerve block anesthesia. Vet Clin North Am Food Anim Pract 2016;32:133–47.
54. Hirsbrunner G, Steiner A. Treatment of infectious arthritis of the radiocarpal joint of cattle with gentamicin-impregnated collagen sponges. Vet Rec 1998;142(15):399–402.
55. Francoz D. Septic arthritis in cattle. In: Anderson DE, Rings DM, editors. Current veterinary therapy - food animal practice. St Louis (MO): Saunders; 2009. p. 259–61.
56. Van Huffel X, Steenhaut M, Imshoot, et al. Carpal arthrodesis as a treatment for chronic septic arthritis in calves and cattle. Vet Surg 1989;18(4):304–11.

Surgical Management of Fractures and Tendons

Rebecca Pentecost, DVM, MS[a],*, Andrew J. Niehaus, DVM, MS[b],
David E. Anderson, DVM, MS[c]

KEYWORDS

- Ruminant • Fracture • Tendon • Surgery

KEY POINTS

- Orthopedic issues are common in ruminants, and many orthopedic issues involve fractures and diseases affecting the tendons.
- Although fractures and tendon pathology can have serious and debilitating consequences, many can have a successful outcome with proper veterinary management.
- Proper fracture management begins with good stabilization at the time the fracture is found.
- Spastic paresis can take on multiple forms, only 1 of which responds well to surgical intervention.

FRACTURES

Fractures occur commonly in cattle and other ruminant patients.[1] Ruminants are excellent surgical candidates because of their ability to tolerate long periods of convalescence, predominance of time spent lying down, rapid bone healing, tolerance for fixation constructs, and relatively low risk of contralateral limb breakdown. Injuries to the axial skeleton, digits, and skull are also reported with some frequency; however, management of these fractures will not be discussed in further detail. Rather, the discussion will focus on long bone fractures.[1] External coaptation remains a valuable treatment option for selected fracture configurations and particularly for distal limb fractures, and it may be used concurrently with surgical management of long bone fractures in ruminants to improve stability and longevity of internal and external fixation constructs.

Fractures occur commonly in neonates and juvenile patients secondary to dystocia or trauma sustained during restraint and handling, and successful surgical treatment is

a Coldwater Animal Clinic, 110 Harvest Drive, Coldwater, OH 45828, USA; b Farm Animal Surgery, Department of Veterinary Clinical Sciences, College of Veterinary Medicine, The Ohio State University, 601 Vernon L. Tharp Street, Columbus, OH 43210-1089, USA; c Department of Large Animal Clinical Sciences, College of Veterinary Medicine, University of Tennessee, 2407 River Drive, Knoxville, TN 37996, USA
* Corresponding author.
E-mail address: pentecost.3@osu.edu

Vet Clin Food Anim 32 (2016) 797–811
http://dx.doi.org/10.1016/j.cvfa.2016.05.012   **vetfood.theclinics.com**
0749-0720/16/$ – see front matter © 2016 Elsevier Inc. All rights reserved.

more likely among younger and lighter patients. The most commonly affected long bone fractures diagnosed include metatarsus/metacarpus (approximately 50%), followed by tibial, radius/ulna, humerus, and femur fractures in order of frequency. Decision making regarding fixation of long bone fractures must include consideration of the cost of treatment, likelihood of successful outcome, perceived potential economic or genetic value of the animal, and the location and type of fracture. Many fractures may be addressed by more than 1 fixation type, with varying degrees of potential success and risk of complications; the owner's perceived economic and sentimental value in conjunction with the availability of specialized equipment and surgeon experience dictates which fixation option is elected.

EMERGENCY TREATMENT

The success of fracture repair is predicated on prompt, aggressive, and appropriate emergency care provided at the site and time of injury. Temporary stabilization of long bone fractures improves prognosis by decreasing the risk of closed fractures becoming open, reduces eburnation of the fracture ends and further fragmentation of fracture fragments, provides pain relief, and improves the ability to handle the patient. Management of wounds, shock, or concurrent morbidities improves the chances of survival and fracture healing. Thorough patient evaluation may reveal life-threatening injuries that require treatment prior to transport. Appropriate resuscitation with intravenous fluids can be initiated prior to transport along with early, aggressive treatment of wounds including debridement, bandaging, and parenteral and regional intravenous perfusion of antibiotics. For neonates, the focus on fracture management should not impede the ingestion of sufficient colostrum during the first hours of life. Failure of transfer of passive immunity provides additional management challenges during fracture repair and increases the risk of morbidity associated with surgical site and systemic infections.

As a general rule, fractures below the level of the midradius or midtibia can be stabilized temporarily with splints or casts. Fractures proximal to this level should not be stabilized prior to transport, as the risk of creating a fulcrum effect with splints or casts increases the risk of complications. Increased muscle and soft tissue around the fracture site provides some inherent support to the limb, and improperly placed splints can worsen outcomes by exacerbating trauma to the soft tissues adjacent to the fracture ends, potentiating injury to important neurovascular structures, and leading to skin perforation. Most cattle will adequately protect the affected limb during transport if handled calmly during loading and if allowed to lie down prior to starting transport.

External coaptation using splints for distal fracture stabilization should include a caudal splint extending at least 1 joint proximal to the fracture. In many cases, a second splint lateral to the fracture provides superior support to the injured limb (**Fig. 1**). Any nonflexible, sturdy material at hand may be used as a splint including boards, broomsticks, or PVC pipe pieces. Initial disinfection or debridement of any wounds occurs first, followed by placement of a padded bandage. The splints extend to the level of the ground, are applied at 90° angles, caudally and laterally, and are held in place with a firmly applied external tape. Splints extend to the midradius or midtibia for injuries located below the carpus or tarsus, respectively. Fractures located proximal to the carpus but distal to the midradius must include a lateral splint extending to the proximal scapula, and fractures located proximal to the tarsus but distal to the midtibia must include a splint extending to the level of the pelvis.

Fiberglass casts provide an alternate method of temporary fracture stabilization for transport. Some fractures may not be amenable to long-term stabilization using

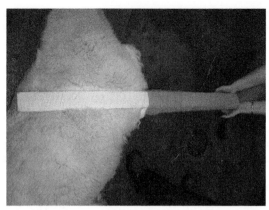

Fig. 1. Fracture of the distal radius in an alpaca is stabilized with a splint. A splint along the caudal aspect of the limb extends from the foot to the elbow; a second laterally applied splint extends from the toe to the proximal scapula.

a cast; however, casts provide adequate support for transport until definitive surgical treatment is performed. Casts are relatively quick and easy to apply, conform to the individual, and require minimal equipment or supplies. As with splints, the cast should extend to the level of the ground (encase the foot), and extend proximal as described earlier based on the location of the fracture.

DIAGNOSTIC IMAGING

Although simple fractures of the metacarpal/metatarsal bones may be accurately diagnosed with physical examination and manipulation of the affected limb alone, radiographs provide useful information for determining if and what type of surgical intervention is indicated. Diagnostic radiographs can be taken through external coaptation to reduce the risk of complications during handling of the injured limb. The minimum dataset includes orthogonal views, although some fractures are best visualized with various oblique images. Images of the unaffected limb provide a template for measurements and preoperative planning for implants. As with other species, use of advanced imaging techniques including computed tomography (CT) or MRI can be used to aid in surgical planning, although the added cost prevents its use in many cases.

PRINCIPLES OF REPAIR

Fracture location, presence and severity of soft tissue and neurovascular trauma, closed or open fracture environment, temperament of the patient, and experience of the surgeon determine which type of surgical fixation is elected. The goal of any fracture fixation method is to provide a means of returning the patient to weight bearing as quickly as possible, maintaining normal joint mobility, and to encourage osteosynthesis and wound healing.

It is important to remember that some fractures may be successfully managed with nonsurgical options. Stall rest, walking blocks, casts, splints, and combinations thereof are feasible options for some fractures and must be considered before incurring the expense and risks associated with surgical fixation.[2] External coaptation provides adequate stabilization against bending forces but is less ideal for oblique, spiral, and comminuted fractures; in these fractures, surgical treatment provides superior outcomes.[3] Additionally, casts cannot provide sufficient immobilization for fractures at or proximal to the midradius or midtibia and decrease the ability to successfully manage open fractures or fractures with extensive soft tissue injuries. Use of certain splints (including Thomas and spica splints) or casts during convalescence can be useful to protect both the fracture and other concurrent modes of fracture fixation by load sharing (**Fig. 2**).

The most commonly elected surgical options include transfixation pin casts, external skeletal fixation, intramedullary pinning, intramedullary interlocking nail, and bone plates. These options can be split into 2 categories: external fixation and internal fixation. Internal fixation tends to offer superior stability and improved ability to reconstruct the fracture, whereas external fixation and transfixation pin casts provide flexibility in application to various fracture types, and can often be placed relatively economically. Transfixation pin casts and external skeletal fixators can be successfully placed and managed in the field, and allow for management of complex fractures not amenable to internal fixation.[4–10] Internal fixation, on the other hand, requires access to more specialized instrumentation, surgeon expertise and experience, and increases the cost of repair, which often limits its use to specialty or referral centers. The advantages, implementation, and potential complications associated with each construct must be considered prior to use in a given case.

EXTERNAL SKELETAL FIXATION

External skeletal fixation (ESF) allows load bearing in the injured limb through the use of an external frame created by placing transcortical pins proximal and distal to the fracture. These transcortical pins are then spanned by a rigid connecting bar. In some cases, the connecting bar may be replaced with alternate materials including

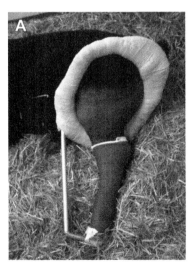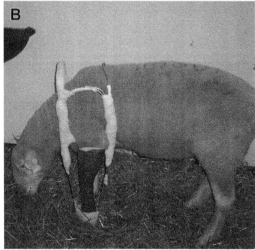

Fig. 2. (*A*) Calf with a Schroeder-Thomas splint applied to the hind limb. A cast extends from the foot to a level proximal to the tarsus. The cast is integrated with the caudal sidebar of the splint. (*B*) A ewe with a Spika splint/cast combination applies to treat a forelimb fracture. The Spika splint has an extension that extends over the shoulder of the patient and reduces abduction of the limb. The configuration of both the Schroeder-Thomas and Spika splint is such that is helps to load-share, thereby reducing the amount of forces experienced by the fractured limb.

polymethyl methacrylate or fiberglass cast tape. The forces created during weight bearing are transferred through the pins to the external frame shielding the fracture. Fixators can have numerous configurations depending on the underlying fracture configuration and fracture location. Type Ia and sometimes Ib fixators are most commonly employed for proximal limb fractures, often in conjunction with other implants.[11] Type II fixators are usually limited to fractures below the stifle or elbow and to fracture configurations that allow bilateral sidebar application. The most robust ESF constructs are Type III and circular constructs.[5,12,13]

Advantages

The advantages of ESF are well described.[14–17] ESF provides early return to function in the affected limb, allows for management of open fractures or wounds, minimizes interference with the fracture healing and associated bone stimulation proteins that are incorporated into the fracture hematoma, allows for fixation of multiple fracture types, provides ease of implant removal, and creates relatively few complications with routine use. The use of ESF has been described in most of the long bones of cattle and other ruminants (**Fig. 3**).[18,19] In extreme cases, transarticular fixators have been used in cases of severe soft tissue trauma, very proximal or distal fracture location that prevents routine fixator placement, or for intentional arthrodesis or ankylosis of a joint.[12,20,21]

Disadvantages

ESF provides less robust fixation compared with bone plates or other means of internal fixation. The less invasive nature of the approach often prevents optimal fracture reduction and reconstruction, interfragmentary compression, and maximum rigidity of stabilization of the affected bone. When placing the transcortical pins, care must be taken to insert them between muscles through fascial planes. Placement through large muscle groups can result in pain and reduced usage of the affected limb. Postoperatively, the ESF construct requires intensive monitoring to ensure that the pins, clamps, and connecting bars are firmly attached and to prevent and treat signs of pin tract infection or pin loosening. Micromotion at the pin–bone interface can lead to pain, decreased load bearing in the affected limb, and increased risk of contralateral

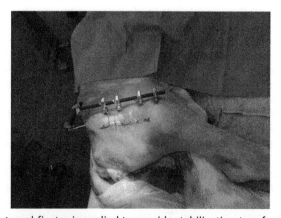

Fig. 3. A Type I external fixator is applied to provide stabilization to a femoral fracture in a neonatal calf. The external fixator is tied to an IM pin that extends from the proximal part of the femur. The fixator prevents migration of the IM pin and the IM pin provides superior neutralization of bending forces.

limb breakdown. Implant failure prior to clinical union of the fracture is another potential complication.

Technique

Dorsal recumbency with the limb suspended from an overhead frame or hoist allows for pin placement in fractures of the radius, ulna, tibia, or metacarpaus/metatarsus, whereas humerus or femur fractures are approached with the patient in lateral recumbency. Marker needles may be placed at the proposed sites for transcortical pin placement and at other important landmarks to identify joints or growth plates. Radiographs are obtained, and the pin sites are evaluated to ensure that pins will be placed in intact cortical bone while avoiding the fracture plane, joints, and fissure lines.

Transcortical pins should be approximately a third of the diameter of the bone in which they are being implanted. For bicortical fixators, midthreaded pins may be used. A minimum of 2 pins should be placed proximal and distal to the fracture although more pins may be used in heavier animals or less stable fracture configurations. Pins should be placed no closer than 1 inch to the fracture plane and should avoid joints or active growth plates.

A 1 cm stab incision is made through the skin down to the level of the bone at the chosen pin site. A pilot hole is then drilled through the bone. Pneumatic orthopedic drills or standard electric or battery-powered drills can be used after appropriate sterilization. Continuous flushing with sterile isotonic solution minimizes thermal damage to the bone during drilling. The hole should be drilled at roughly 80% of the diameter of the desired pin size. As the drill bit is removed from the bone, it is easy for adjacent soft tissue to slide and obscure the hole. A hypodermic needle or small pin may be used to mark the hole between removing the drill bit and insertion of the pin. For bicortical pin placement, the pin is then advanced through the bone. As the pin exits the bone on the opposite side, a second stab incision is created in the skin to allow further advancement of the pin until the threads are fully engaged at both cortices.

Traditional sidebars and clamps can be used to connect the transcortical pins. Sidebars are typically made of stainless steel, but aluminum and carbon frames are also available. The sidebar should be placed as close as possible to the fracture without impinging on the skin and soft tissue overlying the bone. The clamps connecting the pins to the sidebars are prone to loosening and failure compared with other aspects of the construct. Traditional sidebar–clamp assemblies are best reserved for patients weighing less than 150 kg. Use in cattle weighing greater than 150 kg increases the risk of failure of the pin-clamp-sidebar unit. Clamps must be examined daily for tightness, position, and evidence of fatigue.

Acrylic polymer sidebars are inexpensive and versatile with some biomechanical advantages compared with standard steel sidebars and clamps. In an in vitro biomechanical study using a Type I ESF configuration (unilateral frame), a 20 mm acrylic sidebar was equal to or stronger than a 4.8 mm steel sidebar in compression, shear, and torsion. Additional studies have shown similar results for 1.91 cm and 2.54 cm acrylic sidebars used in Type II and Type III configurations. The authors have successfully extrapolated these data to clinical cases. Contrary to traditional sidebars, acrylic sidebars cannot be adjusted after hardening and must be replaced if the configuration is not as desired. A tubing mold is placed through the pins maintaining a distance of at least 10 mm between the tubing and the underlying skin. The acrylic is poured into the tubing mold and allowed to harden. The intense exothermic nature of the acrylics requires particular attention to prevention of thermal injury to the underlying skin and bone. Rinsing the implanted pins with sterile isotonic fluids during the exothermic period helps dissipate heat. The acrylic must be prepared in sufficient volume to avoid layering, air pockets, or cracking in the sidebar, which leads to weakness in the construct and the potential for catastrophic failure. Acrylic sidebars are inherently stiff and brittle and must be closely monitored for signs of failure. Removal is achieved by using obstetric wire to cut the acrylic in sections around the pins.

TRANSFIXATION PIN CASTS

Transfixation pin casts (TPCs) make use of many of the same principles as ESF constructs. Transcortical pins are placed proximal to the fracture similar to the ESF; following pin placement, fiberglass cast tape is used to create a cast that encases the foot and extends proximal to the transfixation pins. During weight bearing, forces are transmitted from the proximal limb, through the transfixation pins to the cast bypassing the injured bone. The distal limb effectively hangs in the cast, which is why this fixation type is sometimes referred to as a hanging limb pin cast. Postoperative management is minimal.

Biomechanically, the construct reduces rotational, compressive, distractional, and sheer forces better than casts without transcortical pins. Distal leg fractures that are inherently unstable may be candidates for transfixation casting.

Transfixation pin casts can be used successfully on fractures below the level of the midradius or midtibia (**Fig. 4**).[4,6–10,19,22] Additionally, TPCs limit joint mobility and can lead to laxity in soft tissue support structures like tendons and ligaments. Open fractures or fractures involving significant soft tissue damage are difficult to manage with TPCs. Cutting holes in the cast aids management of underlying wounds, but complications are common. As with any type of cast, monitoring and prevention of cast sores must be undertaken.

Transcortical pins are placed following the same guidelines as described for ESF pin placement. At least 2 pins should be placed proximal to the fracture, and some surgeons advocate placement of the pins at divergent angles. A double layer of stockinette is placed over the foot extending proximal to the pins. Additional gauze padding may be placed between the toes if desired and over pressure points such as the accessory carpal bone, the calcaneus, and under the dewclaws. Cast padding or resin-impregnated foam is then placed on the limb prior to casting. The padding protects bony protuberances in an effort to minimize the formation of cast sores. An

A   **B**

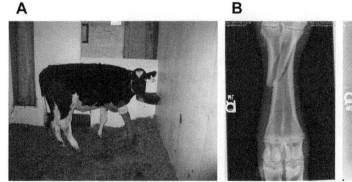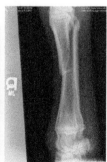

Fig. 4. (*A*) Heifer with a right metacarpal fracture after being hit by a moving vehicle. Transfixation pins were placed through the distal radius, because fracture lines extended to the proximal metacarpus. (*B*) Preoperative dorsopalmar and palmarolatera–dorsomedial oblique radiographic projections of the right metacarpus from the heifer in (*A*). Note the fracture lines extending to the proximal aspect of the metacarpus.

extra layer of cast padding or thick felt should be placed at the proximal limit of the cast to prevent against cast sores at the proximal end. Fiberglass casting tape is then placed, encasing the foot and extending proximal to the transcortical pins. Ending the cast just above the proximal pin sites will create a stress riser at the proximal pins and predispose to pin site fractures. Lamination of the cast occurs when the initial deep layers of the cast are allowed to dry before the more superficial layers are completely applied. Doing so will cause the superficial layers of the cast to not bond properly with the deeper layers. Lamination of the cast weakens the construct and predisposes to cast failure. Once the cast has been applied, the cast material must be allowed to harden completely before the patient uses the cast.

TENDON SURGERY

Surgical diseases involving tendons in ruminants include contracted tendons, tendon laxity, tendon lacerations, and septic tenosynovitis. Spastic paresis is a neuromuscular disease involving the hind limbs in cattle. Although it does not involve tendon pathology per se, one of the surgical methods described to correct this condition involves transection of a portion of the Achilles tendon and will be discussed here.

FLEXOR TENDON CONTRACTURE

Animals that have flexor tendon contracture are unable to fully extend their limbs (**Fig. 5**). Front limbs involving the carpus and fetlock and hind limbs involving the fetlocks can be affected. The condition is more commonly seen affecting the front legs. The name "contracted tendons" is a misnomer, because the inability to extend the legs is due to more than restriction provided by the flexor tendons and should be more properly termed "flexural deformity." In addition to restriction provided by the flexor tendons, ligamentous structures and joint capsule can also provide resistance to full extension. This condition is seen in all species of domesticated ruminants. The condition is most frequently observed as a congenital defect and it is often presumed to be due to uterine malpositioning as it is commononly associated with high birthweights. Acquired contracture can be observed with chronic lameness.

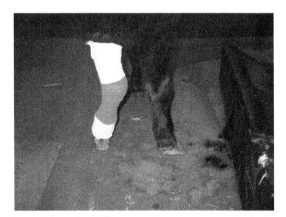

Fig. 5. Calf with bilateral front limb flexor tendon contracture (right leg more severe than left). The calf has been treated with a splint applied to the right forelimb. Note that the splint is unable to achieve full extension of the limb. The calf has also been treated with bilateral toe extensions.

Treatment for animals with tendon contracture varies from conservative to surgical. If the patient is ambulatory, exercise is beneficial. Physical therapy (forced extension) of the leg may help to stretch out restrictive soft tissue structures. Splints applied to the leg in extension can also help to provide pressure over longer periods of time. Care needs to be taken to provide adequate padding to prevent sores caused by the splints. Toe extensions can be applied, which increase the forces applied to the flexor tendons when the animal bears weight on its leg (**Fig. 6**). In order for toe extensions to be effective, the animal must have relatively mild contracture; in severe cases where the dorsal aspect of the toe breaks over the vertical plane, toe extensions will cause the animal's toe to roll over when it attempts to stand, making the condition worse. Although oxytetracycline administration has been effective in foals to decrease contracture,[23] it does not seem to have the same efficacy in calves.[24]

The prognosis is guarded for calves that do not respond to nonsurgical therapy. Surgical therapy for tendon contracture involves transection of the flexor tendons at the level of the midmetacarpus or metatarsus. Flexor tenotomy proximal to the carpus may be employed for cases of contracture involving the carpus. The surgical procedure involves transection of all of the structures that are palpably taught when the leg is forced into extension. Often after all of the taught tendonous structures are transected, the leg still does not achieve normal extension, and these legs may require joint capsule transection to achieve full extension. Care should be taken to ensure integrity of the neurovascular structures on the caudal aspect of the leg; stretching of these structures may result in compromise to blood flow to the distal limb.

SPASTIC PARESIS

Spastic paresis, also known as "Elso Heel," is a progressive neuromuscular disorder of cattle. It was first described by Hamoir in 1922 as an abnormal contractility of the gastrocnemius muscle in a calf in Belgium. Ten years later, the term spastic paresis was coined to describe this neuromuscular disorder.[25] The prevalence of the disease seems to be increasing, especially in the club calf breeds.

Usually signs of the disease occur in young cattle (weeks to months of age). The hallmark clinical sign is hyperextension of the hock. When standing, the affected leg is frequently extended caudally, and if both hind legs are affected, the calf may periodically switch the leg that it holds behind (**Fig. 7**). The extensor tone is normal when the calf is down and relaxed but becomes excessive when the calf stands and

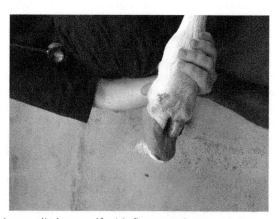

Fig. 6. Toe extension applied to a calf with flexor tendon contracture.

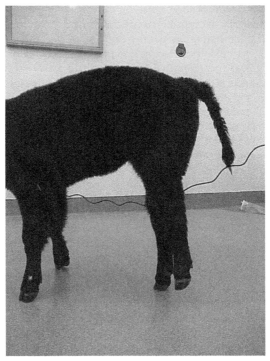

Fig. 7. Calf with spastic paresis. Note the calf is holding left hind leg abducted and caudally. The tail head is also elevated. This calf probably has a mixed (gastrocnemius and quadriceps involvement) form of the condition.

attempts to bear weight. The leg is advanced in an abducted, swinging motion, because the hock and stifle are extended. The base of the tail is often elevated. Eventually muscle atrophy and loss of body condition can occur as affected calves begin to have difficulty ambulating.

The exact etiology and pathogenesis has not been established, but several theories have been proposed. Spastic paresis is thought to be caused by overstimulation of the gastrocnemius and possibly the superficial digital flexor muscle causing a rigid extension of the hock. Studies of affected calves have revealed a total absence of inflammatory processes. No histologic lesions are seen in the peripheral nervous system or musculature.[26] Most researchers agree that the disease has an inherited component, but the mechanism of inheritance has not been established.

Medical therapy for treatment of spastic paresis is not widely used and has only been shown to be effective in the early stages of disease. Supplementation with tryptophan has been shown to decrease the clinical signs in certain cases. Tryptophan, an essential amino acid, is a precursor of a neurotransmitter postulated to be deficient in cases of spastic paresis (serotonin). Lithium, a drug used to treat manic–depressive psychoses, has also been advocated in the treatment of bovine spastic paresis, but the mechanism of action is unknown.[26]

Surgical correction should be viewed as a salvage procedure, with the goal to be to increase animal comfort and ambulation in the hopes of allowing the animal to be fattened for slaughter. Several cases in the authors' practice have been corrected with aspirations of providing enough soundness to compete in exhibition. However, the client should be made aware that although most animals improve following surgical therapy, the spasticity often does not resolve completely. Surgical correction of conformational defects for show also raises ethical concerns. Because of the likely inherited nature of the disease, correction should not be performed on animals to allow them to be used for breeding purposes.

Two surgical options have been described for treatment of spastic paresis, tibial neurectomy and partial tenotomy of the extensors of the hock (gastrocnemius and superficial digital flexor). Tibial neurectomy is aimed at decreasing innervation to these muscle groups, while the tenotomy procedure physically eliminates the tension applied to the calcaneus and also the counterforce on the muscle decreasing reflex stimulation.

To perform a tibial neurectomy, the calf should be placed in lateral recumbency under general anesthesia with the affected leg uppermost. A 15 to 20 cm incision is made at the caudal aspect of the stifle between the semitendinosis and the biceps femoris muscles. Alternatively, an approach can be made through an incision between the 2 bellies of the biceps femoris. Care is taken not to mistake the more cranially running peroneal nerve for the tibial nerve. The peroneal nerve can be identified as it courses over the lateral head of the gastrocnemius muscle. This nerve must be preserved. Electrostimulation of the nerve can be performed intraoperatively to verify the nerve is the tibial nerve prior to transection. As the tibial nerve is stimulated, gastrocnemius contraction resulting in hock extension should occur. A 3 cm section of the tibial nerve is excised.[27]

The tenotomy procedure can be performed with the patient under general anesthesia or heavy sedation and a local block. This procedure can also be performed standing, although one of the authors (AJN) prefers lateral recumbency. Following sedation and proper restraint, the leg above the calcaneus is prepared for aseptic surgery. A 7 cm incision is made directly over the Achilles tendon on the lateral aspect with the distal end of the incision approximately 2 cm proximal to the calcaneus. The deep and superficial tendons of the gastrocnemius muscle (lateral) are identified and separated from the superficial digital flexor tendon (medial). A tendon knife (bistoury) is used to transect the tendons (**Fig. 8**). Both gastrocnemius tendons are completely transected. Care must be taken to not inadvertently incise the tendon of

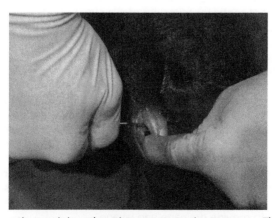

Fig. 8. Calf with spastic paresis is undergoing gastrocnemius tenotomy. The incision is made immediately proximal to the calcaneus on the lateral aspect of the limb. The tendon of the gastrocnemius muscle has been separated from the other structures in the leg. A bistoury has been inserted and is being use to transect the tendon of the gastrocnemius muscle.

the superficial digital flexor that runs in intimate apposition. In severe cases of spastic paresis, a partial tenotomy of the superficial digital flexor may be required in addition to the gastrocnemius tenotomy. Exercise should be restricted for 2 weeks to avoid catastrophic rupture of the superficial digital flexor tendon due to increased tension on the remaining tendinous structure.[27]

The success rates of both the neurectomy and tenotomy are good. The gastrocnemius tenotomy is technically easier to perform and is associated with less catastrophic complications when compared with tibial neurectomy. Complications associated with surgical correction of spastic paresis include surgical infection, hemorrhage, gastrocnemius rupture, and a dropped hock. Peroneal nerve paralysis can also result if failure to properly identify the peroneal nerve during a tibial neurectomy occurs. Due to possible complications, ideally surgery should only be performed on 1 leg at a time for cases of bilateral spastic paresis.[27]

Another form of spastic paresis involving the quadriceps muscle unit has recently been described. This form of spastic paresis causes the affected calf to hold its leg in a more cranially oriented position, and the affected animal has an arched back. It will ambulate by advancing its leg in an abducted motion. This type of spastic paresis does not respond to tibial neurectomy or tenotomy of the gastrocnemius muscle.[28,29] A mixed form of spastic paresis exhibiting characteristics of both gastrocnemius and quadriceps forms is also possible. This form seems to respond partially to surgical intervention; however, is not as responsive as the gastrocnemius form. According to a recent retrospective study, the quadriceps form and the mixed form of spastic paresis accounted for 20% and 47% of cases respectively.[30]

SEPTIC TENOSYNOVITIS

Tendon sheathes can become infected and may require surgical management. Tendon sheaths can act as a conduit that allows for easy spread of sepsis. Because the inflammation involves the tendon, these animals are painful when the tendon is moved. The aims of surgical therapy are similar to that of an abscess: provide drainage of the septic structure, lavage, and antibiotic delivery to the site of infection.

The common digital flexor tendon sheath is the most commonly affected structure, and it usually becomes infected secondary to foot lesions. The discussion here will be limited to treatment of septic tenosynovitis of this structure. The deep digital flexor attaches to the flexor process of third phalanx in the hoof. Hoof ulcers frequently occur over this process (Rulterholtz ulcers) and allow for ascension of environmental organisms. Affected animals present with severe lameness and are reluctant to bear weight on the affected leg. Swelling is usually evident traveling from the foot proximally, through the fetlock area, possibly extending to the hock or carpus. The animals will also be painful on palpation of the affected area. Ultrasound examination of this area will reveal increased fluid around surrounding the flexor tendons. Although examination of the hoof will reveal a painful lesion on one of the toes, because pathology involves structures common to both sides of the digit, affected animals often will not respond to therapy by elevation of the affected toe with a block on the opposite toe.

Although acute cases may respond to medical therapy, consisting of antibiotics and anti-inflammatories, many cases are chronic by the time they are presented to a veterinarian, and these cases will require aggressive therapy. The affected tendon sheath should be opened to provide drainage and lavage.

A Bier block (regional intravenous anesthesia) is useful to provide anesthesia to the affected region. A tourniquet is placed on the limb proximal to the affected area to isolate the vasculature. Local anesthetic is injected in a vein distal to the tourniquet.

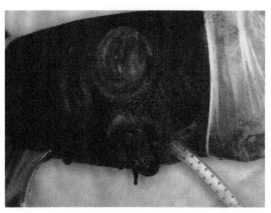

Fig. 9. A Jackson-Pratt drain has been inserted into the common digital flexor tendon sheath of a cow that has septic tenosynovitis. The drain is used to provide daily lavage of the septic structure.

Local distribution of the local anesthetic occurs and provides anesthesia to the structures distal to the tourniquet (see Edmonson MA: Local, Regional, and Spinal Anesthesia in Ruminants, in this issue).

Ultrasound examination of the tendon sheaths can be useful to provide the optimum location to open the sheath, ideally an area where the fluid pocket is the most superficial, disrupting the least amount of healthy tissue. A longitudinal incision should be made into the sheath. At least 2 areas on the sheath should be opened to provide for through-and-through lavage. The distal aspect of the sheath may already be open (at the foot) providing for drainage. A large bore drain can be inserted into the septic structure to maintain patency of the portals and provide for long-term lavage over the next several days (**Fig. 9**).

Delivery of antibiotics to the site of infection is another goal of surgical therapy. Systemic antibiotics should be picked based on a high volume of distribution, which will favor therapeutic tissue levels at the site of infection. Often one is limited in antibiotic selection in ruminants because of US Food and Drug Administration (FDA) regulations.

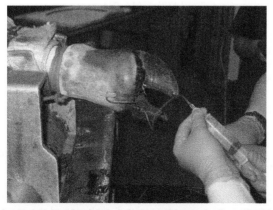

Fig. 10. Regional intravenous anesthesia is being administered to anesthestize the fetlock distally on a cow. A tourniquet has been placed proximally to the fetlock isolating the distal vasculature. 20 mL of 2% lidocaine are being injected into the dorsal common digital vein.

Antibiotics administered locally can be given at a much lower dose but yet achieve higher tissues levels at the site of infection. Intravenous regional limb perfusion (RLP) of antibiotics is a useful technique and has been shown to achieve superior tissue levels of antimicrobials. It is convenient to perform RLP at the same time as the Bier block, utilizing the same intravenous access and tourniquet (**Fig. 10**). Ideally the tourniquet should stay in place for 30 minutes.

SUMMARY

Orthopedic issues are common in ruminants and can result in severe, debilitating lameness. Prognosis will be predicated on the diagnosis and specific structures involved. Often the chronicity of the problem prior to initiating veterinary treatment will determine the outcome. It is important to be able to diagnose the problem in a timely fashion and be able to initiate proper therapy in a timely manner to maximize the chances for a success.

Long bone fractures result in instability and pain that will prohibit weight bearing in many instances. Fracture management should begin early with support of the affected limb to prevent against worsening of the fracture, damage to collateral soft tissue structure or neurovascular compromise. Different techniques for fracture fixation exist and the ideal method to employ in any given case will depend on fracture configuration, soft tissue damage, and health of the patient. Many of these cases can have a successful outcome if managed properly.

Tendon disorders may require surgical management to restore the animal to normal function. Flexural deformities, tendon lacerations, and septic tenosynovitis are a few examples of conditions involving tendons or associated structures that are indications for surgical intervention. Prognosis will depend largely on the diagnosis and the chronicity of the problem. Spastic paresis is becoming more prevalent in certain cattle populations and although its pathogenesis does not involve tendon pathology, one of the reported treatments for the condition involves tenotomy of the gastrocnemius tendon.

REFERENCES

1. Ferguson JG. Management and repair of bovine fractures. Compend Contin Educ Pract Vet 1982;4:S128–35.
2. Bani Ismail ZA, Hawkins JF, Al-Majali AM. External coaptation for the treatment of long bone fractures in cattle: a retrospective study of 35 cases (1996-2001). Pol J Vet Sci 2007;10(4):279–84.
3. Denny HR, Sridhar B, Weaver BM, et al. The management of bovine fractures: a review of 59 cases. Vet Rec 1988;123(11):289–95.
4. Baxter GM, Wallace CE. Modified transfixation pinning of compound radius and ulna fracture in a heifer. J Am Vet Med Assoc 1991;198(4):665–8.
5. Bilgili H, Kurum B, Captug O. Use of a circular external skeletal fixator to treat comminuted metacarpal and tibial fractures in six calves. Vet Rec 2008; 163(23):683–7.
6. Hamilton GF, Tulleners EP. Transfixation pinning of proximal tibial fractures in calves. J Am Vet Med Assoc 1980;176(8):725–7.
7. Kofler J, Wetchy G, Schoffmann G. Transfixation pinning and casting of a comminuted metacarpal fracture in a 870 kg bull. Vet Surg 2014;43(8):1014–9.
8. Mulon PY. Correction of a severe torsional malunion of the metacarpus in a calf by transverse osteotomy, transfixation pinning and casting. Vet Comp Orthop Traumatol 2010;23(1):62–5.

9. St-Jean G, Clem MF, DeBowes RM. Transfixation pinning and casting of tibial fractures in calves: five cases (1985-1989). J Am Vet Med Assoc 1991;198(1):139–43.
10. St Jean G, Debowes RM. Transfixation pinning and casting of radial-ulnar fractures in calves: a review of three cases. Can Vet J 1992;33(4):257–62.
11. Yamagishi N, Devkota B, Takahashi M. Outpatient treatment for humeral fractures in five calves. J Vet Med Sci 2014;76(11):1519–22.
12. Aithal HP, Amarpal, Kinjavdekar P, et al. Management of fractures near the carpal joint of two calves by transarticular fixation with a circular external fixator. Vet Rec 2007;161(6):193–8.
13. Aithal HP, Kinjavdekar P, Amarpal, et al. Management of tibial fractures using a circular external fixator in two calves. Vet Surg 2010;39(5):621–6.
14. Richardson DW, Nunamaker DM, Sigafoos RD. Use of an external skeletal fixation device and bone graft for arthrodesis of the metacarpophalangeal joint in horses. J Am Vet Med Assoc 1987;191(3):316–21.
15. Palmer RH, Hulse DA, Hyman WA, et al. Principles of bone healing and biomechanics of external skeletal fixation. Vet Clin North Am Small Anim Pract 1992;22(1):45–68.
16. Braden TD, Brinker WO, Little RW, et al. Comparative biomechanical evaluation of bone healing in the dog. J Am Vet Med Assoc 1973;163(1):65–9.
17. Behrens F, Searls K. External fixation of the tibia. Basic concepts and prospective evaluation. J Bone Joint Surg Br 1986;68(2):246–54.
18. Kaneps AJ. Orthopedic conditions of small ruminants. Llama, sheep, goat, and deer. Vet Clin North Am Food Anim Pract 1996;12(1):211–31.
19. Kaneps AJ, Schmotzer WB, Huber MJ, et al. Fracture repair with transfixation pins and fiberglass cast in llamas and small ruminants. J Am Vet Med Assoc 1989;195(9):1257–61.
20. Anderson DE, St Jean G, Desrochers A. Repair of open, comminuted fractures of the radius and ulna in a calf with a transarticular type II external skeletal fixator. Agri Pract 1994;15(9):24–8.
21. Toombs JP. Transarticular application of external skeletal fixation. Vet Clin North Am Small Anim Pract 1992;22(1):181–94.
22. Lundvall RL. Observations on the treatment of fractures of the long bones in large animals. J Am Vet Med Assoc 1960;137:308–12.
23. Madison JB, Garber JL, Rice B, et al. Effect of oxytetracycline on metacarpophalangeal and distal interphalangeal joint angles in newborn foals. J Am Vet Med Assoc 1994;204(2):246–9.
24. Metzner M, Baumgart I, Klee W. Effect of infusion of 60 mg/kg oxytetracycline on forelimb flexor tendon contracture in calves. Vet Rec 2007;160(5):166–7.
25. Vlaminck L, De Moor A, Martens A, et al. Partial tibial neurectomy in 113 Belgian blue calves with spastic paresis. Vet Rec 2000;147(1):16–9.
26. Ledoux JM. Bovine spastic paresis: etiological hypotheses. Med Hypotheses 2001;57(5):573–9.
27. Ducharme NG. Spastic paresis (Elso Heel). In: Farm animal surgery. St Louis (MO): Saunders; 2004. p. 349–50, 501–503.
28. De Vlamynck C, Pille F, Vlaminck L. Bovine spastic paresis: current knowledge and scientific voids. Vet J 2014;202(2):229–35.
29. Touati K, Muller P, Gangl M, et al. Spastic paresis of femoral quadriceps muscle: a new clinical form in Belgian White Blue calves. Ann de Medecine Veterinaire 2003;147(4):261–5.
30. De Vlamynck C, Pille F, Vlaminck L. Long term outcome of conservative management or surgical treatment of bovine spastic paresis: 79 cases. Vet Surg 2016;45(2):187–93.

Surgical Management of the Teat and the Udder

Pierre-Yves Mulon, Dr Vet

KEYWORDS

- Teat • Laceration • Milk flow disorders • Surgery • Cattle

KEY POINTS

- Lacerations of the teat should be treated as emergency, and first intention repair should be attempted under sedation in lateral or dorsal recumbency.
- Surgeons should pay attention to the atraumatic manipulation of the tissue and the anatomic reconstruction using small-diameter absorbable suture material.
- Hand milking should be prohibited for 10 days postoperatively after laceration repair; prognosis is overall good.
- Ultrasound evaluation of the teat allows an excellent understanding of the internal lesions and should be performed before planning any elective surgery.
- Milk outflow impairment originating from the rosette of Fürstenberg or the streak canal is best treated using minimally invasive surgery (theloscopy).

Teats are extremely sensitive to trauma, and even the smallest trauma can lead to severe disturbances in milk outflow. Management of teat trauma is critical for the future of the cow in the herd. Minimal dysfunction of the normal physiologic barriers (the teat wall or streak canal) may lead to chronic inflammation or infection of the gland, resulting in premature culling of the animal as worst-case scenario.[1] Teats are well exposed to trauma.[2] Enlargement of the udder after calving puts the teat at risk of self-inflected injury. Trauma can also originate from other cows in the herd, hazardous/sharp objects in the barn, or even the milking machine. Teat disorders are divided into 2 types: external (not covered) and internal (covered).[3] Whether the lesion is acute or chronic, appropriate actions should be taken to preserve the function of the teat and the teat canal.

ANATOMY OF THE TEAT AND THE UDDER

The udder is divided into 4 quarters. Each has its independent gland that produces milk. The milk excreted by the acini travels through ducts of increasing sizes that coalesce into a large lactiferous sinus (gland cistern).[4] The gland cistern is separated from

The author has nothing to disclose.
Department of Large Animal Clinical Sciences, College of Veterinary Medicine, University of Tennessee, 2407 River Drive, Knoxville, TN 37996, USA
E-mail address: pymulon@gmail.com

the teat cistern by the annular ring. The most distal barrier to the teat is the streak canal, and it is through this that milk is evacuated from the teat. The proximal aspect of the streak canal is called the rosette of Fürstenberg (**Fig. 1**). Blood is supplied to the udder primarily by the external pudendal artery traveling through the inguinal ring, and secondarily by the mammary branch of the ventral perineal artery.[5,6] Blood return is mainly via the cranial epigastric vein and secondarily by the external pudendal vein. The vascularization is extremely dense and ramified within the whole udder. Two vascular plexus are present at the proximal and distal extremities of the teat: close to the annular ring and around the streak canal. Those 2 plexus are connected with longitudinal vessels lying immediately underneath the submucosa of the teat. The teat wall is composed of 5 layers. The mucosa is a double-layered epithelium firmly attached to the submucosal layer. Immediately underneath the submucosa lies a conjunctive layer followed by a smooth muscle layer. The entire teat is protected from the outside by a stratified squamous epithelium (skin). On a study of 148 quarters of 38 cows, the rear teats were shorter and thicker than front teats, whereas teat canal length and teat wall thickness did not differ by quarter.[7] The teat mucosa ends at the rosette of Fürstenberg. The streak canal (ductus papillaris mammae) is an invagination of the teat skin and is composed of a stratified squamous epithelium in which the stratum corneum produces keratin. The netlike integrated elastic system containing smooth muscular fibers at the level of the streak canal functions as a sphincter.

DIAGNOSIS OF SURGICAL CONDITIONS
Clinical Examination

Milk flow impairment is a common cause for presentation of lactating cows to the veterinarian and warrants a thorough evaluation of the teat. Palpation of the udder and teat will allow the clinician to determine whether a portion of the teat and udder is inflamed, fibrotic, and/or painful. Careful attention to the palpation of the teat by gently rolling it between the thumb and index finger may allow one to locate the site of the lesion. Wearing examination gloves during the evaluation is recommended. Whenever possible, a California Mastitis Test (CMT) should be performed on all quarters to assess for possible subclinical mastitis. If stripping milk by hand is impossible, it is the author's opinion that it is more beneficial to first perform an ultrasound examination rather than to blindly try to force a cannula into the streak canal to avoid iatrogenic damage to the teat (**Fig. 2**). Even with a negative CMT, a milk sample should be

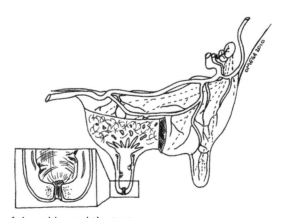

Fig. 1. Anatomy of the udder and the teat.

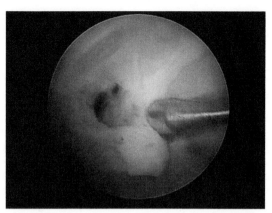

Fig. 2. Theloscopic evaluation of an injured rosette of Fürstenberg. The teat probe for canal measurement has been carefully inserted through the streak canal. A traumatic secondary opening is present laterally to the normal streak canal as a result of a previous forced intro-duction of a metallic milking probe (teat cannula). An enlarged fibrous mass is also present near the rosette.

submitted for bacteriologic culture before attempting surgery. Physical examination gives often limited information on the extension of the lesion and better comprehen-sion of the lesion is gained through imaging.

Ultrasonography of the Teat and the Udder

Ultrasound is the first complementary technique that should be performed to further evaluate teat disorders.[8] It necessitates a 5- to 10-MHz linear probe like the rectal probe used for the reproduction work. With the teat cleaned with alcohol and then covered with acoustic gel, the probe is gently apposed longitudinally on the teat (**Fig. 3**).

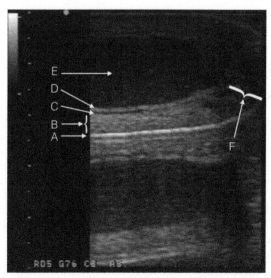

Fig. 3. Ultrasonography of a normal teat. (A) Skin; (B) muscular and conjunctival layer; (C) blood vessel; (D) teat cistern mucosa; (E): teat cistern lumen; (F) streak canal.

From the skin to the teat cistern, echogenicity will appear as follows:

Skin: hyperechoic
Muscular and conjunctive layer: homogenous and mildly echoic
Vessels: hypoechoic
Submucosa and mucosa: hyperechoic
Milk: variable; the milk appears more hyperechoic as the somatic cell count increases

By orientating the probe transversally, a cross-section of the teat is obtained. The distribution of the blood vessel is well determined. It is always recommended to apply the ultrasound probe on the opposite side of the lesion to avoid compressing it during the examination.

Referencing images of the normal teats will help to better define ultrasonographic lesions on the injured teats and aid better understanding of the abnormality. Ultrasonography provides the diagnostic precision necessary to diagnose fibrotic lesions on the rosette of Fürstenberg, fibrotic lesions of the teat wall, fibrosis of the gland, presence of a varicose vein, and the communication between glandular tissue and teat cisterns in conjoined teats.

Radiography of the Teat

Twenty to 30 mL of radiopaque contrast solution (50% diatrizoate sodium) is aseptically infused into the teat cistern via the streak canal, and a radiograph is taken.[2] The cassette should be placed between the quarters in order to avoid superimposition of other teats. Front-quarter radiographs can be obtained easily, but the rear quarters are best imaged with the hind limb elevated in a claw-trimming chute. This examination was performed on a regular basis before the refinement of the ultrasound technology. Single-contrast radiographs allow determination of the site and length of obstruction. In cases of conjoined teats, radiography can be used to demonstrate the independence and the distribution of the glandular tissue. An initial radiograph is taken after the infusion of the conjoined supernumerary teat, followed by a second radiograph after the infusion of the anatomically appropriate teat.

Theloscopy

Theloscopy, endoscopy of the teat, can be accomplished by the insertion of a small-diameter rigid endoscope (theloscope) into the streak canal. This surgical procedure can be either diagnostic or therapeutic and will be discussed later.

RESTRAIN AND ANESTHESIA

Adequate restraint and anesthesia are mandatory before conducting any type of teat surgery, including theloscopy. Standing surgery can be performed for minor procedures such as blind opening of the streak canal. The cow is restrained in a chute and sedated. Local anesthesia using an infusion of lidocaine hydrochloride 2% is performed. For surgeries requiring suturing, placing the cow in lateral or dorsal recumbency under sedation offers a better immobilization of the patient and allows delicate tissue manipulation. Xylazine hydrochloride administered at 0.1 mg/kg intravenously or at 0.2 mg/kg intramuscularly (IM) offers adequate sedation in most cases. The legs and head are secured to maintain the safety of the surgeon throughout the procedure. The use of a tilt table will elevate the surgical field from the ground and allow the surgeon to operate while standing. Local anesthesia of the teat is performed with subcutaneous infiltration of lidocaine hydrochloride 2% around the base of the teat (ring block) (**Fig. 4**). Care should be taken not to penetrate the rich vascular plexus

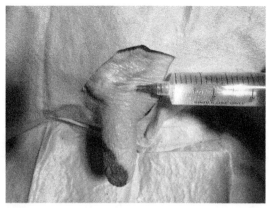

Fig. 4. Local anesthesia: subcutaneous infiltration of lidocaine 2% at the base of the teat to perform a ring block.

at this level. Additional anesthesia with infusion of lidocaine within the teat cistern can also be performed to provide anesthesia to the teat mucosa.

TRAUMATIC TEAT LACERATIONS

Teat lacerations are the result of external trauma. The presence of a sharp object in the environment, self-inflected trauma during rising, and trauma by another cow are possible causes of traumatic teat lacerations. Laceration of the teat is a surgical emergency, and appropriate care should be provided as soon as possible to ensure the best prognosis for return to production. The management of teat lacerations must commence as soon as possible. The tissue of the udder and teats is extremely reactive and sensitive to inflammation, and mitigating the acute inflammatory response should be a principle of teat repair. Administration of a nonsteroidal anti-inflammatory drug (NSAID) should be administered immediately. Applying a cold hydrotherapy on the injured teat will counteract inflammation and reduce the wound contamination.[2,3,9–16] Any wound on a teat should be considered contaminated due to the nature of the trauma. All teat trauma carries the risk of mastitis even if the teat wall is not completely breached. Antibiotics will be necessary, and it is best to start as soon as possible. The use of procaine penicillin (22,000 IU/kg IM) is sufficient to ensure adequate protection in most cases.

Defining the Laceration

The shape, location, and length vary greatly with teat lacerations (**Fig. 5**). The evaluation of the laceration should include its location and its conformation, but also the depth of the wound. Lacerations are described in **Box 1**.

Surgical Repair of Teat Laceration

After a thorough cleaning and adequate surgical preparation and draping, the first surgical step is the debridement of the wound. The wound should be considered highly contaminated with organic particles trapped within large fibrinous clots. The margins of the wound can be excised, but it is better to be conservative in this action to allow for proper reconstruction. Regular washing of the wound with sterile isotonic saline–containing antibiotics is recommended to allow tissue irrigation as well as mechanical debridement.

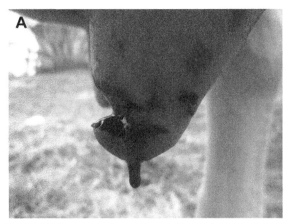
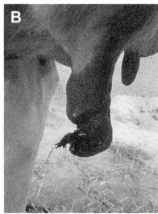

Fig. 5. (*A*) Transverse laceration on the distal end of the teat involving the streak canal. (*B*) Complex laceration of the teat involving the distal portion of the teat cistern. Gross contamination is present.

Diffuse bleeding of connective tissue is often present at the end of surgical debridement, but excessive bleeding must be controlled to maintain adequate hemostasis during the reconstruction phase. Once debridement is completed, anatomic reconstruction is undertaken. Identification of the different layers is important to assure an adequate anatomic repair (**Fig. 6**). Suturing layer by layer is needed using a small-diameter absorbable suture material (USP 4-0 to 3-0). For vertical laceration, the mucosa is sutured using a continuous suture pattern with a 3-mm bite interval. For transverse lacerations, the mucosa is sutured with a simple interrupted suture pattern to prevent any stenosis at the suture level. An interval of 3 mm between bites ensures proper sealing of the suture. Wound lavage with saline is performed between each suture. The submucosa and associated connective tissue are sutured using the same suture material using the same principle for suture patterns as for the mucosa. The interval between bites for this level could be wider and up to 5 mm. After a proper wound lavage, the skin is then sutured. The skin is sutured with a nonabsorbable monofilament small-diameter suture material (USP 3-0 to 2-0) using interrupted suture patterns (eg, simple, cruciate, horizontal mattress, angle suture). In an in vitro study evaluating the tensile strength of multiple suture materials commonly used in teat surgery, Nichols and Anderson[17] demonstrated that polydioxanone's loss of tensile strength over time was not influenced by the contact media, even in contaminated milk. Poliglecaprone was determined to be an inappropriate choice of suture

---

Box 1
Different types of lacerations

- Superficial (intact teat cistern)/deep (communication with the teat cistern with milk drainage from the wound)

- Longitudinal (oriented with the long axis of the teat)/transverse (transects the teat)

- Linear/complex (eg, y shape)

- Proximal (near the base of the teat)/distal (near the tip of the teat)

- Involvement of any vascular plexus and/or the streak canal

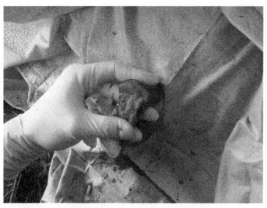

Fig. 6. Same cow pictured in **Fig. 5B**. End of the surgical debridement of the wound. Anatomic structures are identified before suturing the teat.

material for teat surgery, and polyglycolic acid did not respond well facing contaminated milk.

If the laceration involves the streak (papillary) canal, reconstruction must be started distally to ensure a perfect anatomic reconstruction of the region. Insertion of a silicone teat in the streak canal is advised to avoid stenosis. The postoperative care in cases where the laceration involves the streak canal is similar to the postoperative care following milk-flow disorders originating from the rosette of Fürstenberg.

Postoperative Care

The postoperative period is as important as the surgery itself. Systemic antibiotic therapy should be continued for at least 3 days in all cases; it may be supplemented by intramammary infusions. NSAID is continued for 24 to 48 hours. The wound should be protected with a bandage. A cow udder harness can be used to further isolate the udder from the environment.

Hand milking should be prohibited for 10 days. During hand milking, an uneven external pressure is applied by the fingers and the palm, inducing an elevation of the pressure inside the teat cistern. This increased pressure may force milk to dissect through the teat closure, which can allow reopening of the streak canal. Milk will follow the path of least resistance, increasing the risk of fistula formation. In contrast, during the milking-machine process, the external pressure on the teat wall is evenly distributed by the liner, and the milk is suctioned from the teat cistern by the negative pressure, limiting the risk of milk infiltration. The farmer should not strip the cow's first stream before milking the affected quarter. Therefore, he should pay special attention to any inflammation of the udder parenchyma to detect any early mastitis.

Mechanical milking is carried out on the day after surgery. Because of the presence of inflammation, the use of a large-diameter teat cup may be an option to facilitate the milking in some cases. It is important to avoid overmilking following teat surgery. After milking, a postmilking teat dip should be performed.

The author recommends removal of any nonabsorbable skin sutures 8 days postoperatively to limit the formation of fibrosis in the tissue.

It is the author's experience that the overall prognosis of teat lacerations is good in both the short and the long term.

Complications

Complications following teat laceration repair include mastitis, partial or complete dehiscence of the wound, fibrosis of the teat, and fistula formation. The development of mastitis in the days following surgery is possible and must be closely monitored and addressed appropriately with targeted medication. Wound dehiscence often results from an overly aggressive debridement, causing too much tension on the margins of the wound/sutures or from a fistula repair for which the fibrotic healing tissue did not have enough suture-holding strength.

Fibrosis along the suture may reduce milking abilities of the teat. Formation of a fistula (**Fig. 7**) can appear within 10 days after surgery if suture of the mucosa or teat wall did not provide sufficient sealing at milking or when hand milking was performed on the teat. The fistula should be allowed to heal by second intention before surgical revision to ensure of the proper suture-holding power of the fibrotic scar tissue. Generally, after 4 to 6 weeks, the wound can be properly reviewed and sutured. With the cow restrained in lateral recumbency, an elliptical incision is performed around the fistula in a longitudinal orientation until the lumen of the teat cistern is encountered. Then, the wound is closed in 3 layers as mentioned previously; identical postoperative care is given to the cow.

CONGENITAL DISORDERS

Congenital disorders include absence of milk for the quarter conjoined supernumerary teats, or true separated supernumerary teats. The latter is often excised at an early age and will not be discussed here.

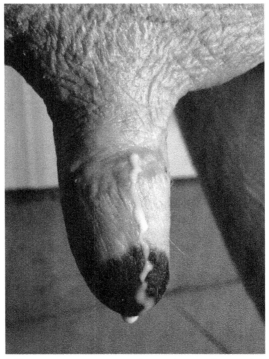

Fig. 7. Teat fistula following a transverse teat laceration on the proximal third of the teat. Milk constantly leaked from the pinhead hole.

Atresia

Heifers with a dry teat should be examined. On physical examination, no lumen can be palpated within the teat. Ultrasonography is the diagnostic imaging procedure of choice to determine if milk is present in the udder cistern or not.[8]

If milk is present in the gland cistern and in the teat cistern, atresia is located at the streak canal level, usually at the skin level. Perforation can be performed with either a large-diameter needle or a No. 11 scalpel blade to reach the streak canal and allow milk outflow.

If milk is present at the proximal aspect of the teat cistern or gland cistern, a circular membrane may be present either in the teat cistern or at the annular ring level. Blind perforation through the streak canal can be performed or a surgical opening of the teat (thelotomy) and resection of the membrane and primary suture of the mucosa can be performed. The author favors the last technique because it allows a better excision of the redundant tissue and minimizes the risk of serious complication, especially for the membranes located close to the annular ring.[2]

If the anatomy of the gland cistern is abnormal with no or minimal milk associated with the absence of teat cistern (confirmed by ultrasonography), the atresia is considered complete, and no surgical treatment should be attempted (**Fig. 8**).

Conjoined Supernumerary Teat

Conjoined supernumerary teats remain undetected until after the first calving because they are intimately attached to the main teat and appear as Siamese teats.[2,9,10] The owner notices a protuberance of various length and size on the base of the normal teat and may mistake it as a congenital fistula.

Each supernumerary teat is connected to independent mammary tissue (separate from the mammary gland of the main teat) (**Fig. 9**). Evaluation of the infectious status of the conjoined teat is important because milk outflow is usually impaired, possibly resulting in subclinical mastitis. Ultrasonographic evaluation offers a clear evaluation of the importance of each teat cistern as well as characterization of the thickness and length of the septum between the cisterns (**Fig. 10**). Comparison of 2 radiographs with infusion of the contrast media only in the conjoined teat initially, followed by infusion of both teats, will outline the independence of the 2 mammary glands.

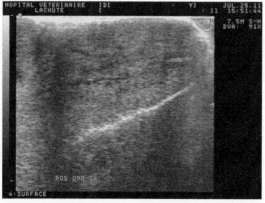

Fig. 8. Ultrasonographic evaluation of a complete fibrosis of the teat. The streak canal appears as a hyperechoic line surrounded by 2 hypoechoic lines at the distal extremity of the teat. The teat is filled by a homogenous echogenic tissue, and no cistern can be identified.

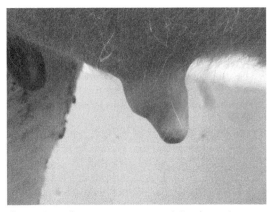

Fig. 9. External conformation of supernumerary conjoined teat in a cow. The supernumerary teat appears as a bulge caudally to the normal teat.

An accurate assessment of the quantities of milk produced by each gland is a good indicator of the relative size of the supernumerary gland and its contribution to the total production of that quarter. It is performed preferentially during milking of the 3 other quarters to allow the milk release through the oxytocin reflex. A teat cannula can be inserted into streak canal, and milk production of each gland can be quantified. Therapeutic options vary from the chemical sclerosis of the supernumerary gland, simple resection of the conjoined teat, to the anastomosis of the 2 cisterns.

If milk production is low, sclerosis of the accessory mammary gland may be considered. The induced inflammatory reactions of varying intensity may require administration of NSAIDs to increase the comfort of the animal.

Conjoined teat resection should be performed if the location and the shape of supernumerary teat prevent proper implementation of the teat cup liner on the main teat. Reduced milk production from the supernumerary gland is important because a recurrent deformation may appear after accumulation of milk. With the cow in lateral recumbency, an elliptical incision is performed around the streak canal until reaching the conjoined teat cistern, and the incision is closed as described for longitudinal teat laceration.

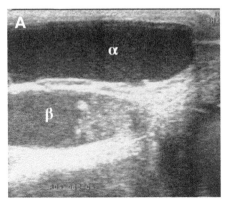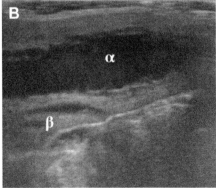

Fig. 10. Ultrasonographic evaluation of different conjoined supernumerary teat. (*A*) Large-diameter accessory teat cistern. (*B*) Small-diameter accessory teat cistern. (α) Principal teat. (β) Conjoined supernumerary teat.

Anastomosis of the 2 cisterns is performed for large conjoined supernumerary teats for which there is significant milk production. As the surgery is elective, food is withheld for 24 to 36 hours before performing the surgery. This surgery is preferably carried out in early lactation, after the complete elimination of colostrum from the udder. A dose of NSAID is administered before surgery, and antibiotic treatment is begun. Sedation is given to the cow, and then the cow is placed in lateral recumbency on the side opposite the teat being operated. The teat is then surgically prepared and a local anesthesia with a ring block is carried out. A teat cannula is placed in each streak canal. An elliptical incision is made around the streak canal of the accessory teat to invade the lumen of the accessory teat. The incision may be extended proximally when the length of the teat allows. Rigorous hemostasis must be carried out before proceeding. Regular tissue perfusion with isotonic crystalloid solution containing antibiotics eliminates blood clots and increases the visibility of the operative field.

The teat cannula inserted in the main teat is then mobilized and directed toward the opening created by the supernumerary teat resection (**Fig. 11**). An incision is then made in the intercisternal septum. It must be sufficiently long to allow the introduction of a jaw of a rongeur into the cistern of the main teat (**Fig. 12**). The jaws of the rongeur are kept clamped for 2 minutes, and then an incision around them is carried out using a scalpel. Significant hemorrhage may occur immediately after creating the window in the septum because it is common that one or more vessels are present within the septum. Hemostasis should be performed carefully. The initial size of the anastomosis

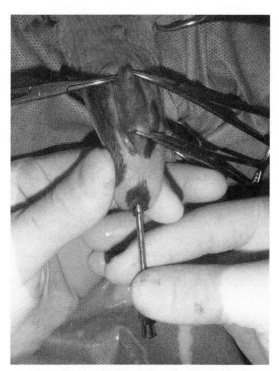

Fig. 11. Thelotomy of the supernumerary conjoined teat after resection of the associated streak canal. A metallic milking probe is inserted through the streak canal of the principal teat and pointed outward to point out the septum between the 2 teat cisterns.

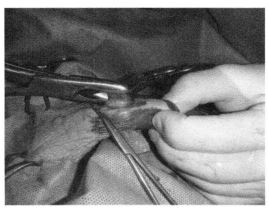

Fig. 12. Septum opening between the supernumerary and principal teat cisterns. A rongeur has been introduced in the principal teat cistern before being firmly tightened to assure hemostasis.

should be as large as possible taking care not to invade the annular ring at the proximal aspect of the teat.

The anastomosis of the 2 cisterns is completed with the suture of the mucosa of the main teat with the mucosa of the conjoined supernumerary teat. To minimize stenosis, 2 semicircular sutures are made using a small-diameter absorbable suture (3-0 USP Metric 3) rather than a single circular suture. The thelotomy wound is then sutured in 3 layers: mucosa, connective tissue, and skin. Passive milking through a teat cannula is favored for 24 hours to avoid manipulation of the teat. It is not unusual to observe pink tainted milk and the presence of small blood clots in the milk postoperatively. Mechanical milking can resume 3 days postoperatively. As for teat laceration, hand milking is traumatic to the repaired teat and is prohibited for 10 days postoperatively. Antibiotic therapy should be continued for 3 days and a second dose of NSAIDs may be given after 24 hours.

Intraoperative complications include severe bleeding that may completely obstruct the surgical field. The presence of large blood clots may migrate in the proximal teat cistern leading to streak canal obstruction. These obstructions may create the appeal of hand milking. Remember that hand milking can cause not only an infiltration of milk in the connective tissue and the creation of a fistula but also postsurgical recurrence of the septal bleeding. If mastitis is present in one of the 2 glands, it should be treated aggressively, and the surgery should be postponed for a few days. Stenosis or occlusion of the anastomosis is possible in the weeks following the procedure.

The prognosis of this type of surgery is good. However, it is important to adequately evaluate the desired teat conformation before making the elliptical incision in order to be sure not to induce any iatrogenic deformity of the operated teat (curve, excessive diameter reduction). Despite the fact that the communication between the 2 cisterns is made as long as possible (**Fig. 13**), stenosis may occur over time.

MILK OUTFLOW DISTURBANCES
Diagnosis

Milk flow disturbances have multiple causes. Anatomic dysfunction of the udder or teat and alteration of the milk ejection reflex (milk letdown) have been determined to be responsible for 16% and 52%, respectively, of poor milkability cases in Switzerland.[18,19] Causes of milk outflow impairment are many. Teat wall–related

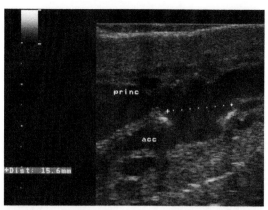

Fig. 13. Postoperative ultrasonographic evaluation of the 15.6-mm-long anastomosis between the principal (princ) and supernumerary (acc) teat cisterns.

problems and pathologic entities at the rosette of Fürstenberg or streak canal level should be differentiated. Milk ejection difficulties are often chronic conditions and single- or multiple-milking probe (teat cannula) introductions have generally been attempted before presentation. It is crucial to collect this information in the history because of the possible worsening of the lesions.

The specific examination of the teat should allow for the differentiation of diffuse or localized fibrosis, fibrosis of the streak canal, and/or the rosette of Fürstenberg, pediculated/free intracisternal masses, and the obstruction of milk flow by impinging varicose veins.

Digital palpation is the first step to establish the diagnosis. However, the distinction between different diseases is not always possible with palpation alone. Ultrasonography and radiography allow the determination and the location of the lesion (see **Fig. 13**; **Fig. 14**). Ultrasonography is very sensitive to determine excessive fibrous tissue or an obstructing mass lesion too close to the rosette of Fürstenberg (**Fig. 15**).[8]

Parietal Fibrosis

Localized fibrosis can be treated by a direct approach of the fibrosis zone with an en-bloc excision or by thelotomy opposite to the area of fibrosis and excision via the teat canal. The choice between the 2 techniques is dependent on the extent of the fibrosis zone. In both cases, an elliptical incision is made with a scalpel blade around the fibrosis so that the area of the mass removal is complete, taking care not to jeopardize functional reconstruction of the teat. The mucosa is then sutured with fine absorbable suture material using a simple continuous pattern.

Surgical correction of circular fibrosis of the teat wall is more challenging. A thelotomy is performed longitudinally over the entire length of the teat. The excision of the circular fibrotic portion is performed by incising the mucosa proximally and distally to the fibrotic area and then separating the fibrous mass from the underlying connective tissue. Reconstruction of the teat starts with the suturing of the mucosa. It may be necessary to moderately undermine the mucosa distally and proximally to successfully suture it, taking advantage of its elastic properties. The circular mucosal lining is sutured with interrupted sutures separated by about 3 mm apart. The mucosa of the longitudinal thelotomy incision is sutured with a simple continuous suture, and the superficial layers are done in a similar fashion as described for lacerations. Postoperative care is similar to that described for surgical treatment of the teat lacerations.

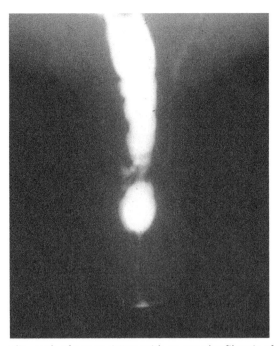

Fig. 14. Contrast radiograph of a teat cistern with an annular fibrosis of the mucosa.

Repeated introduction of a metal milking probe (teat cannula) can generate a significant inflammatory response that may lead to very extensive fibrosis of the interior wall of the teat. Fibrotic tissue resection is mandatory to re-create a lumen allowing the flow of milk. However, the mucosal defect may be too large to permit accurate mucosal reconstruction (**Fig. 16**). In these cases, a silicone prosthesis in the lumen of the teat cistern may be necessary to maintain patency. The prosthesis is then used as a stent to maintain an appropriate teat cistern diameter during re-epithelialization

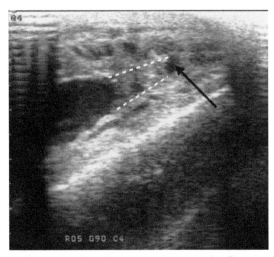

Fig. 15. Ultrasonographic evaluation of a teat with an annular fibrosis of the mucosa illustrated by the 2 yellow dotted lines. The arrow points out the distal end of the teat cistern.

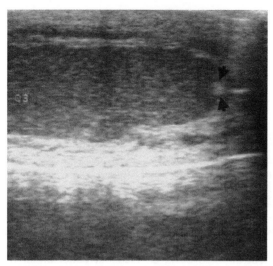

Fig. 16. Ultrasonographic evaluation of a cow suffering milking difficulties. A hyperechoic mass (*arrowheads*) is present at the rosette of Fürstenberg.

of the mucosa. The prosthesis is left in place approximately 8 weeks and then a second operation is performed opposite to the first thelotomy for the removal of the prosthesis.

The 2 most common complications are migration of the prosthesis during milking and production of exuberant granulation tissue leading to a recurrence of the initial condition. The success rate associated with the introduction of the prosthesis is 40% to 50%.

Fibrosis of the Streak Canal and the Rosette of Fürstenberg

The partial or complete obstructions whose origin is the papillary duct (streak canal) or the Fürstenberg rosette represent a real therapeutic challenge because this anatomic structure is sensitive to the slightest inflammation. Using a teat knife to blindly perform 3 to 4 incisions at a 30° angle may temporarily improve milk ejection. However, the use of theloscopy offers the possibility of very accurate manipulation of lesions and allows the surgeon to operate under direct vision and limiting unnecessary iatrogenic trauma.

In the author's opinion, theloscopy is best performed under sedation with the cow restrained in lateral recumbency either on a tilt table or on the floor, despite a previous description of it being performed on a cow restrained in a claw-trimming chute.[20–22] After standard surgical preparation and anesthesia of the teat, 2 procedures are performed: the retrograde step with the theloscope inserted through the streak canal in direction of the annular ring (**Fig. 17**) and the normograde step with the theloscope inserted in the lateral teat wall in looking in the direction of the rosette of Fürstenberg (**Fig. 18**). A teat clamp is applied at the annular ring level to stop the continuous filling of the teat cistern by milk. Retrograde theloscopy is performed first by gently introducing the sleeve with the blunt trocar through the streak canal. The trocar is removed, and the theloscope is introduced. The normograde theloscopy is conducted by the retrograde insertion of a sharp trocar through the streak canal. The sharp trocar is then forced through the lateral teat wall at the proximal third of the length. The sleeve is slid over the trocar, and the theloscope is inserted in a normograde fashion after trocar removal, allowing a complete evaluation of the rosette of Fürstenberg and entry of the streak canal. Masses or proliferative fibrous tissue around the rosette of

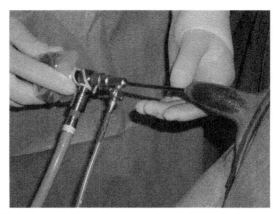

Fig. 17. Retrograde theloscopy through the streak canal. The theloscope points toward the proximal aspect of the teat. A teat clamp has been installed proximally at the annular ring.

Fürstenberg are best trimmed using an Eisenhut cutter under direct visualization (**Fig. 19**). After completion of the normograde theloscopy, the skin of the teat wall may be sutured with one single suture using small-diameter suture material.

With all abnormality involving the streak canal or the Fürstenberg rosette, the immediate postoperative period is crucial to the success of the surgery. It is recommended that the teat be stented for 9 days. To do this, a silicone teat insert is inserted via the streak canal and left in place with a bandage. The silicone insert is changed 2 to 3 days apart depending on milk production, udder congestion, and cow comfort. The milk is drained by passive milking at each bandage change. This rest promotes good healing of the mucosa forming the rosette of Fürstenberg and allows the streak canal to heal at a fixed diameter because the smooth muscle fibers forming the streak canal sphincter cannot crush the silicone insert within the canal. Silicone teat inserts may be replaced by wax teat inserts after the 9 days to allow the stretched streak canal to contract again. The wax teat inserts are sterilely changed after each milking for another 10 days. Alternatively, a custom-made silicone cannula can also be inserted through the streak canal and sutured to the teat wall. An advantage of this method is that it allows for passive milking as often as needed without remanipulating the streak canal

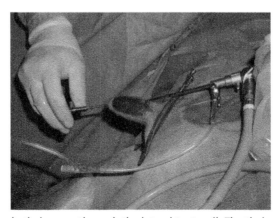

Fig. 18. Normograde theloscopy through the lateral teat wall. The theloscope points at the rosette of Fürstenberg. An Eisenhut cutter has been introduced through the streak canal.

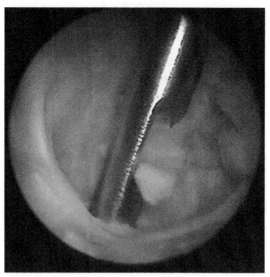

Fig. 19. Theloscopic view of the distal end of the teat cistern. An Eisenhut cutter is used to trim the fibrous tissue around the rosette of Fürstenberg.

(**Fig. 20**). This treatment should be considered only in the absence of mastitis. The interval in which the silicone teat insert is changed will vary depending on milk production and the possible development of infection during treatment. Increased surveillance by the owner is required for the proper management.

Surgical Excision of Intracisternal Masses

The presence of polyps and lactoliths in the lumen of the teat is infrequent (**Fig. 21**). These pedunculated masses located distally in teat cistern can induce milk flow disturbances during milking and need to be removed. Blind removal of those masses using a Hugs teat tumor extractor or a Cornell teat curette may allow the removal of the tissue. However, it is the author's opinion that performing a theloscopy or conducting a

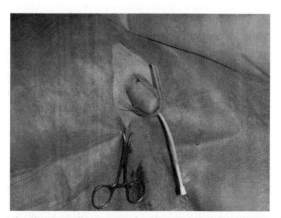

Fig. 20. Custom-made silicone milking cannula. The silicone tube is inserted in the streak canal, and the wings are sutured to the teat wall. This device allows passive milking without manipulation within the canal. The yellow plug inserted in the end can be removed before milking. (*Courtesy of* Dr Nichols, Université de Montréal, St-Hyacinthe, Québec, Canada.)

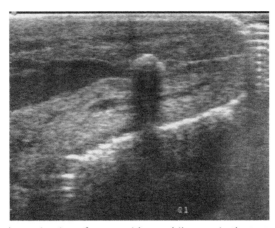

Fig. 21. Ultrasound examination of a cow with a mobile mass in the teat cistern. The hyperechoic crescent-shaped structure just proximal to the streak canal acted as a valve during milking, obstructing the opening of the rosette of Fürstenberg.

longitudinal thelotomy helps ensure the complete excision of the mass while minimizing iatrogenic trauma to the teat mucosa during blind attempts to grasp the mass.

Surgical Correction of Varicose Vein

Changes in the muscular to elastic tissue ratio have been described in the veins of the udder.[23] Veins may appear more dilated and tortuous, eventually developing valvular dysfunction over time and becoming a varicose vein.[2,9,10] Dilated varicose veins can impair milk flow by reducing the lumen diameter at the proximal teat. A reduced lumen diameter at the proximal teat has been described if the varicose vein develops at the annular ring level or on the teat itself. Three treatment options are described: sclerotherapy, ligation associated with sclerotherapy, and phlebectomy.[24] Sclerotherapy is performed by the injection of 25% dextrose in the vein after blood drainage and the application of 2 hemostatic forceps obstructing the 2 extremities of the vein for 10 to 15 minutes. Sclerotherapy can also be conducted in conjunction with ligation of the vein. Small skin incisions are performed over the ligation sites, and blunt dissection allows vein isolation and ligation with 2-0 absorbable suture material. Phlebectomy, an en-bloc resection of the vein, can be performed along its pathway paying attention to ligate and remove the enlarged collateral vein at the same time. In a study of 22 cows suffering milk outflow difficulties related to varicose vein, Lardé and colleagues[24] reported good overall prognosis with no significant difference between the treatment options. Sclerotherapy alone or associated with ligation was associated with recurrence of the varicose vein in 3 cows.

MASTECTOMY

Acute gangrenous and chronic unresponsive mastitis are the most common indication of radical mastectomy in cattle. Two techniques have been described: en-bloc resection of the udder, and more recently, physiologic mastectomy. The en-bloc resection of the udder should be performed under general anesthesia. An elliptical incision is made around the mammary gland at about one-third of the length in order to preserve the skin for closure. Subcutaneous dissection is conducted in order to separate the gland from the abdominal wall (**Fig. 22**). Strict attention to hemostasis should be paid throughout the procedure. The external pudendal artery and vein are identified

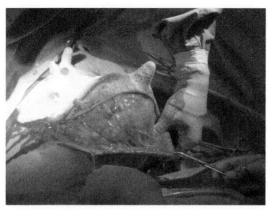

Fig. 22. Radical mastectomy under general anesthesia in a heifer suffering from papillary ductal carcinoma. The skin incisions have been made as close as possible to the teat due to the poor development of the udder.

and ligated, as are the mammary vein and the ventral perineal artery and vein. After transection of the fascial attachments of the suspensory apparatus to completely free the udder, Penrose drains are placed, and the skin is sutured using appropriate tension-relieving technique. Prognosis associated with the surgical procedure appears to be good as a salvage procedure for nonproducing animals.

Physiologic mastectomy has been developed as a salvage procedure for production animals. It is performed in the standing position. Using a conventional paralumbar fossa laparotomy on the ipsilateral side of the infected quarter, the external pudendal vessels entering the inguinal canal are located and carefully dissected in order to place ligatures around them using large nonabsorbable material. Ligation of the perineal artery and vein has also been described.[25] This procedure is typically an inexpensive salvage procedure.

REFERENCES

1. Beaudeau F, Fourichon C, Frankena K, et al. Impact of udder disorders on culling of dairy cows. Vet Res 1994;25:223.
2. Couture Y, Mulon PY. Procedures and surgeries of the teat. Vet Clin North Am 2005;21(1):173–204.
3. Nichols S. Diagnosis and management of teat injury. In: Anderson DE, Rings DM, editors. Current veterinary therapy—food animal practice. St Louis (MO): Saunders; 2009. p. 398–406.
4. Barone R. Mamelles de la vache. In: Barone R, editor. Anatomie comparée des mammifères domestiques—tome quatrième Splanchnologie II. 2nd edition. Paris: Vigot; 1990. p. 475–87.
5. Budras KD, Habel RH. The udder with blood vessels, lymphatic system, nerves, and development. In: Budras KD, Habel RH, editors. Bovine anatomy an illustrated text. Hannover (Germany): Schlütersche; 2003. p. 90–1.
6. Paulrud CO. Basic concept of the bovine teat canal. Vet Res Commun 2005;29: 215–45.
7. Weiss D, Weinfurtner M, Bruckmaier RM. Teat anatomy and its relationship with quarter and udder milk flow characteristics in dairy cows. J Dairy Sci 2004; 87(10):3280–9.

8. Franz S, Floek M, Hofmann-Parisot M. Ultrasonography of the bovine udder and teat. Vet Clin North Am Food Anim Pract 2009;25(3):669–85.
9. Mulon PY, Desrochers A. Les affections traumatiques du trayon et leur traitement chirurgical. Bulletin de la SNGTV 2007;41:71–8.
10. Mulon PY, Desrochers A. Correction chirurgicale des trayons accessoires chez la vache laitière. Bulletin de la SNGTV 2007;42:71–6.
11. Steiner A. Teat surgery. In: Fubini SL, Ducharme NG, editors. Farm animal surgery. St Louis (MO): Saunders; 2004. p. 408–19.
12. Steiner A. Teat surgery. In: Fubini SL, Ducharme NG, editors. Food animal surgery. 1st edition. St Louis (MO): WB Saunders; 2004. p. 414–8.
13. Bailey JV. Principles of reconstructive surgery. In: Auer JA, Stick JA, editors. Equine surgery. 3rd edition. St Louis (MO): Saunders; 2006. p. 254–68.
14. Ghamsari SM, Taguchi K, Abe N, et al. Effect of different suture patterns on wound healing of the teat in dairy cattle. J Vet Med Sci 1995;57:819–24.
15. Ducharme NG, Arighi M, Horney D, et al. Invasive teat surgery in dairy cattle I. Long-term follow-up and complications. Can Vet J 1987;28:757–62.
16. Ducharme NG, Arighi M, Horney D, et al. Invasive teat surgery in dairy cattle II. Long-term follow-up and complications. Can Vet J 1987;28:763–7.
17. Nichols S, Anderson DE. Breaking strength and elasticity of synthetic absorbable suture materials incubated in phosphate-buffered saline solution, milk, and milk contaminated with Streptococcus agalactiae. Am J Vet Res 2007;68(4):441–5.
18. Belo CJ, Schlegel S, Moll J, et al. Milk ejection disorders in Swiss dairy cows: a field study. J Dairy Res 2009;76:222–8.
19. Cable CS, Peery K, Fubini SL. Radical mastectomy in 20 ruminants. Vet Surg 2004;33:263–6.
20. Geishauser T, Querengässer K, Querengässer J. Teat endoscopy (theloscopy) for diagnosis and therapy of milk flow disorders in dairy cows. Vet Clin North Am 2005;21(1):205–25.
21. Bleul UT, Schwantag SC, Bachofner C, et al. Milk flow and udder health in cows after treatment of covered teat injuries via theloresectoscopy: 52 cases (2000–2002). J Am Vet Med Assoc 2005;226:1119–23.
22. Allen AJ, Barrington GM, Parish SM. Physiologic mastectomy via flank laparotomy. Vet Clin North Am Food Anim Pract 2008;24(3):511–6.
23. Linzell JL. Valvular incompetence in the venous drainage of the udder. J Physiol 1960;153:481–91.
24. Lardé H, Nichols S, Desrochers A, et al. Milk flow obstruction caused by varicose vein of the teat in dairy cattle. Vet Surg 2013;42:885–91.
25. Belbis G, Quentin X, Périé P, et al. Traitement chirurgical par ligatures vasculaires des infections graves de la mamelle chez la vache. Bulletin des GTV 2011;62:53–60.

Index

Note: Page numbers of article titles are in **boldface** type.

Vet Clin Food Anim 32 (2016) 833–848
http://dx.doi.org/10.1016/S0749-0720(16)30057-3
0749-0720/16/$ – see front matter

vetfood.theclinics.com